Gastric Cancer

Editor

STEVEN F. MOSS

GASTROENTEROLOGY
CLINICS OF NORTH AMERICA

www.gastro.theclinics.com

June 2013 • Volume 42 • Number 2

ELSEVIER

1600 John F. Kennedy Boulevard ● Suite 1800 ● Philadelphia, Pennsylvania, 19103-2899
http://www.theclinics.com

GASTROENTEROLOGY CLINICS OF NORTH AMERICA Volume 42, Number 2
June 2013 ISSN 0889-8553, ISBN-13: 978-1-4557-7091-5

Editor: Kerry Holland
Developmental Editor: Donald Mumford

Gastroenterology Clinics of North America (ISSN 0889-8553) is published quarterly by Elsevier Inc., 360 Park Avenue South, New York, NY 10010-1710. Months of issue are March, June, September, and December. Business and Editorial Offices: 1600 John F. Kennedy Blvd., Suite 1800, Philadelphia, PA 19103-2899. Customer Service Office: 6277 Sea Harbor Drive, Orlando, FL 32887-4800. Periodicals postage paid at New York, NY and additional mailing offices. Subscription prices are $305.00 per year (US individuals), $153.00 per year (US students), $508.00 per year (US institutions), $335.00 per year (Canadian individuals), $617.00 per year (Canadian institutions), $423.00 per year (international individuals), $211.00 per year (international students), and $617.00 per year (international institutions). Foreign air speed delivery is included in all *Clinics* subscription prices. All prices are subject to change without notice. **POSTMASTER**: Send address changes to *Gastroenterology Clinics of North America*, Elsevier Health Sciences Division, Subscription Customer Service, 3251 Riverport Lane, Maryland Heights, MO 63043. Telephone: 1-800-654-2452 (U.S. and Canada); 314-447-8871 (outside U.S. and Canada). Fax: 314-447-8029. E-mail: journalscustomerservice-usa@elsevier.com (for print support); journalsonlinesupport-usa@elsevier.com (for online support).

Reprints. For copies of 100 or more, of articles in this publication, please contact the Commercial Reprints Department, Elsevier Inc., 360 Part Avenue South, New York, New York 10010-1710. Tel. (212) 633-3813, Fax: (212) 462-1935, E-mail: reprints@elsevier.com.

Gastroenterology Clinics of North America is also published in Italian by Il Pensiero Scientifico Editore, Rome, Italy; and in Portuguese by Interlivros Edicoes Ltda., Rua Commandante Coelho 1085, 21250 Cordovil, Rio de Janeiro, Brazil.

Gastroenterology Clinics of North America is covered in *MEDLINE/PubMed (Index Medicus)*, *Excerpta Medica*, *Current Contents/Clinical Medicine*, *Science Citation Index*, *ISI/BIOMED*, and *BIOSIS*.

Printed and bound by CPI Group (UK) Ltd, Croydon, CR0 4YY
Transferred to digital print 2013

Contributors

EDITOR

STEVEN F. MOSS, MD
Professor, Department of Medicine, Warren Alpert Medical School of Brown University;
Program Director, Gastroenterology Fellowship Training Program at Rhode Island
Hospital/Brown University; Director of Endoscopy, Providence VA Medical Center,
Providence, Rhode Island

AUTHORS

JAFFER A. AJANI, MD
Department of Gastrointestinal Medical Oncology, The University of Texas MD Anderson
Cancer Center, Houston, Texas

ANDREW M. BLAKELY, MD
Department of Surgery, Warren Alpert Medical School of Brown University, Providence,
Rhode Island

MARIELA A. BLUM, MD
Department of Gastrointestinal Medical Oncology, The University of Texas MD Anderson
Cancer Center, Houston, Texas

PELAYO CORREA, MD
Professor, Division of Gastroenterology, Vanderbilt University Medical Center, Nashville,
Tennessee

CATHERINE DE MARTEL, MD, PhD
International Agency for Research on Cancer, Lyon, France

WOLFGANG FISCHBACH, MD, PhD
Professor, Department of Internal Medicine and Palliative Care Unit, Klinikum
Aschaffenburg – Academic Teaching Hospital of the University of Würzburg,
Am Hasenkopf, Aschaffenburg, Germany

DAVID FORMAN, BA, PhD, FFPHM
International Agency for Research on Cancer, Lyon, France

BJORN GUSTAFSSON, MD, PhD
Department of Cancer Research and Molecular Medicine, Norwegian University of
Science and Technology, Trondheim, Norway

RYU ISHIHARA, MD
Department of Gastrointestinal Oncology, Osaka Medical Center for Cancer and
Cardiovascular Diseases, Osaka, Japan

MARK KIDD, PhD
Department of Surgery, Yale University School of Medicine, New Haven, Connecticut

JERZY LASOTA, MD
Laboratory of Pathology, NCI/NIH, Bethesda, Maryland

MARKKU MIETTINEN, MD
Laboratory of Pathology, NCI/NIH, Bethesda, Maryland

THOMAS J. MINER, MD
Associate Professor of Surgery, Associate Residency Program Director in Surgery, Director of Surgical Oncology, Department of Surgery, Warren Alpert Medical School of Brown University, Providence, Rhode Island

IRVIN M. MODLIN, MD, PhD, DSc
Department of Surgery, Yale University School of Medicine, New Haven, Connecticut

RICHARD M. PEEK Jr, MD
Departments of Medicine and Cancer Biology, Vanderbilt University, Nashville, Tennessee

MARTYN PLUMMER, PhD
International Agency for Research on Cancer, Lyon, France

STEVEN M. POWELL, MD
Associate Professor of Medicine, Division of Gastroenterology/Hepatology, Department of Medicine, University of Virginia, Charlottesville, Virginia

MURRAY B. RESNICK, MD, PhD
Vice Chief and Director of Anatomical Pathology, Professor of Pathology, Department of Pathology, Rhode Island Hospital, Providence, Rhode Island

KAZUKI SUDO, MD
Department of Gastrointestinal Medical Oncology, The University of Texas MD Anderson Cancer Center, Houston, Texas

TAKASHI TAKETA, MD
Department of Gastrointestinal Medical Oncology, The University of Texas MD Anderson Cancer Center, Houston, Texas

VICTORIA P.Y. TAN
Clinical Assistant Professor, Department of Medicine, University of Hong Kong, Hong Kong

NORIYA UEDO, MD
Department of Gastrointestinal Oncology, Osaka Medical Center for Cancer and Cardiovascular Diseases, Osaka, Japan

DUSHANT S. UPPAL, MD, MSc
Fellow, Division of Gastroenterology/Hepatology, Department of Medicine, University of Virginia, Charlottesville, Virginia

ROOPMA WADHWA, MD, MHA
Department of Gastrointestinal Medical Oncology, The University of Texas MD Anderson Cancer Center, Houston, Texas

BENJAMIN C.Y. WONG
Clinical Professor, Department of Medicine, University of Hong Kong, Hong Kong

LYDIA E. WROBLEWSKI, PhD
Department of Medicine, Vanderbilt University, Nashville, Tennessee

EVGENY YAKIREVICH, MD, DSc
Assistant Professor of Pathology, Department of Pathology, Rhode Island Hospital, Providence, Rhode Island

KENSHI YAO, MD
Department of Endoscopy, Fukuoka University Chikushi Hospital, Fukuoka, Japan

Contents

treatment option for potential cure and can be beneficial in the palliation of advanced disease. Several neoadjuvant chemotherapy regimens have been recently evaluated as potential adjuncts to surgery. This review describes the current role of surgical therapy in staging, resection, and palliation of gastric cancer.

Gastric cancer (GC) is a major health burden throughout the world, especially in certain endemic regions. GC is commonly diagnosed at an advanced stage because of the lack of early detection strategies and is usually associated with a dismal outcome. For patients with localized GC (LGC), surgery is the best cure: cure rates are highly associated with the surgical pathology stage. Adjunctive therapies improve the cure rates by about an additional 10%. Therefore, a multimodality approach is highly recommended for all patients with LGC. This article highlights some of the therapeutic advances made against GC and features important ongoing trials.

Gastric marginal zone B-cell lymphoma of mucosal-associated lymphoid tissue (MALT) is the predominant entity within the primary gastrointestinal lymphomas. *Helicobacter pylori* represents the decisive pathogenetic factor for gastric MALT lymphoma. The goal of treating gastric MALT lymphoma should be complete cure. The first choice of treatment is *H pylori* eradication. Patients with histologically persistent residual lymphoma after successful *H pylori* eradication and normalization of endoscopic findings should be managed by a watch-and-wait strategy. Patients who do not respond to *H pylori* eradication should be referred for radiation or chemotherapy.

Gastric neuroendocrine neoplasms of the stomach can be divided into the usually well-differentiated, hypergastrinemia-dependent type I and II lesions and the more aggressively behaving gastrin-independent type III lesions. Studying menin and its complex interrelationship with gastrin may provide insight into tumor biology at the clinical level and in terms of basic cell biology (eg, the role of the epigenome in neuroendocrine cell proliferation), and lead to potential consideration of other targets that are known candidates for molecular-based therapies in other adenocarcinomas.

Gastrointestinal stromal tumors (GISTs) are the most common mesenchymal tumor of the gastrointestinal tract. Soon after GIST was recognized as a tumor driven by a KIT or platelet-derived growth factor receptor muta-tion, it became the first solid tumor target for tyrosine kinase inhibitor therapies. More recently, alternative molecular mechanisms for GIST path-ogenesis have been discovered. These are related to deficiencies in the succinate dehydrogenase complex, NF1-gene alterations in connection with neurofibromatosis type 1 tumor syndrome, and mutational activation of the BRAF oncogene in very rare cases.

GASTROENTEROLOGY
CLINICS OF NORTH AMERICA

NOW AVAILABLE FOR YOUR iPhone and iPad

Preface

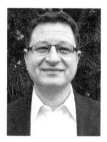

Steven F. Moss, MD
Editor

Gastric cancer is the second most common cause of cancer mortality worldwide. Although the incidence of this disease is on the decline in the United States, it still remains one of our most common gastrointestinal neoplasms and is especially prevalent among immigrants and the socioeconomically deprived in the United States.

Recent years have seen major advances in our understanding of the pathogenesis of gastric cancer, especially regarding the importance of *Helicobacter pylori* and its associated inflammatory response. This has resulted in the emergence of adjuvant oncologic therapies of proven benefit for advanced cases as a method of treatment, in addition to surgery.

In view of this recent progress in the field, I am delighted to have had the opportunity to invite some outstanding colleagues to contribute their expertise on all aspects of gastric cancer. This edition of *Gastroenterology Clinics of North America* is the first to be devoted to this topic for many years and is therefore much needed in that it provides a thorough, authoritative, and clinically practical approach for the management of gastric malignancy in 2013 and beyond.

Most articles focus on gastric adenocarcinoma, as this is by far the most common type of gastric malignancy. The overview is provided by Pelayo Correa, whose observations on the gradual progression of the gastric preneoplastic process from chronic gastritis through intestinal metaplasia and dysplasia highlighted the importance of a slow and chronic inflammatory process in the etiology of gastric cancer. This conceptual framework, made in the 1970s—before anyone had appreciated a possible infectious etiology, predated the rediscovery of *H pylori*. Our current understanding of how *H pylori* and its associated inflammatory response drive gastric carcinogenesis derives from intensive research in the last 2 decades. These insights, particularly regarding putative bacterial oncogenes, inflammatory-driven neoplasia, and the role of bone marrow–derived cell recruitment to the sites of chronic inflammation, have led to the development of new paradigms in cancer pathobiology that are now being applied to tumors outside of the stomach .

Throughout this monograph, a notable theme is the heterogeneity of gastric cancer—including tumors of different subsites, histopathology, etiology, pathogenesis, and biological behavior. Dissecting this complexity is important, as evidenced

Gastroenterol Clin N Am 42 (2013) xiii–xiv
http://dx.doi.org/10.1016/j.gtc.2013.02.002
0889-8553/13/$ – see front matter © 2013 Published by Elsevier Inc.

gastro.theclinics.com

by the diverse treatment modalities now available. Fortunately, the evidence base from which to select appropriate endoscopic, surgical, and oncologic therapies is growing rapidly and increasingly serves as the basis for rational interdisciplinary clinical decision-making. Colleagues from Southeast Asia, where gastric cancer is especially prevalent, have provided us with their views on chemopreventive programs and with specific practical state-of-the-art advice based on their experience with advanced endoscopic techniques to impact outcome in high-risk populations.

Although mainly focused on gastric adenocarcinoma, this edition of *Gastroenterology Clinics of North America* also includes articles that cover gastric neuroendocrine or carcinoid tumors, gastrointestinal stromal tumors, and marginal zone B-cell ("MALT") lymphomas. Once considered very rare, increasing recognition of these entities by endoscopists and pathologists and recent elucidation of their underlying biology and cellular and molecular pathogenesis have led to much progress in the management of these neoplasms, including the development of specific, highly targeted therapies with impressive cure rates.

In highlighting recent developments in gastric neoplasia, we present here an updated overview of all aspects of gastric cancer that should be of interest to all practicing gastroenterologists as well as to other specialists seeking to improve the management of the many patients with stomach cancer.

Steven F. Moss, MD
Department of Medicine
Warren Alpert Medical School of Brown University
Rhode Island Hospital
593 Eddy Street, APC 414
Providence, RI 02903, USA

E-mail address:
Steven_moss@brown.edu

Gastric Cancer: Overview

Pelayo Correa, MD

KEYWORDS

- Gastric cancer • *Helicobacter pylori* • Etiology • Epidemiology • Host factors
- Precancerous cascade • Prevention • Early detection

KEY POINTS

- Gastric cancer represents a major health burden worldwide.
- The cause of gastric cancer is multifactorial, although infection with *Helicobacter pylori* is considered to be the primary cause.
- Infection with *H pylori* is very prevalent; it has been estimated that at least 50% of adults worldwide harbor the infection.
- The early stages of gastric cancer are usually asymptomatic or associated with nonspecific symptoms, such as dyspepsia.
- Strategies addressing cancer prevention are based on eradication of *H pylori* infection, recommendations on dietary changes to increase daily intake of fresh fruits and vegetables, and reduction in salt consumption.

INTRODUCTION

Gastric cancer is a major health burden worldwide. It is the second cause of cancer deaths after lung cancer.[1,2] More than 90% of the tumors are adenocarcinomas, the main focus of this review. The prognosis is dismal, with an average 5-year survival rate of less than 20%, mainly because of late diagnosis, because the early stages are clinically silent. Only a few countries, especially Japan, have set up extensive programs of early detection. If the tumor is detected and treated before it invades the muscular layer of the stomach, the 5-year survival rate can reach 90%.[3] The highest incidence rates are reported for East Asia (Korea, Mongolia, Japan, and China) with annual incidence rates between 40 and 60 per 100,000 inhabitants. In Latin America, pockets of high risk are reported in the Andes Mountains, with rates between 20 and 30 per 100,000,[1] in contrast to the much lower rates reported for the coastal and river valley regions.[4] Lower rates are found in Africa (~0.3 to 3 per 100,000, and in affluent populations of North America). The incidence rate in African Americans

Conflicts of Interest: The author has no conflicts of interest to declare.

Division of Gastroenterology, Vanderbilt University Medical Center, 1030C MRB IV, 2215B Garland Avenue, Nashville, TN 37232, USA

E-mail address: pelayo.correa@vanderbilt.edu

Gastroenterol Clin N Am 42 (2013) 211–217
http://dx.doi.org/10.1016/j.gtc.2013.01.002   **gastro.theclinics.com**

is about double that seen in white American. In general, the incidence rate for men is double that for women.[1]

In recent decades, there has been a gradual decrease in gastric cancer rates in many populations. It has been proposed that this decrease reflects trends in food handling, especially refrigeration and the abundance of fresh fruit and vegetables in the diet, as well as a decrease in the use of tobacco and dietary salt. However, not all types of gastric cancer are declining; tumors of the cardia and esophagogastric junction are becoming more frequent. Recently, an unexplained increase in gastric cancer incidence in younger individuals, mostly less than 40 years of age, has been reported.[5]

ETIOLOGY

The cause of gastric cancer is multifactorial, although infection with *Helicobacter pylori* is considered to be the primary cause; its effects are modulated by microbial, environmental, and host factors.

Gastric cancer is one of a few types of neoplasms directly linked to an infectious agent. In 1994, the International Agency for Research on Cancer (IARC) classified infection with *H pylori* as a class I human carcinogen for gastric cancer.[6] The same infectious agent is recognized as the primary cause of gastric mucosa-associated lymphoid tissue (MALT) lymphoma.

H pylori is a gram-negative bacterium capable of colonizing the gastric mucosa and eliciting an immune response in the host. The infection is predominantly acquired in early infancy and remains present for life if not treated with antibiotics. One type of gastritis associated with the infection, namely multifocal atrophic gastritis, may be linked to the precancerous process. Nonatrophic antral gastritis is not associated with the precancerous process but may be linked to duodenal ulcer. Reactive oxygen species (ROS) may be generated by the infection and may induce DNA mutations. *H pylori* is also able to induce hypermethylation of DNA, especially the CpG islands, thereby silencing genes associated with tumor suppression. A study on subjects infected with *H pylori* reported that a population at high risk for gastric cancer from the Colombian Andes (Tuquerres) had significantly greater hypermethylation of the *RPRM* gene (a tumor suppressor gene) in the gastric mucosa compared with those in a low-risk population on the Pacific coast (Tumaco).[7]

H pylori strains vary considerably in their pathogenicity and carcinogenicity. More virulent strains carry the cytotoxic-associated gene *cagA*, encoding an oncogenic protein that can be injected directly into gastric epithelial cells by a type IV secretion system.[8,9] Most strains in East Asia and in the high-risk area of the Colombian Andes are *cagA* positive. After entering the cytoplasm of the gastric epithelial cells, CagA becomes phosphorylated in motifs that contain the EPIYA sequences and starts a chain of molecular events linked to carcinogenesis. The EPIYA sequences are classified as A, B, C, or D according to the amino acids flanking them. The number and type of EPIYA motifs vary in different *H pylori* strains. In western countries, *H pylori* strains contain EPIYA motifs A, B, and C. In East Asia, the strains contain the D motif instead of the C motif.[10] Strains with more than 3 EPIYA motifs induce significantly more gastric atrophy, intestinal metaplasia, and gastric cancer. In vivo and in vitro studies have shown that CagA induces disruption of intercellular junctions, loss of epithelial polarity, increased proliferation, reduced apoptosis, and eventually carcinogenicity.[11] Another virulence-associated gene is *vacA*, which induces cytoplasmic vacuoles, pores in the cell membrane, and apoptosis.[12] Although all *H pylori* strains contain the *vacA* gene, genetic variations determine its functional activity and cancer risk. The *vacA* gene has genetic variations in the *s* (signal) region, which can be s1a, s1b, s1c, or s2. The middle region shows alleles that can be m1 or m2 and the intermediate region can be i1 or i2. Strains *vacA* s1/m1 or *vacA*s1/m1/i1 convey a higher risk of progression and cancer than strains vacA s2/m2 or vacA s2/m2/i2.

Some adhesion proteins of the membrane have been linked to higher virulence. One of them is BabA (blood-group antigen-binding adhesin) encoded by the gene *babA*, not present in all strains. BabA adheres to the antigen Lewis[b], present in the epithelial cell membrane. Infections with *H pylori* strains *babA2*-positive are associated with greater cancer risk.

The Infectious Agent

Infection with *H pylori* is very prevalent; it has been estimated that at least 50% of adults worldwide harbor the infection. However, a small minority (less than 1%) ever develop gastric cancer. *H pylori* has been a member of the human microbiota since time immemorial. Both species, *Homo sapiens* and *H pylori*, migrated together out of Africa approximately 60,000 years ago and populated most of the world. Throughout millennia, gradual transformations of the bacterial genome have resulted in several prototypes, including hpEurope, hpAfrica1 (including hspWest Africa and hspSouth Africa), hpAfrica2 and hpSahul (Oceania).[13,14] In Colombia, the inhabitants who live at high altitude in the Andes Mountains (Tuquerres) are mestizos (admixture of Amerindian and European); they have a high risk of gastric cancer and are infected with *H pylori* of the European prototype. By contrast, inhabitants of the Pacific coast, who are predominantly of Africa origin, carry a prevalence of approximately 30% European and 70% African *H pylori* strains. Independent of geographic location, patients infected with European prototype strains have more severe gastric premalignant lesions and oxidative damage than those infected with African prototype strains.[15] These findings show that although *cagA* and *vacA* are associated with virulence, they are not the only genes linked to virulence and carcinogenicity. They also indicate that migrants from Europe and Africa brought with them their original *H pylori* strains.

Epstein-Barr Virus

The presence of Epstein-Barr virus (EBV) has been found in between 5% and 16% of gastric cancers, implying that it may possibly play a causative role. The virus is more frequently found in men than in women, in tumors of the cardia or gastric body and in tumors found in gastrectomy specimens. It is very prevalent ($\sim$90%) in gastric lymphoepitheliomas (carcinomas with lymphoid stroma).[16]

Environmental Factors

Tobacco use has been found to be a risk factor for gastric cancer and precancerous lesions.[17] High dietary salt consumption increases cancer risk.[18] Consumption of processed meat has also been associated with a high cancer risk.[19] No clear association has been found with alcohol consumption. Consumption of fresh fruits and vegetables has been associated with reduced cancer risk.

Host Factors

Several studies have reported an association between cancer risk and genetic polymorphisms of genes linked to the inflammatory response, such as the interleukins *IL1B*, *IL1RN*, *IL10*, and tumor necrosis factor-α, *TNF*.[20–22] Several of these are tumor suppressors of gastric acid secretion, which may facilitate bacterial colonization of the gastric corpus. The *IL1B-511T* allele is a risk factor for gastric adenocarcinoma.

CLINICAL CHARACTERISTICS

The early stages of gastric cancer are usually asymptomatic or associated with nonspecific symptoms such as dyspepsia. Advanced stages may be accompanied by persistent abdominal pain, anorexia, and weight loss. Ulcerated tumors may be associated with hematemesis. Persistent vomiting may be a sign of pyloric stenosis. The lack of specific symptoms may lead to a delayed diagnosis. Approximately 80% of patients are diagnosed at advanced stages in most countries where no early detection programs are in place.

CLASSIFICATION SYSTEMS

The location of the tumor dictates the anatomic classification: (1) cardial, (2) distal. It is frequently difficult to assign the location of origin in tumors of the gastroesophageal junction as esophageal or gastric, especially when the tumor has reached a considerable size. The occurrence of distal tumors has decreased in recent decades; in contrast, the occurrence of proximal tumors has increased, especially in industrialized countries, apparently related to gastroesophageal reflux. Adenocarcinomas of the cardia display aggressive behavior, invading the gastric and esophageal walls and metastasizing to local lymph nodes; the 5-year survival rate is around 14% in the United Sates. The American Joint Commission on Cancer Classification (AJCC) decided to classify tumors of the gastroesophageal junction and those involving the proximal 5 cm of the stomach as esophageal carcinomas.[23]

The degree of invasion dictates the classification of gastric cancer as early or advanced. Early cancers are limited to the mucosa and submucosa, irrespective of lymph node metastasis. Beyond those layers, tumors are classified as advanced. Five year survival rates are 85% to 100% for early cancers and 5% to 20% for advanced cancers. Advanced cancer cases are classified according to the gross morphology as Bormann groups: (1) polyploid, (2) ulcerated with well-defined borders, (3) ulcerated with ill-defined borders, (4) infiltrating diffuse without evidence of mass or ulceration, which is frequently called linitis plastica.

Histologic Classification

The most frequently used classification is the Lauren classification,[24] which recognizes 2 types: intestinal (with intercellular junctions) and diffuse (without intercellular junctions), representing 2 different nosologic entities. Both types are associated with H pylori infection. Other classifications, more complex and of limited use, are proposed by the World Health Organization and the Japanese Endoscopic Society.[25,26] The intestinal type adenocarcinoma is so named because it forms glands or tubules lined by epithelium resembling the intestinal mucosa. It is the most frequent type found in all high incidence populations and its incidence has decreased in recent decades. It displays cohesion among tumor cells. Diffuse carcinoma cells lack cohesion and invade tissues independently or in small clusters. Signet ring cell carcinomas are classified as diffuse. Their tumor cells contain abundant cytoplasmic mucin that displaces the nucleus toward the periphery. Some classifications include the term colloid carcinomas for tumors with excessive mucus secretion, intracellular and/or extracellular. A small proportion of tumors are mixed, with intestinal and diffuse components. For statistical purposes, they are included in the intestinal type category.

The Precancerous Cascade

Before cancer becomes clinically apparent, a prolonged precancerous process takes place, with well-defined sequential stages: chronic active gastritis → chronic atrophic gastritis → intestinal metaplasia, first complete or small intestinal type and then incomplete or colonic → dysplasia (also called intraepithelial neoplasia), and finally invasive carcinoma. The process is initiated and sustained by infection with H pylori. Although the bacterial colonies remain in the gastric lumen, they induce an inflammatory process in the gastric mucosa that usually lasts for decades and may lead to gland loss (atrophy). The process is multifocal and is first seen in the incisura angularis and extends with time to the anterior and posterior gastric walls. Subsequently, the gastric epithelium is replaced by cells with intestinal phenotype (intestinal metaplasia). The metaplastic cells first display a small intestinal complete phenotype but, with time, they have a tendency to develop focal areas of large intestinal (incomplete or colonic) phenotype. Complete metaplastic cells are eosinophilic absorptive enterocytes with a well-developed brush border alternating with well-developed goblet cells; colonic metaplastic cells lack a brush border and have multiple irregular intracytoplasmic mucus vacuoles. Dysplasia is first low-grade and later develops foci of high-grade with increasing degrees of nuclear polymorphism and irregular architecture, which increase the cancer risk. In Japan, high-grade dysplasia is classified as intramucosal carcinoma. As the process advances, genetic abnormalities accumulate, such as mutations in the APC, TP53, and Kras genes. Hypermethylation and microsatellites may also be observed.

PREVENTION AND EARLY DETECTION

Strategies addressing cancer prevention are based on eradication of H pylori infection, recommendations on dietary changes to increase the daily intake of fresh fruits and vegetables and reduce salt consumption. Patients with extensive atrophic or metaplastic changes in the gastric mucosa have increased cancer risk. In these patients, periodic endoscopic surveillance is recommended.[27] If incomplete metaplasia or dysplasia are diagnosed, such surveillance is necessary. If the lesions are clearly identified topographically, endoscopic resection is a valid strategy. In Japan, endoscopic resection of such lesions leads to 5-year survival rates up to 90%.[3] An active search for serologic markers of high cancer risk is under way in Japan. So far, besides low pepsinogen levels as markers of corpus atrophy, accepted markers are not generally are available.

ACKNOWLEDGMENTS

This work was supported by grant P01-CA28842 from the National Cancer Institute.

REFERENCES

1. Ferlay J, Shin HR, Bray F, et al. GLOBOCAN 2008 v2.0, cancer incidence and mortality worldwide: IARC CancerBase No. 10 [Internet]. Lyon (France): International Agency for Research on Cancer; 2010. Available at: http://globocan.iarc.fr. Accessed October 4, 2012.
2. Jemal A, Bray F, Center MM, et al. Global cancer statistics. CA Cancer J Clin 2011;61:69–90.
3. Miyahara R, Niwa Y, Matsuura T, et al. Prevalence and prognosis of gastric cancer detected by screening in a large Japanese population: data from a single institute over 30 years. J Gastroenterol Hepatol 2007;22:1435–42.
4. Correa P, Cuello C, Duque E, et al. Gastric cancer in Colombia. III. Natural history of precursor lesions. J Natl Cancer Inst 1976;57:1027–35.

5. Anderson WF, Camargo MC, Fraumeni JF Jr, et al. Age-specific trends in incidence of noncardia gastric cancer in US adults. JAMA 2010;303:1723–8.

6. IARC monographs on the evaluation of carcinogenic risks to humans. Schistosomes, liver flukes and *Helicobacter pylori*. International Agency for Research on Cancer. Lyon (France): IARC Press; 1994.

7. Schneider BG, Peng DF, Camargo MC, et al. Promoter DNA hypermethylation in gastric biopsies from subjects at high and low risk for gastric cancer. Int J Cancer 2010;127:2588–97.

8. Censini S, Lange C, Xiang Z, et al. cag, a pathogenicity island of *Helicobacter pylori*, encodes type I-specific and disease-associated virulence factors. Proc Natl Acad Sci U S A 1996;93:14648–53.

9. Covacci A, Censini S, Bugnoli M, et al. Molecular characterization of the 128-kDa immunodominant antigen of *Helicobacter pylori* associated with cytotoxicity and duodenal ulcer. Proc Natl Acad Sci U S A 1993;90:5791–5.

10. Higashi H, Tsutsumi R, Fujita A, et al. Biological activity of the *Helicobacter pylori* virulence factor CagA is determined by variation in the tyrosine phosphorylation sites. Proc Natl Acad Sci U S A 2002;99:14428–33.

11. Hatakeyama M. *Helicobacter pylori* and gastric carcinogenesis. J Gastroenterol 2009;44:239–48.

12. Cover TL, Blanke SR. *Helicobacter pylori* VacA, a paradigm for toxin multifunctionality. Nat Rev Microbiol 2005;3:320–32.

13. Achtman M, Azuma T, Berg DE, et al. Recombination and clonal groupings within *Helicobacter pylori* from different geographical regions. Mol Microbiol 1999;32:459–70.

14. Falush D, Wirth T, Linz B, et al. Traces of human migrations in *Helicobacter pylori* populations. Science 2003;299:1582–5.

15. de Sablet T, Piazuelo MB, Shaffer CL, et al. Phylogeographic origin of *Helicobacter pylori* is a determinant of gastric cancer risk. Gut 2011;60:1189–95.

16. Murphy G, Pfeiffer R, Camargo MC, et al. Meta-analysis shows that prevalence of Epstein-Barr virus-positive gastric cancer differs based on sex and anatomic location. Gastroenterology 2009;137:824–33.

17. IARC monographs on the evaluation of carcinogenic risks to humans. Tobacco smoke and involuntary smoking. International Agency for Research on Cancer. Lyon (France): IARC Press; 2004.

18. Joossens JV, Hill MJ, Elliott P, et al. Dietary salt, nitrate and stomach cancer mortality in 24 countries. European Cancer Prevention (ECP) and the INTERSALT Cooperative Research Group. Int J Epidemiol 1996;25:494–504.

19. Gonzalez CA, Jakszyn P, Pera G, et al. Meat intake and risk of stomach and esophageal adenocarcinoma within the European Prospective Investigation Into Cancer and Nutrition (EPIC). J Natl Cancer Inst 2006;98:345–54.

20. Camargo MC, Mera R, Correa P, et al. Interleukin-1beta and interleukin-1 receptor antagonist gene polymorphisms and gastric cancer: a meta-analysis. Cancer Epidemiol Biomarkers Prev 2006;15:1674–87.

21. Loh M, Koh KX, Yeo BH, et al. Meta-analysis of genetic polymorphisms and gastric cancer risk: variability in associations according to race. Eur J Cancer 2009;45:2562–8.

22. Persson C, Canedo P, Machado JC, et al. Polymorphisms in inflammatory response genes and their association with gastric cancer: a HuGE systematic review and meta-analyses. Am J Epidemiol 2011;173:259–70.

23. Edge SB, Byrd DR, Compton CC, editors. AJCC cancer staging manual. New York: Springer-Verlag; 2009.

24. Lauren P. The two histological main types of gastric carcinoma: diffuse and so-called intestinal-type carcinoma. An attempt at a histo-clinical classification. Acta Pathol Microbiol Scand 1965;64:31–49.
25. Japanese Gastric Cancer Association. Japanese classification of gastric carcinoma: 3rd English edition. Gastric Cancer 2011;14:101–12.
26. Bosman FT, Carneiro F, Hruban RH, et al, editors. WHO classification of tumours of the digestive system. Lyon (France): International Agency for Research on Cancer; 2010.
27. Correa P, Piazuelo MB, Wilson KT. Pathology of gastric intestinal metaplasia: clinical implications. Am J Gastroenterol 2010;105:493–8.

Gastric Cancer
Epidemiology and Risk Factors

Catherine de Martel, MD, PhD, David Forman, BA, PhD, FFPHM*,
Martyn Plummer, PhD

KEYWORDS

- Gastric cancer • Epidemiology • Risk factors • Helicobacter • Cardia • Noncardia

KEY POINTS

- There is a 10-fold international variation in the occurrence of gastric cancer, with rates in men double those of women.
- Globally, rates are declining by approximately 2.5% per annum but this is compensated by growth of and aging in the population.
- *Helicobacter pylori* infection is the major risk factor for noncardia gastric cancer and is now regarded by some as a necessary cause of such tumors.
- The best route to control noncardia gastric cancer would be through eradication of *H pylori*, although further research is required to evaluate such a strategy.
- Cardia gastric cancer is not associated with *H pylori* but is associated with cigarette smoking, increased body mass index, and with high socioeconomic status.

INTRODUCTION

Gastric cancer has long been one of the world's major cancers and remains one of the major causes of malignant disease morbidity and mortality. This article provides an overview of current understanding regarding the epidemiology of gastric cancer. A global picture is presented of incidence and mortality patterns and this is then followed by a consideration of the major identified risk factors. It is now apparent that the most important of these risk factors is infection with the bacteria *Helicobacter pylori* and this is, therefore, discussed in some detail with other factors. It is now clear that there is heterogeneity in the epidemiology of gastric cancer according to its location within the stomach with a distinction between cancers arising in the proximal cardia region and those arising more distally (noncardia). As a consequence, and where the data and literature allow, the epidemiology is reviewed in relation to each of these 2 groupings.

Conflict of Interests: Nil.
International Agency for Research on Cancer, 150 Cours Albert Thomas, 69372 Lyon Cedex 08, France
* Corresponding author.
E-mail address: formanD@iarc.fr

DESCRIPTIVE EPIDEMIOLOGY
Incidence and Mortality: Worldwide Estimates

GLOBOCAN 2008[1,2] provides the most recent figures available for the worldwide cancer burden. Almost 1 million new cases of gastric cancer (988,000 cases; 7.8% of all cancers) were estimated to have occurred globally in 2008, making it the fourth most common malignancy in the world, after cancers of the lung (1.68 million cases; 12.7% of all cancers), breast (1.31; 10.9%), and colorectum (1.24; 9.8%). More than 73% (728,000 cases) of gastric cancer cases occur in Asia, and almost half the world's total (47%) gastric cancer occurs in China (**Fig. 1**). Europe contributes nearly 15% of the global burden (146,000 cases), whereas Central and South America contribute a further 7% (65,000 cases) (see **Fig. 1**).

A global map of male age-standardized incidence rates using GLOBOCAN 2008 data (**Fig. 2**) shows that the highest rates occur in Eastern and South Eastern Asia, Eastern Europe, and parts of Central and South America. High rates are also evident in some countries in Africa and Southern Europe. The equivalent global map of female incidence rates (data not shown) is almost identical except that, in any given country, female rates are approximately half those seen in male rates.

Gastric cancer is the second leading cause of cancer death worldwide (738,000 deaths, 9.7% of all cancer deaths) after lung cancer (1.38 million deaths; 18.2% of all cancer deaths). Because prognosis following a diagnosis of gastric cancer is usually poor, the pattern of mortality is very similar to that for incidence and the proportional breakdowns of the 2 indicators by continent do not seem substantially different (see **Fig. 1**). For this reason, global maps of incidence and mortality are also very similar (data not shown). The above estimates represent the figures for cases of adenocarcinoma, the most common histologic type of gastric cancer. The authors recently estimated a worldwide total of lymphomas of gastric origin in 2008 to be 18,000 (ie, less than 2% of the number of adenocarcinomas).[3] Other gastric malignant histologies would be less common than this.

The summarized GLOBOCAN 2008 results present the best available estimates of the worldwide burden of gastric cancer. Because many assumptions are made in deriving these estimates and, in some cases, the observed data on which they are based are of suboptimal quality, it is important to consider also more reliable incidence information available from high-quality population-based cancer registries. Such information is provided in **Fig. 3**, which shows recent age-standardized incidence rates, by sex, from almost 50 cancer registries around the world, all of which have met the quality standards for publication in the definitive publication: Cancer Incidence in Five Continents.[4,5] The geographic distribution of these cancer registries reflects population coverage by high-quality cancer registration and there is a clear and notable deficit of such information from countries in Africa, Asia, and Central and South America.

Fig. 3 shows several important features of the descriptive epidemiology of gastric cancer. There is an approximate 10-fold variation in incidence rates ranging from, in men, around 60 per 100,000 in Japan and Korea to less than 6 per 100,000 in US whites, Jordan, and Saudi Arabia. Some part of the extremely high rates in Japan and Korea may be due to intensive radiographic or endoscopic surveillance programs and the detection of very small lesions that may rarely be diagnosed in other populations[6] but, even excluding these countries, one can still observe more than a fivefold variation in male incidence with rates over 30 per 100,000 in Belarus, the Russian Federation, and Costa Rica. Restricting attention to Europe, there is considerable variation between the highest rates, generally in Eastern European countries, and the lowest, in Scandinavian countries, Switzerland, and France. There is also wide

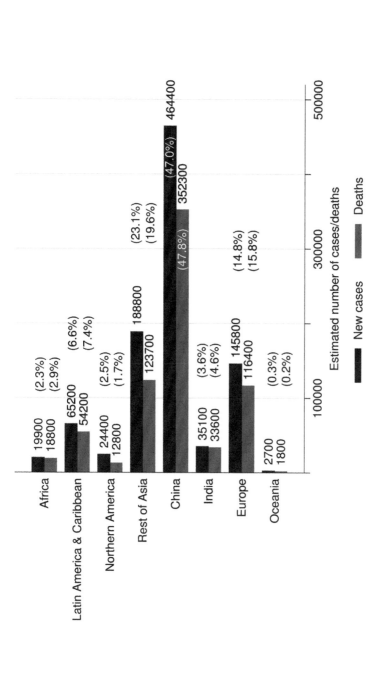

Fig. 1. Estimated number of new cases of and deaths from gastric cancer (proportion of global fraction) for 2008, both sexes combined, by world region. (*From* Ferlay J, Shin HR, Bray F, et al. GLOBOCAN 2008 v2.0, Cancer Incidence and Mortality Worldwide: IARC CancerBase No. 10 [Internet]. Lyon (France): International Agency for Research on Cancer; 2010. Available at: http://globocan.iarc.fr. Accessed January 7, 2013.)

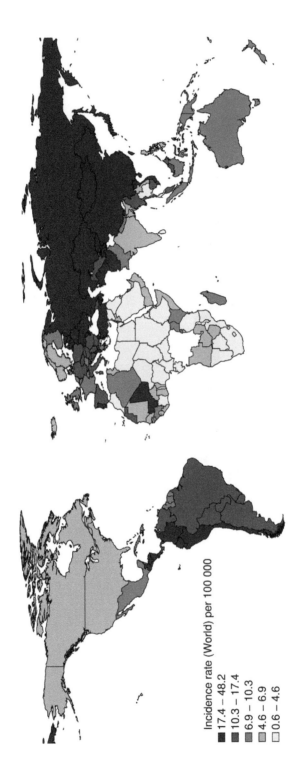

Fig. 2. World map showing estimated 2008 male age-standardized (world) incidence rates per 100,000 by country for gastric cancer. (*From* Ferlay J, Shin HR, Bray F, et al. GLOBOCAN 2008 v2.0, Cancer Incidence and Mortality Worldwide: IARC CancerBase No. 10 [Internet]. Lyon (France): International Agency for Research on Cancer; 2010. Available at: http://globocan.iarc.fr. Accessed January 7, 2013.)

Incidence rate (World) per 100 000

- 17.4 – 48.2
- 10.3 – 17.4
- 6.9 – 10.3
- 4.6 – 6.9
- 0.6 – 4.6

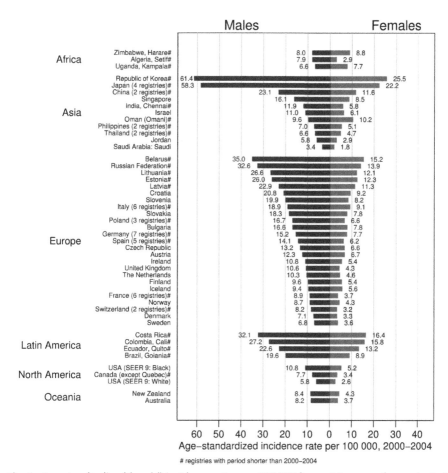

Fig. 3. Age-standardized (world) incidence rates per 100,000 for gastric cancer from selected cancer registries, 2000–2004, by sex. (*Data from* Curado MP, Edwards B, Shin HR, et al. Cancer incidence in five continents, vol. IX. Lyon (France): IARC; 2007. IARC Scientific Publications No 160. Updated with more recent data from cancer registries where available.)

variation within Asia and other interesting heterogeneities between, for example, countries within South America and between white and black US populations. **Fig. 3** also shows the worldwide consistency in the approximate 2:1 male/female ratio in incidence rates. The rank order of countries within each continent is more or less the same for both sexes. Although etiologic explanations can be proposed for the geographic distribution between populations,[7,8] the sex ratio difference in risk is more complex to understand.[9]

Incidence and Mortality: Trends Over Time

Cancer registry data from specific populations can also be used to analyze trends over time. **Fig. 4** provides such data from a group of registries selected to be representative of different world regions and different underlying incidence rates. Time trends in corresponding national rates of mortality are shown alongside those for incidence. As with the previous figures, the trends for women in each population (see **Fig. 4**B) are substantively the same as those for men (see **Fig. 4**A) but with reduced rates. The

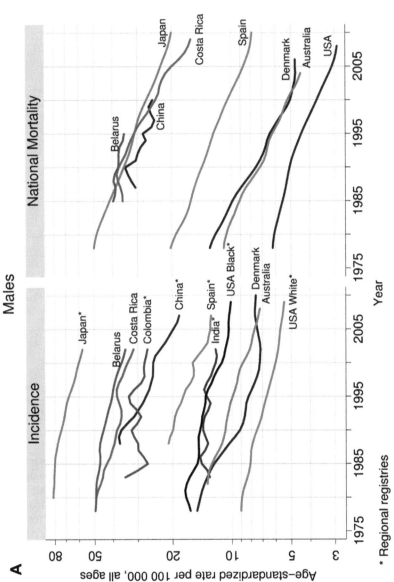

Fig. 4. Age-standardized (World) incidence and mortality rates in selected populations, 1978–2010. (*A*) male; (*B*) female. (*Data from* Curado MP, Edwards B, Shin HR, et al. Cancer incidence in five continents, vol. IX. Lyon (France): IARC; 2007. IARC Scientific Publications No 160. Updated with more recent data from cancer registries where available; and the World Health Organization. WHO mortality database. Available at: http://www. dep.iarc.fr/WHOdb/WHOdb.htm. Accessed January 8, 2013.)

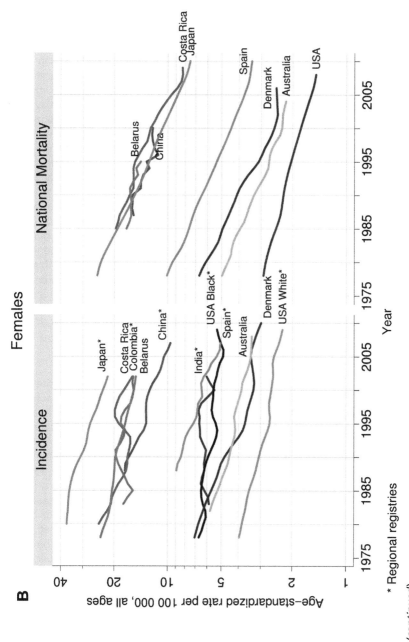

Fig. 4. (continued)

time span considered is usually from around 1980 to around 2010, depending on the availability of data. Over this 30-year period, and after making allowance for some sporadic year-to-year fluctuations, the tendency is toward a marked decline in age-standardized incidence and mortality apparent in nearly all populations. This marked decline in age-standardized incidence and mortality is irrespective of whether the population is at the high (eg, Japanese men) or low (eg, white US women) end of the risk spectrum. The one exception would seem to be incidence rates among the Indian population, which have remained relatively constant at around 15 per 100,000 in men and 6 per 100,000 in women. For those populations with long-running series, the extent of decline seems slightly greater in magnitude for mortality than for incidence, indicating that the former may be a result of a combined effect of improved survival with reduction in underlying risk. However, the extent of and consistency in risk reduction between apparently heterogeneous populations are quite remarkable and perhaps indicates a reduction in exposure to a globally ubiquitous risk factor such as *H pylori*. The downward trajectory in gastric cancer incidence worldwide is responsible for the substantive change in its ranking against other major cancers since the first global estimates were produced for 1975.[10] At this time, gastric cancer represented the most common neoplasm worldwide.

Analysis of these and other cancer registry data over time has provided an average Estimated Annual Percentage Change in gastric cancer incidence of -2.5% per annum.[11] One can apply this to GLOBOCAN 2008 estimates of the likely burden of gastric cancer in 2030, taking account of known changes in population demographics (ie, the growth in the population and the changes in its age structure). On this basis, the current global annual burden of gastric cancer, 988,000 new cases in 2008, is estimated to increase by a small extent to 991,000 new cases by 2030. Thus, the substantial decline in gastric cancer incidence rate is, more or less, balanced by the demographic changes in the world's population and, unless the Estimated Annual Percentage Change can be decreased still further, the absolute burden of this neoplasm will remain static.

Distribution by Subtype: Cardia Versus Noncardia

There is increasing interest in the distribution of gastric cancer by subsite of the stomach, in particular, the distinction between cancers originating in the most proximal cardia region and those originating more distally (noncardia). This interest is driven in part by evidence suggesting that these 2 categories may have different etiologies.[12] There have also been reports indicating that gastric cardia cancers have been increasing in incidence in recent decades,[13,14] thus providing a contrasting trend from that observed for gastric cancer overall. It has recently been estimated that, for 2008, approximately 88% of gastric cancers globally would likely originate from regions other than the cardia, thus implying a current annual burden of 118,000 cardia and 880,000 noncardia cancers.[3] **Fig. 5** shows cardia cancer incidence rates, derived from Cancer Incidence in Five Continents data, for the same populations as shown in **Fig. 4**. Some populations, such as those from Japan and China, which have high rates of gastric cancer overall, also have relatively high rates of cardia cancer. These high rates of cardia cancer were, however, also the case for certain populations, such as from Denmark and among USA whites that have low rates of gastric cancer overall. As a proportion of the total gastric cancer incidence, the contribution from the cardia is, therefore, much higher in such low-risk populations.

Because gastric cardia cancers are not readily distinguished from lower esophageal adenocarcinomas, there has undoubtedly been some variation in pathologic practice in the organ to which these cancers have been assigned for classification purposes. Such variation may be present both between countries and over different time periods,

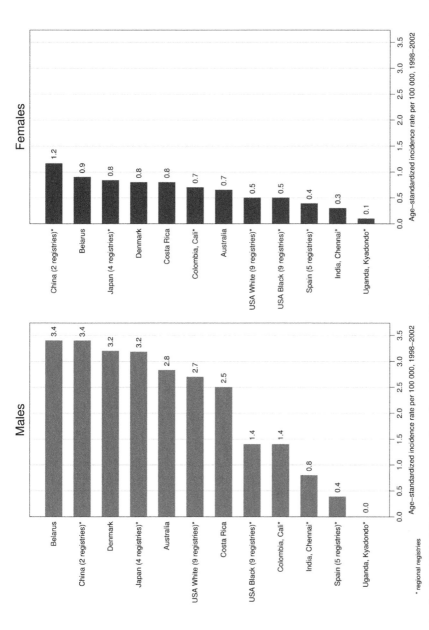

Fig. 5. Age-standardized (World) incidence rates of cardia gastric cancers (ICD-10 C16.0) from selected cancer registries, 1998–2002, by sex. (*Data from* Curado MP, Edwards B, Shin HR, et al. Cancer incidence in five continents, vol. IX. Lyon (France): IARC; 2007. IARC Scientific Publications No 160.)

thereby complicating interpretation of geographic and secular trends. Comparisons within the same populations over the same time period may, therefore, be more informative. Thus within the SEER cancer registries in the United States, white men had higher rates of cardia cancer than black men in contrast to the inverse pattern for gastric cancer overall. Comparisons by sex (see **Fig. 5**) also show that male cardia cancer rates were 3 to 4 times greater than those in women, indicating a somewhat larger excess than the 2:1 ratio for gastric cancer overall. In looking at these rates of cardia cancer, it should be noted that most cancer registry data sets include many gastric cancer notifications where the subsite is unspecified. Thus, for the registries shown in **Fig. 5**, more than 20% of gastric cancers (and often more than 50%) will not be specified regarding a cardia/noncardia location.

Migrant Studies

Migration studies show that first-generation migrants coming from countries with high incidence to countries of low incidence share the risk of their country of origin but that the incidence rate decreases in the following generation.[15] This decrease is particularly important for women.[16] The global picture suggests that environmental factors acting early in life have a crucial role in gastric carcinogenesis.

RISK FACTORS FOR GASTRIC CARCINOMA
Helicobacter pylori

H pylori is a spiral Gram-negative bacterium that colonizes the stomach. Although most infections are asymptomatic, H pylori is associated with chronic gastritis, peptic ulcer disease, gastric B-cell mucosa-associated lymphoid tissue lymphoma, and gastric adenocarcinoma. It is thought that H pylori was once ubiquitous in the human population, but in many populations its prevalence is declining in successive birth cohorts and it is now rare among children in Western Europe, North America, Oceania, and Japan.[17] The risk of H pylori infection is associated with low socioeconomic status, particularly overcrowding and poor sanitation,[18,19] so the gradual disappearance of H pylori in these populations may be a byproduct of economic development. The widespread use of antibiotics may also have played a role. It is noteworthy that the reduction in H pylori prevalence generally matches the decline in gastric cancer incidence and mortality.

In 1994, an expert working group convened by the International Agency for Research on Cancer (IARC) classified infection with H pylori as carcinogenic to humans, based on its association with gastric adenocarcinoma and mucosa-associated lymphoid tissue lymphoma.[20] This conclusion was confirmed in 2009 by a second IARC working group,[21] with the added precision that H pylori causes noncardia gastric carcinoma, because the risk of H pylori infection seems to be limited to the distal part of the stomach. The authors recently estimated that 75% of noncardia gastric cancers worldwide are attributable to H pylori.[3] However, it now seems that the strength of the association between gastric cancer and H pylori may have been underestimated, because of inaccurate assessment of H pylori infection status. Indeed, it has been hypothesized that H pylori is a necessary cause of gastric cancer.[22]

Almost all of the epidemiologic evidence on the relationship between H pylori and gastric cancer comes from serologic assessment of anti-H pylori immunoglobulin G (IgG) antibodies. It is now widely accepted that retrospective serologic assessment of H pylori infection in gastric cancer cases has poor sensitivity, so that case-control studies systematically underestimate the strength of the association. This problem is caused by atrophic gastritis, a precancerous lesion, which leads to a reduction in the burden of *H pylori* infection and a subsequent reduction in IgG antibody titers to the extent that an *H pylori* infection may become serologically undetectable. For this reason, most of the evidence base for the carcinogenicity of *H pylori* comes from prospective studies.

The most comprehensive relative risk estimates for *H pylori* and gastric cancer come from a pooled analysis of 12 prospective studies, which included 762 cases of noncardia gastric cancer and 2250 controls. The pooled odds ratio (OR) was 2.97 (95% CI 2.34–3.77) for *H pylori* infection.[23] The same study included 274 cases of cardia gastric cancer and 827 controls with an OR of 0.99 (95% CI 0.40–1.77) for *H pylori* infection. When the pooled analysis was restricted to cases occurring at least 10 years after the blood draw used for *H pylori* diagnosis, the OR increased to 5.93 (95% CI 3.41–10.3) for noncardia cancer but reduced to 0.46 (95% CI 0.23–0.90) for cardia cancer. This subgroup analysis underscores both the difference between cardia and noncardia cancer and the need to account for the effect of gastric carcinogenesis on *H pylori* measurement, even in prospective studies. Further follow-up of the individual studies contributing to this pooled analysis is reviewed in the IARC Monographs, volume 100, part B,[21] and did not change the substantive conclusions.

The cag pathogenicity island

H pylori is genomically highly diverse and this diversity may contribute to the clinical outcome of the infection. Several genetic factors associated with *H pylori* colonization (*babA, sabA, alphAB, hopZ*) and virulence (*cagA, vacA*) have been identified.[21] The genetic marker that has attracted the most attention in epidemiologic studies is the presence of the *cag* pathogenicity island, a DNA sequence of 40 kbp that is present in 70% of *H pylori* strains in Europe and North America, but is ubiquitous in Asia and most of Africa.[21] The CagA protein encoded by the *cagA* gene within the *cag* pathogenicity island is highly immunogenic, which allows the serologic detection of an infection with a *cag*-positive *H pylori* strain by the presence of anti-CagA antibodies. CagA-positive strains are associated with higher risk of gastric cancer than Cag-negative strains. A meta-analysis of 16 cohort and case-control studies including 778 cases of noncardia gastric cancer and 1409 matched controls found an elevated risk of CagA-positive *H pylori* infections, with an OR of 2.01 (95% CI 1.21–3.32) for CagA-positivity among all *H pylori*-infected individuals.[24]

The *cag* pathogenicity island is also associated with precancerous gastric lesions. Plummer and colleagues[25] analyzed a cross-sectional endoscopic survey of 2145 individuals from Venezuela, in which both the presence of *H pylori* DNA and the presence of the *cagA* gene were determined by polymer chain reaction on gastric biopsies. Infection with *cagA*-positive *H pylori* strains but not *cagA*-negative strains was associated with severity of precancerous lesions. Using individuals with normal gastric mucosa or superficial gastritis as controls, the OR for dysplasia was 15.5 (95% CI 6.4–37.2) for *cagA*-positive *H pylori* compared with 0.90 (95% CI 0.37–2.17) for *cagA*-negative *H pylori*. Gonzalez and colleagues[26] analyzed a follow-up study of 312 individuals from Spain with an average of 12.8 years of follow-up between 2 endoscopies, also using polymer chain reaction detection and genotyping of *H pylori*. The relative risk for progression of precancerous lesions was 2.28 (95% CI 1.13–4.58) for *cagA*-positive strains compared with *cagA*-negative strains.

Enzyme-linked immunobsorbent assay versus immunoblot

The standard laboratory method for assessing *H pylori* antibodies in epidemiologic studies is enzyme-linked immunobsorbent assay (ELISA). The few studies that have compared ELISA with immunoblot have consistently found stronger OR for noncardia gastric cancer with immunoblot assays. These studies are summarized in **Table 1**.

Two case-control studies have used immunoblot indirectly, as an exclusion criterion. Ekstrom and colleagues[27] analyzed a case-control study of gastric cancer including 231 noncardia cases and 238 controls using ELISA to measure H pylori infection. The authors excluded both cases and controls from the "H pylori negative" exposure group if they were positive for anti-CagA antibodies by immunoblot, on the basis that this was a marker of past infection that was no longer detectable by ELISA. This exclusion increased the OR for H pylori from 2.2 (95% CI 1.4–3.6) to 21.0 (95% CI 8.3–53.4). Brenner and colleagues[22] analyzed a case-control study including 57 noncardia gastric cancer cases and 360 controls, applying several exclusion criteria to minimize the bias of retrospective assessment of H pylori infection, including the exclusion of participants who were H pylori negative by ELISA, but CagA positive by immunoblot. These exclusions increased the OR from 3.7 (95% CI 1.7–7.9) to 18.3 (95% CI 2.4–136.7). However, the exclusions also reduced the number of noncardia gastric cancer cases from 57 to 33 with a corresponding loss of power; despite the dramatic increase in OR, the confidence interval is still consistent with the original estimate of 3.7.

These results are limited by the retrospective nature of the H pylori measurements and the extensive data manipulation used during the analysis. However, increased OR with immunoblot have been observed in 3 prospective studies using the same commercial test (Helicoblot 2.1; Genelabs Diagnostics, Singapore). Siman and colleagues[28] revisited the prospective study reported by Siman and colleagues[29] after a further 8 years of follow-up, increasing the number of noncardia gastric cancer cases from 27 to 67. The original study used ELISA and reported an OR of 11.1 (95% CI 2.4–71.8); the follow-up analysis used immunoblot, with an OR of 17.8 (95% CI 4.2–74.8). Mitchell and colleagues[30] reported results for both ELISA and immunoblot in a prospective study of 67 cases. The OR was 2.3 (95% CI 0.9–5.8) using ELISA compared with 10.6 (95% CI 2.4–47.4) using immunoblot. Finally, Gonzalez and colleagues[31] reported a prospective study of 88 cases from 10 European countries. The OR using ELISA was 6.81 (95% CI 3.0–15.1) compared with 21.4 (95% CI 7.1–64.4) using immunoblot.

Taken together, these results suggest that epidemiologic studies using ELISA to measure H pylori infection may have underestimated the relative risk of H pylori infection because of misclassification of the exposure status, and they raise the possibility that H pylori may be a necessary cause of noncardia gastric cancer. Gonzalez and colleagues[31] note that the H pylori prevalence of 93% they observed in noncardia

Table 1
Studies of noncardia gastric cancer comparing H pylori assessment by ELISA and by immunoblot

Study	Country	Design	No. of Cases[a]	ELISA OR	95% CI	Immunoblot OR	95% CI
Ekstrom et al,[27] 2001	Germany	Retrospective	231 (182)	2.2	1.4–3.6	21.0	8.3–53.4
Brenner et al,[22] 2004	Sweden	Retrospective	57 (33)	3.7	1.7–7.9	18.3	2.4–136.7
Siman et al,[29] 1997	Sweden	Prospective	27	11.1	2.4–71.8	—	—
Siman et al,[28] 2007	Sweden	Prospective	67	—	—	17.8	4.2–74.8
Mitchell et al,[30] 2008	Australia	Prospective	34	2.3	0.9–5.8	10.6	2.4–47.4
Gonzalez et al,[31] 2012	Europe	Prospective	88	6.81	3.0–15.1	21.4	7.1–64.4

[a] Brackets indicate the number of cases in the immunoblot analysis after applying exclusion criteria.

gastric cancer cases is similar to the sensitivity of the immunoblot test to past infection (92%) and so the results are compatible with an underlying 100% prevalence in cases.

H pylori eradication trials

H pylori infection is persistent if untreated, but it may be eradicated by a combination of 2 antibiotics and a proton pump inhibitor.[32] Trials of H pylori eradication for the prevention of gastric cancer face an important logistical problem that gastric carcinogenesis is a long process, requiring decades of follow-up. Hence eradication trials have concentrated on progression and regression of precancerous lesions as a primary endpoint and have low power to detect differences in gastric cancer incidence or mortality, even when these data are collected as secondary outcomes.[21] An exception is the Shandong Intervention Trial, which, after 15 years of follow-up, shows a significant reduction in gastric cancer incidence in the group receiving H pylori treatment (3.0% vs 4.6%, OR = 0.61, 95% CI 0.38–0.96) and a similar but nonsignificant reduction in gastric cancer mortality (hazard ratio 0.67, 95% CI 0.36–1.28).[33] In a review of H pylori eradication trials, Roesler and colleagues[32] conclude that there is a point of no return in the development of precancerous gastric lesions, beyond which H pylori eradication is ineffective in reducing the risk of subsequent gastric cancer. Thus, despite the overwhelming evidence that H pylori causes gastric cancer, there is still doubt over whether large-scale eradication programs in adults would be effective in reducing gastric cancer incidence, even in high-risk populations.

A slightly different issue is the use of H pylori eradication in the management of early gastric cancer (EGC), an in situ carcinoma which, in Japan and Korea, is treated by endoscopic resection. One nonrandomized study[34] and one randomized trial[35] of H pylori eradication after endoscopic resection of EGC have shown reduced incidence of metachronous EGC. However, these findings have not been reproduced.[36] Irrespective of the implications for clinical management of EGC, these results raise the possibility that H pylori is involved in the most advanced stages of gastric carcinogenesis, in apparent contradiction with the "point-of-no-return" hypothesis for gastric cancer prevention.

Other Risk Factors

Socioeconomic status (SES) and surrogate factors for SES

Less developed countries share a greater burden of gastric cancer than more developed countries, where both incidence and mortality are currently decreasing, due in part to the slow disappearance of H pylori that accompanied progressive access to better living conditions in people born after World War II. Furthermore, within any country or population, noncardia gastric cancer is most often seen in lower socioeconomic groups and has been associated with many risk factors that act as surrogate for lower SES, mainly low income, lower education, number of siblings, crowding, and lower occupational activity.[37,38] Hence, higher SES is inversely associated with noncardia gastric cancer, whereas it is strongly associated with cardia gastric cancer and esophageal adenocarcinoma. To be noted, many factors involved in gastric cancer epidemiology are also associated with SES and probably confound some of the observed associations, as is especially true for H pylori infection, as seen in a large European multicenter study, where adjustment for the presence of the bacterium makes the effect of SES in noncardia gastric cancer totally disappear (**Table 2**).[39] Other factors, such as fruit and vegetable consumption, cigarette smoking, and physical activity, may also confound any observed association with SES.

Table 2
Main risk factors for gastric cancer by anatomic location

Risk Factor	Noncardia (Distal) Gastric Cancer RR (95% CI)	Cardia Gastric Cancer RR (95% CI)	Source of Data
Helicobacter pylori serology			
IgG antibodies positive	**2.97 (2.34–3.77)**	0.99 (0.72–1.35)	Pooled analysis of nested
IgG-positive and serum drawn >10 y before cancer	**5.93 (3.41–10.3)**	**0.46 (0.23–0.90)**	case-control studies HCCG 2001
Higher socioeconomical status			
University degree vs lowest education level (adjusted for *H pylori* infection)	1.51 (0.81–2.78)	**2.38 (1.12–5.0)**	EPIC study Nagel et al,[39] 2007
Cigarette smoking			
Current vs never	**1.60 (1.41–1.80)**	**1.87 (1.31–2.67)**	Meta-analysis Ladeiras-Lopes et al,[40] 2008
Alcohol drinking			
Current vs never	1.07 (0.91–1.26)	0.94 (0.78–1.13)	Meta-analysis
Heavy vs never	1.17 (0.78–1.75)	0.99 (0.67–1.47)	Tramacere et al,[44,45] 2012
Obesity			
BMI 25 to 30	1.16 (0.94–1.43)	**1.40 (1.16–1.68)**	Meta-analysis
BMI >30	1.26 (0.89–1.78)	**2.06 (1.63–2.61)**	Yang et al,[58] 2009
Diet			
Fruits (highest vs lowest category)	**0.61 (0.44–0.84)**	**0.58 (0.38–0.89)**	Meta-analysis Lunet et al,[48] 2007
Vegetables (highest vs lowest category)	**0.75 (0.59–0.95)**	**0.63 (0.50–0.79)**	

Statistically significant associations are shown in bold.
Abbreviation: RR, Relative risk estimates.

Tobacco and alcohol

Smoking is an established cause of gastric cancer, but seems to act as a moderate risk factor, compared with other tobacco-related cancers. A meta-analysis including only prospective studies (cohorts, case-cohorts, and nested case-control studies) showed a summary risk estimate of gastric cancer of 1.62 (1.50–1.75) in male smokers and a summary risk estimate of gastric cancer of 1.20 (1.01–1.43) in female smokers, compared with never smokers.[40] This and other meta-analyses have shown that the risk for stomach cancer increases significantly with increasing number of cigarettes per day, pack-years, or duration of smoking.[41] The risk for gastric cancer has also been generally found to be lower in former smokers than in current smokers.

Gastric cancers may show a slightly different effect in response to smoking according to subsite, although the literature shows some heterogeneity. A meta-analysis yielded summary relative risks of 1.87 (95% CI 1.31–2.67) for cardia cancers and 1.60 (95% CI 1.41–1.80) for noncardia cancers based on 9 cohort studies (see **Table 2**).[40]

Very few studies have effectively investigated the role of tobacco while controlling for *H pylori*. If *H pylori* is a necessary cause of gastric cancer, then smoking must act as a cofactor rather than an independent risk factor. Hence, it is interesting to note that smoking and CagA-positive *H pylori* strains seem to act synergistically in increasing the risk of noncardia cancer. In smokers, the relative risk in subjects infected with CagA-positive or CagA-negative strains were 16.6 (95% CI 4.3–64.2) and 9.2 (95% CI 2.7–31.9), respectively, compared with nonsmokers without detected *H pylori* infection, whereas in non-smokers, the same relative risks were 6.1 (95% CI 2.3–16.5) and 2.4 (95% CI 0.8–6.9), respectively, compared with nonsmokers without detected *H pylori* infection.[42]

A possible relationship between alcoholic beverage consumption and risk for stomach cancer has long been hypothesized, but in most prospective studies, the relative risk was not significantly elevated.[43] However, in the few studies that distinguished between anatomic locations, a slightly stronger association was found for noncardia than for cardia gastric cancer (see **Table 2**).[44,45]

Food and nutrition

In 2007, an expert panel convened by the World Cancer Research Fund (WCRF) and the American Institute for Cancer Research graded nutritional risk factors for cancer on a 5-level scale, according to the strength of the evidence (convincing, probable, suggestive, inconclusive, and unlikely).[46] According to this panel, no dietary risk factor for gastric cancer belongs to the level 1 (convincing), but a few belong to level 2 (probable). Probable protective factors are nonstarchy vegetables, including specifically allium vegetables as well as fruits. Probable risk factors are salt and also salt-preserved foods. All other dietary factors show limited level of evidence (levels 3 or 4).

Fruits and vegetables In a meta-analysis based on 17 case-control studies and 5 cohort studies and looking at all stomach cancers irrespective of anatomic location, the WCRF expert panel found that the estimated effect for the highest versus the lowest level of intake was significantly protective in case-control studies, but weak and nonsignificant in cohort studies (relative risk 0.98; 95% CI 0.91–1.06 for non-starchy vegetables and relative risk 0.95; 95% CI 0.89–1.02 for fruit).[46] Furthermore, the protective effect for fruit intake was stronger in studies performed in Asia than in the United States and Europe. For instance, the European Prospective Investigation into Cancer and Nutrition (EPIC) study did not find any evidence of association with fresh fruit intake or with total vegetable intake, even though a protective effect of total vegetables and onion and garlic (allium vegetables) was suggested for the intestinal type.[47]

One meta-analysis published in 2007 has investigated noncardia versus cardia gastric cancer separately in relation to fruit and vegetable consumption. The summary data showed that higher fruit or vegetable intake was associated with a decreased risk of gastric cancer for both cardia and noncardia cancer location (see **Table 2**), but seemed to have a more clear-cut protective effect on intestinal cancer types.[48] Again to be noted, except for one study included in the meta-analysis, all individual risk estimates were obtained using a case-control design.

Salt and salted preserved food According to the WCRF expert panel, a dose response relationship between salt consumption and gastric cancer incidence is substantially supported by the literature. For instance, the increase in relative risk for total salt use is estimated around 8% per gram per day from 2 cohort studies. Similar increased risks are found when salt consumption is measured in different ways (ie, salt added at the table and salted or salty food). Two recent meta-analyses, the first one including only prospective studies, have confirmed these results, showing summary relative risks of 1.68 (95% CI 1.17–2.41) and 1.22 (95% CI 1.17–1.27) for high-salt versus low-salt intake.[49,50] Cardia and noncardia were not investigated separately in any of these reviews, but 2 interesting subgroup analyses or separate findings should be mentioned. First, salt consumption was a particularly strong predictor of gastric cancer in studies conducted in Japanese populations. Of note, a recent population study in Norway did not find any effect of a high consumption of dietary salt on gastric cancer risk.[51] Second, in the few studies that controlled for *H pylori*, the effect of salt appeared to be independent of the CagA status. However, the association was found to be stronger in the presence of *H pylori* infection with atrophic gastritis.[52,53]

A few other recent studies have brought some more insight on the broad subject of diet in regard to gastric cancer. First the EPIC has published data suggesting that flavonoids (phenolic compounds that occur widely in plant-based foods such as fruit and vegetables, tea, wine, and cocoa products) are associated with a significant 20% reduction of gastric cancer risk in women.[54] Second, a recent meta-analysis has suggested a 50% higher risk of gastric cancer associated with intake of pickled vegetables/food and perhaps stronger associations in China and Korea.[55]

Vitamin C Few studies were able to evaluate accurately the effect of vitamin C on the risk of gastric cancer. Within the EPIC cohort, higher plasma vitamin C levels were associated with a lower risk of cancer and did not seem to be limited to a particular anatomic subsite or histologic subtype.[56] In contrast, dietary vitamin C showed no significant association with cancer risk. The WCRF expert panel was not able to draw any conclusions about Vitamin C based on available evidence.[46]

Body Mass Index and Physical Activity

Overweight and obesity have been associated with increased risk of many cancers.[57] A recent meta-analysis has shown an elevated risk for cardia gastric cancer with a summary relative risk estimate of 1.4 (95% CI 1.16–1.68) in overweight subjects (body mass index [BMI] 25–30), and 2.06 (95% CI 1.63–2.61) in obese subjects (BMI >30) (see **Table 2**).[58] However, no increased risk has been found for noncardia gastric cancer in several different population-based cohorts.[57,59,60]

Conversely, regular physical activity seems to be associated with a decreasing risk of noncardia gastric cancer. Among many studies that have looked at physical activity in patients with cancer, 2 recent prospective studies specifically targeted gastric cancer, and both found a protective association.[59,61]

Epstein-Barr Virus

Epstein-Barr virus (EBV) is present in approximately 10% of gastric cancers. There is strong mechanistic evidence that EBV is a cause of gastric cancer. EBV DNA is present in tumor cells in monoclonal form and transforming EBV cells are expressed in the tumor cell.[21] However, epidemiologic evidence for an association between EBV and gastric cancer is weak, because of the difficulty of controlling for confounding by *H pylori*. For this reason, the same working group that concluded that *H pylori* causes noncardia gastric cancer did not conclude that EBV causes gastric cancer.[21]

Genetic Factors

Up to 3% of the total gastric cancer burden is thought to be the result of an inherited predisposition syndrome.[62] Among them, inherited gastric cancers of the diffuse type are generally referred to as hereditary diffuse gastric cancer (HDGC). The identification of a germline inactivating mutation in the gene encoding for E-cadherin (CDH1) in a Maori family from New Zealand was the start point to understand HDGC pathogenesis.[63] In HDGC families, carriage of the abnormal E-cadherin gene confers more than an 80% lifetime risk of developing gastric cancer, leading to recommended genetic testing, screening, and often prophylactic total gastrectomy to carriers of CDH1 mutation.[62]

Other inherited predisposition syndromes are shown in **Table 3** and include Lynch syndrome, which shows an intestinal histology in 90% of the cases, and carries a lifetime risk of around 10% for gastric cancer (of note, this risk is much higher for colorectal or endometrial cancer); hereditary breast and ovarian cancer syndrome because of germline BRCA1 and BRCA2 mutations; Li-Fraumeni syndrome due to germline p53 mutations; and the much rarer familial adenomatous polyposis, Peutz-Jeghers, and juvenile polyposis syndromes associated with germline mutations in the APC gene, SMAD4 and BMPR1A genes, and STK11 gene, respectively.[64]

Other Miscellaneous Factors

Pernicious anemia, an autoimmune disorder characterized by atrophic damage restricted to the gastric body mucosa (gastric atrophy type A), confers an excess risk of developing gastric adenocarcinoma, with an incidence rate similar to that seen in gastric atrophy caused by H pylori (gastric atrophy type B).[65] This excess risk seems to be independent of H pylori infection, although the potential interaction between infection and pernicious anemia has not yet been thoroughly studied.

Prior gastric surgery for benign disorders (mainly gastric ulcer) has been established as a risk factor for subsequent development of adenocarcinoma well before the discovery of H pylori. It is not clear if a prior gastric surgery is itself increasing the risk of cancer in the remnant stomach (acting synergically with H pylori through mechanical adverse effects of the surgery, ie, bile reflux) or if it is merely a surrogate for long-term H pylori infection with the more aggressive CagA strains.[66,67]

Ionizing radiation has been proved to increase the risk of many cancers, including gastric carcinoma.[68] The best evidence comes from the longitudinal study including 38,576 atomic-bomb survivors in Hiroshima and Nagasaki, Japan, followed up between 1980 and 1999.[69] For a person-years weighted mean dose of 1.6 Gy, the relative risk was 1.71 (95% CI 1.27–2.30) compared with the lowest dose, with a significant dose response trend ($P = .009$).

Table 3
Inherited predisposition syndromes for gastric cancer

Cancer Syndrome	Gene	Population Frequency	Gastric Cancer Risk
Hereditary diffuse gastric cancer (HDGC)	CGH1	Very rare	>80%
Hereditary breast/ovarian cancer	BRCA1/2	1/40 to 1/400	2.6–5.5%
Lynch syndrome	MLH1, MSH2, MSH6, PMS2, Epcam	1/440	6–13%
Li-Fraumeni syndrome	p53	1/5000	2.8%
Familial adenomatous polyposis	APC	1/10,000 to 1/15,000	0.5%–2%
Juvenile polyposis	SMAD4, BMPR1A	1/16,000 to 1/100,000	21%
Peutz-Jeghers syndrome	STK11	1/25,000 to 1/250,000	29%

From Chun N, Ford JM. Genetic testing by cancer site: stomach. Cancer J 2012;18(4):355–63.

SUMMARY

Gastric cancer is one of the major malignancies in the world, although there is significant international variation in its occurrence with rates in the areas of highest incidence being 10 times greater than in areas of lowest incidence. In general, male rates are double the female rates. Those countries where data are available over time show declining incidence rates with an estimated annual percentage change of −2.5% per annum. In terms of absolute numbers, however, the decline in incidence is compensated by growth of and aging in the population leading to a relatively small predicted net change over the next decades. The global pattern of cardia cancer is not the same as that for noncardia gastric cancer.

Infection with H pylori is the major risk factor for noncardia gastric cancer and is now regarded by some as a necessary cause of such tumors. Many epidemiologic studies have shown evidence of a strong association between infection and noncardia cancer. The magnitude of this association may have been substantially underestimated in most studies using ELISA rather than immunoblot technology. CagA-positive strains of H pylori may show a stronger association with noncardia gastric cancer than negative strains. There is not clear evidence yet that population-based eradication of H pylori results in a reduced risk of gastric cancer. Tobacco smoking is another risk factor for noncardia cancer. Although its effect is quite modest, it may act synergistically with H pylori, especially the most virulent CagA strains. Many studies and meta-analyses indicate that elevated consumption of fruit and vegetables protects against noncardia cancer, although evidence for this relationship is less compelling in prospective cohort studies.

Cardia gastric cancer does not show an association with H pylori and may even be associated with an absence of infection. Like noncardia cancer, it is associated with cigarette smoking and elevated fruit and vegetable consumption seems protective. However, unlike noncardia cancer, there seems to be positive associations with increased BMI and with high socioeconomic status.

The best route to the control of noncardia gastric cancer would seem to be through the eradication of H pylori, although further research is required to evaluate such a strategy. Tobacco control and dietary guidance to increase fruit and vegetable intake may be effective to some extent and, of course, would be beneficial for control of other diseases. Cardia cancer is currently much less significant in global terms but it may be increasing in incidence and may also be a part of the spectrum of cancers that are obesity related.

ACKNOWLEDGMENTS

We thank Joannie Lortet-Tieulent for support in providing the figures and Katiuska Veselinovic for preparing the manuscript.

REFERENCES

1. Ferlay J, Shin HR, Bray F, et al. Estimates of worldwide burden of cancer in 2008: GLOBOCAN 2008. Int J Cancer 2010;127:2893–917.
2. Ferlay J, Shin HR, Bray F, et al. GLOBOCAN 2008 v2.0, Cancer Incidence and Mortality Worldwide: IARC CancerBase No. 10 [Internet]. 2010. Lyon (France): International Agency for Research on Cancer; 2010. Available from: http://globocan.iarc.fr. Accessed January 7, 2013.
3. de Martel C, Ferlay J, Franceschi S, et al. The global burden of cancers attributable to infections in the year 2008: a review and synthetic analysis. Lancet Oncol 2012;13(6):607–15.

4. Curado MP, Edwards B, Shin HR, et al. Cancer incidence in five continents, vol. IX. Lyon (France): IARC; 2007. IARC Scientific Publications No 160.
5. Parkin DM, Ferlay J, Curado MP, et al. Fifty years of cancer incidence: CI5 I-IX. Int J Cancer 2010;127:2918–27.
6. Schlemper RJ, Itabashi M, Kato Y, et al. Differences in diagnostic criteria for gastric carcinoma between Japanese and western pathologists. Lancet 1997; 349:1725–9.
7. An international association between Helicobacter pylori infection and gastric cancer. The EUROGAST Study Group. Lancet 1993;341:1359–62.
8. Joossens JV, Hill MJ, Elliott P, et al. Dietary salt, nitrate and stomach cancer mortality in 24 countries. European Cancer Prevention (ECP) and the INTERSALT Cooperative Research Group. Int J Epidemiol 1996;25:494–504.
9. Sipponen P, Correa P. Delayed rise in incidence of gastric cancer in females results in unique sex ratio (M/F) pattern: etiologic hypothesis. Gastric Cancer 2002;5:213–9.
10. Parkin DM, Stjernsward J, Muir CS. Estimates of the worldwide frequency of twelve major cancers. Bull World Health Organ 1984;62:163–82.
11. Bray F, Jemal A, Grey N, et al. Global cancer transitions according to the Human Development Index (2008-2030): a population-based study. Lancet Oncol 2012; 13:790–801.
12. McColl KE, Going JJ. Aetiology and classification of adenocarcinoma of the gastro-oesophageal junction/cardia. Gut 2010;59:282–4.
13. Devesa SS, Blot WJ, Fraumeni JF Jr. Changing patterns in the incidence of esophageal and gastric carcinoma in the United States. Cancer 1998;83: 2049–53.
14. Botterweck AA, Schouten LJ, Volovics A, et al. Trends in incidence of adenocarcinoma of the oesophagus and gastric cardia in ten European countries. Int J Epidemiol 2000;29:645–54.
15. Haenszel W. Report of the working group on studies of cancer and related diseases in migrant populations. Int J Cancer 1969;4:364–71.
16. Kamineni A, Williams MA, Schwartz SM, et al. The incidence of gastric carcinoma in Asian migrants to the United States and their descendants. Cancer Causes Control 1999;10:77–83.
17. Herrera V, Parsonnet J. Helicobacter pylori and gastric adenocarcinoma. Clin Microbiol Infect 2009;15:971–6.
18. Palli D, Galli M, Caporaso NE, et al. Family history and risk of stomach cancer in Italy. Cancer Epidemiol Biomarkers Prev 1994;3:15–8.
19. Rothenbacher D, Bode G, Berg G, et al. Helicobacter pylori among preschool children and their parents: evidence of parent-child transmission. J Infect Dis 1999;179:398–402.
20. IARC Working Group on the Evaluation of Carcinogenic Risks to Humans. Schistosomes, liver flukes and Helicobacter pylori. IARC Monogr Eval Carcinog Risks Hum 1994;61:1–241.
21. Proceedings of the IARC Working Group on the Evaluation of Carcinogenic Risks to Humans. Biological Agents. A review of human carcinogens. IARC Monogr Eval Carcinog Risks Hum 2012;100(Pt B):1–441.
22. Brenner H, Arndt V, Stegmaier C, et al. Is Helicobacter pylori infection a necessary condition for noncardia gastric cancer? Am J Epidemiol 2004;159:252–8.
23. Helicobacter and Cancer Collaborative Group. Gastric cancer and Helicobacter pylori: a combined analysis of 12 case control studies nested within prospective cohorts. Gut 2001;49:347–53.

24. Huang J, Zheng G, Sumanac K, et al. Meta-analysis of the relationship between cagA seropositivity and gastric cancer. Gastroenterology 2003;125:1636–44.

25. Plummer M, van Doorn LJ, Franceschi S, et al. Helicobacter pylori cytotoxin-associated genotype and gastric precancerous lesions. J Natl Cancer Inst 2007;99:1328–34.

26. Gonzalez CA, Figueiredo C, Lic CB, et al. Helicobacter pylori cagA and vacA genotypes as predictors of progression of gastric preneoplastic lesions: a long-term follow-up in a high-risk area in Spain. Am J Gastroenterol 2011;106: 867–74.

27. Ekstrom AM, Held M, Hansson LE, et al. Helicobacter pylori in gastric cancer established by CagA immunoblot as a marker of past infection. Gastroenterology 2001;121:784–91.

28. Siman JH, Engstrand L, Berglund G, et al. Helicobacter pylori and CagA sero-positivity and its association with gastric and oesophageal carcinoma. Scand J Gastroenterol 2007;42:933–40.

29. Siman JH, Forsgren A, Berglund G, et al. Association between Helicobacter pylori and gastric carcinoma in the city of Malmo, Sweden. A prospective study. Scand J Gastroenterol 1997;32:1215–21.

30. Mitchell H, English DR, Elliott F, et al. Immunoblotting using multiple antigens is essential to demonstrate the true risk of Helicobacter pylori infection for gastric cancer. Aliment Pharmacol Ther 2008;28:903–10.

31. Gonzalez CA, Megraud F, Buissonniere A, et al. Helicobacter pylori infection assessed by ELISA and by immunoblot and noncardia gastric cancer risk in a prospective study: the Eurgast-EPIC project. Ann Oncol 2012;23:1320–4.

32. Roesler BM, Costa SC, Zeitune JM. Eradication treatment of helicobacter pylori infection: its importance and possible relationship in preventing the development of gastric cancer. ISRN Gastroenterol 2012;2012:935410.

33. Ma JL, Zhang L, Brown LM, et al. Fifteen-year effects of Helicobacter pylori, garlic, and vitamin treatments on gastric cancer incidence and mortality. J Natl Cancer Inst 2012;104:488–92.

34. Uemura N, Mukai T, Okamoto S, et al. Effect of Helicobacter pylori eradication on subsequent development of cancer after endoscopic resection of early gastric cancer. Cancer Epidemiol Biomarkers Prev 1997;6:639–42.

35. Fukase K, Kato M, Kikuchi S, et al. Effect of eradication of Helicobacter pylori on incidence of metachronous gastric carcinoma after endoscopic resection of early gastric cancer: an open-label, randomised controlled trial. Lancet 2008;372: 392–7.

36. Maeheta Y, Nakamura S, Fujisawa K, et al. Long-term effect of Helicobacter pylori eradication on the development of metachronous gastric cancer after endoscopic resection of early gastric cancer. Gastrointest Endosc 2012;75:39–46.

37. Hemminki K, Zhang H, Czene K. Socioeconomic factors in cancer in Sweden. Int J Cancer 2003;105:692–700.

38. Power C, Hypponen E, Smith GD. Socioeconomic position in childhood and early adult life and risk of mortality: a prospective study of the mothers of the 1958 British birth cohort. Am J Public Health 2005;95:1396–402.

39. Nagel G, Linseisen J, Boshuizen HC, et al. Socioeconomic position and the risk of gastric and oesophageal cancer in the European Prospective Investigation into Cancer and Nutrition (EPIC-EURGAST). Int J Epidemiol 2007;36:66–76.

40. Ladeiras-Lopes R, Pereira AK, Nogueira A, et al. Smoking and gastric cancer: systematic review and meta-analysis of cohort studies. Cancer Causes Control 2008;19:689–701.

41. IARC Working Group on the Evaluation of Carcinogenic Risks to Humans. Personal habits and indoor combustions. Volume 100 E. A review of human carcinogens. IARC Monogr Eval Carcinog Risks Hum 2012;100:1–538.
42. Brenner H, Arndt V, Bode G, et al. Risk of gastric cancer among smokers infected with Helicobacter pylori. Int J Cancer 2002;98:446–9.
43. IARC Working Group on the Evaluation of Carcinogenic Risks to Humans. Alcohol consumption and ethyl carbamate. IARC Monogr Eval Carcinog Risks Hum 2010; 96:3–1383.
44. Tramacere I, Pelucchi C, Bagnardi V, et al. A meta-analysis on alcohol drinking and esophageal and gastric cardia adenocarcinoma risk. Ann Oncol 2012;23: 287–97.
45. Tramacere I, Negri E, Pelucchi C, et al. A meta-analysis on alcohol drinking and gastric cancer risk. Ann Oncol 2012;23:28–36.
46. Wiseman M. The second World Cancer Research Fund/American Institute for Cancer Research expert report. Food, nutrition, physical activity, and the prevention of cancer: a global perspective. Proc Nutr Soc 2008;67:253–6.
47. Gonzalez CA, Pera G, Agudo A, et al. Fruit and vegetable intake and the risk of stomach and oesophagus adenocarcinoma in the European Prospective Investigation into Cancer and Nutrition (EPIC-EURGAST). Int J Cancer 2006;118: 2559–66.
48. Lunet N, Valbuena C, Vieira AL, et al. Fruit and vegetable consumption and gastric cancer by location and histological type: case-control and meta-analysis. Eur J Cancer Prev 2007;16:312–27.
49. D'Elia L, Rossi G, Ippolito R, et al. Habitual salt intake and risk of gastric cancer: a meta-analysis of prospective studies. Clin Nutr 2012;31:489–98.
50. Ge S, Feng X, Shen L, et al. Association between habitual dietary salt intake and risk of gastric cancer: a systematic review of observational studies. Gastroenterol Res Pract 2012;2012:808120.
51. Sjodahl K, Jia C, Vatten L, et al. Salt and gastric adenocarcinoma: a population-based cohort study in Norway. Cancer Epidemiol Biomarkers Prev 2008;17: 1997–2001.
52. Peleteiro B, Lopes C, Figueiredo C, et al. Salt intake and gastric cancer risk according to Helicobacter pylori infection, smoking, tumour site and histological type. Br J Cancer 2011;104:198–207.
53. Shikata K, Kiyohara Y, Kubo M, et al. A prospective study of dietary salt intake and gastric cancer incidence in a defined Japanese population: the Hisayama study. Int J Cancer 2006;119:196–201.
54. Zamora-Ros R, Agudo A, Lujan-Barroso L, et al. Dietary flavonoid and lignan intake and gastric adenocarcinoma risk in the European Prospective Investigation into Cancer and Nutrition (EPIC) study. Am J Clin Nutr 2012;96: 1398–408.
55. Ren JS, Kamangar F, Forman D, et al. Pickled food and risk of gastric cancer– a systematic review and meta-analysis of English and Chinese literature. Cancer Epidemiol Biomarkers Prev 2012;21:905–15.
56. Jenab M, Riboli E, Ferrari P, et al. Plasma and dietary vitamin C levels and risk of gastric cancer in the European Prospective Investigation into Cancer and Nutrition (EPIC-EURGAST). Carcinogenesis 2006;27:2250–7.
57. Lukanova A, Bjor O, Kaaks R, et al. Body mass index and cancer: results from the Northern Sweden Health and Disease Cohort. Int J Cancer 2006;118:458–66.
58. Yang P, Zhou Y, Chen B, et al. Overweight, obesity and gastric cancer risk: results from a meta-analysis of cohort studies. Eur J Cancer 2009;45:2867–73.

59. Sjodahl K, Jia C, Vatten L, et al. Body mass and physical activity and risk of gastric cancer in a population-based cohort study in Norway. Cancer Epidemiol Biomarkers Prev 2008;17:135–40.

60. Kuriyama S, Tsubono Y, Hozawa A, et al. Obesity and risk of cancer in Japan. Int J Cancer 2005;113:148–57.

61. Leitzmann MF, Koebnick C, Freedman ND, et al. Physical activity and esophageal and gastric carcinoma in a large prospective study. Am J Prev Med 2009;36: 112–9.

62. Fitzgerald RC, Hardwick R, Huntsman D, et al. Hereditary diffuse gastric cancer: updated consensus guidelines for clinical management and directions for future research. J Med Genet 2010;47:436–44.

63. Guilford P, Hopkins J, Harraway J, et al. E-cadherin germline mutations in familial gastric cancer. Nature 1998;392:402–5.

64. Chun N, Ford JM. Genetic testing by cancer site: stomach. Cancer J 2012;18: 355–63.

65. Annibale B, Lahner E, Bordi C, et al. Role of Helicobacter pylori infection in pernicious anaemia. Dig Liver Dis 2000;32:756–62.

66. Leivonen M, Nordling S, Haglund C. Does Helicobacter pylori in the gastric stump increase the cancer risk after certain reconstruction types? Anticancer Res 1997;17:3893–6.

67. Mezhir JJ, Gonen M, Ammori JB, et al. Treatment and outcome of patients with gastric remnant cancer after resection for peptic ulcer disease. Ann Surg Oncol 2011;18:670–6.

68. IARC Working Group on the Evaluation of Carcinogenic Risks to Humans. Radiation. IARC Monogr Eval Carcinog Risks Hum 2012;100:7–303.

69. Sauvaget C, Lagarde F, Nagano J, et al. Lifestyle factors, radiation and gastric cancer in atomic-bomb survivors (Japan). Cancer Causes Control 2005;16: 773–80.

Genetics/Genomics/Proteomics of Gastric Adenocarcinoma

Dushant S. Uppal, MD, MSc, Steven M. Powell, MD*

KEYWORDS

- Gastric cancer • Molecular genetics • Hereditary gastric cancer • Genomics
- Proteomics

KEY POINTS

- Hereditary diffuse gastric cancer can be caused by epithelial cadherin mutations for which genetic testing is available.
- Inherited cancer predisposition syndromes can be associated with gastric cancer.
- Chromosomal and microsatellite instability occur in gastric cancers.
- Several consistent genetic and molecular alterations have been identified in gastric cancers.
- Biomarkers and molecular profiles are being discovered with potential for diagnostic, prognostic, and treatment guidance implications.

INTRODUCTION

Gastric adenocarcinomas comprise the vast majority of malignant tumors arising from the stomach. Although other histopathologic forms of stomach tumors exist, they are rare in occurrence. Gastric cancer (GC) remains a significant worldwide health burden. GCs exhibit heterogeneity in clinical, biologic, and genetic aspects. The complexity of the genetics involved in gastric adenocarcinoma is reflected in the temporal, regional, and gender variation in GC incidence rates. A better understanding of these phenomena through molecular and genetic studies of gastric tumor genesis is anticipated to provide important insights into cancer development in general and lead to earlier diagnosis and better management options.

INHERITED SUSCEPTIBILITY
Familial Clustering

Most cases of GC appear to occur sporadically, without an obvious hereditary component. Familial clustering has been observed in approximately 12% of gastric carcinoma

Division of Gastroenterology/Hepatology, Department of Medicine, University of Virginia, 1300 Jefferson Park Avenue, Charlottesville, VA 22908, USA
* Corresponding author. Division of Gastroenterology/Hepatology, University of Virginia Health Systems, 1300 Jefferson Park Avenue, Box 800708, Charlottesville, VA 22908-0708.
E-mail address: smp8n@virginia.edu

Gastroenterol Clin N Am 42 (2013) 241–260
http://dx.doi.org/10.1016/j.gtc.2013.01.005
0889-8553/13/$ – see front matter © 2013 Elsevier Inc. All rights reserved.

cases, with a dominant inheritance pattern.[1] Notably, Napoleon Bonaparte apparently suffered from GC involving most of his stomach and may have had other family members (ie, his father and sister) afflicted as well.[2,3] In the Swedish Family Cancer Database, when a parent presented with gastric carcinoma, offspring showed an increased risk of the concordant carcinoma, with a Standardized Incidence Ratio (SIR) of 1.59, only at ages older than 50 years.[4] The increased risk from sibling GC probands (SIR of 5.75) was noted for those diagnosed before age 50 years. Taken together, these findings suggest that some of the familial risk factors are likely to be environmental, siblings being at a higher risk than offspring-parent pairs, consistent with the transmission patterns of *Helicobacter pylori* infection.

Case-control studies have observed consistent (up to threefold) increases in risk for GC among relatives of patients with GC.[5] A population-based control study found an increased risk of developing GC among first-degree relatives of affected patients (odds ratio [OR] = 1.7 with an affected parent, OR = 2.6 with an affected sibling), with the risk increasing (OR up to 8.5) if more than one first-degree relative was affected.[6] Interestingly, a higher risk was noted in individuals with an affected mother versus an affected father. Studies have shown a slight trend toward increased concordance of GCs in monozygotic twins compared with dizygotic twins.[7] A genomic analysis of 170 affected sib-pairs from 142 Japanese families with GC yielded several chromosomal regions, with the strongest linkage at 2q33-35, harboring potential susceptibility genes.[8]

Inherited Predisposition Syndromes

Inherited predisposition cancer syndromes are thought to comprise only 1% to 3% of all GCs.[9] Several genetic susceptibility traits with an inherited predisposition to GC development exist. Some are well-characterized clinically with their underlying genetic alterations being unveiled and are described in this article.

Hereditary diffuse gastric cancer

Three large Maori families with an obvious autosomal dominant, highly penetrant inherited predisposition to the development of GC, having sufficient power with which to perform productive linkage studies, revealed linkage to the epithelial cadherin (*E-cadherin*)/*CDH1* locus on 16q22.1 in 1998.[10] Further analysis of these families demonstrated association of GC development with germline mutations in the *E-cadherin* (*CDH1*) gene. Since then, multiple germline *E-cadherin* mutations have been reported in more than 100 families throughout the world.[11] The CDH1 gene mutations have been scattered across the 16 exons this gene encompasses, with approximately 70% being truncating and 30% missense in nature.[12,13] Moreover, there have even been large deletions of the E-cadherin gene identified in a small percentage (4%) of hereditary diffuse gastric cancer (HDGC) families, likely involving nonallelic homologous recombination in Alu repeat regions.[14]

The first definition of the hereditary diffuse GC trait, which is the only inherited cancer syndrome dominated by GC, was made in 1999.[15] The ages of onset for diffuse GC in subjects harboring germline *E-cadherin* mutations ranged from 14 to older than 70 years. The cumulative risk estimate for advanced GC by 80 years of age was estimated to be 67% for men and 83% in women with wide confidence intervals, as these were based on 11 HDGC families.[16] The mean age at GC diagnosis was 40 years in this study. Additionally, female *CDH1* mutation carriers had a high risk of developing lobular breast cancers with a lifetime risk of 60% by the age of 80 years. The incomplete penetrance of germline *E-cadherin* mutations was seen in several obligate carriers, who remained unaffected even in their eighth and ninth decades of life. Variable penetrance is suggested in the larger HDGC families and a later onset of the youngest cases in more recent HDGC families, most in their late 20s to early 30s.[11,17] A founder (common ancestry) mutation was observed in 4 Newfoundland families with penetrance of symptomatic GC by 75 years of age, being 40% for men and 63% for women.[18] Whether this incomplete penetrance is due to the stochastic nature of the second allele alteration or perhaps to the presence of phenotype-altering alleles at other genetic loci, remains to be determined. Indeed, allele-specific monoclonal *CDH1* promoter hypermethylation or loss of heterozygosity was found in early GC lesions from mutation carriers.[19,20]

Importantly, 12 of 18 asymptomatic gene carriers who underwent prophylactic gastrectomy had occult cancer, often seen as tiny clusters of signet ring cells within and underlying the mucosa. Only one of these individuals had a diffuse GC detected endoscopically with random biopsies before gastrectomy, indicating the ineffectiveness of this type of surveillance for these lesions. Indeed, no lesions were identified endoscopically or radiologically in 6 CDH1 gene carriers, yet all 6 had early-stage (TMN stage T1a) multifocal signet ring cell GC found on pathology examination after prophylactic gastrectomy.[21]

A study of 42 families diagnosed with HDGC trait by having at least 2 members affected had an *E-cadherin* mutation identified in 40% of cases.[22] If the clinical criteria were more stringent to include 1 GC occurring before 50 years of age, then more than half the cases had *E-cadherin* mutations detected. When large deletions were screened in addition to point mutations and small frameshift mutations, 46% of 160 high-risk families were found to have a germline E-cadherin gene alteration.[14] Furthermore, a study of 25 "sporadic" diffuse GCs identified 1 case with a germline *E-cadherin* mutation and none in 14 intestinal-type GCs.[23] Germline *CDH1* mutations were found in approximately 7% of sporadic diffuse GC cases diagnosed before the age of 50 years.[24] No germline mutations of this gene were detected in apparent "sporadic" diffuse GC cases with a mean age of 62 years in Great Britain.[25]

The first consensus guidelines for the clinical diagnosis and management of familial GC were developed in 1999,[26] then updated in 2010.[9] Management algorithms have been formulated, highlighting genetic testing and counseling based on collective experience and the literature to date. Genetic counseling for a kindred manifesting a strong predisposition toward development of diffuse GCs is imperative to ensure appropriate management. Once a gene carrier of an *E-cadherin* mutation reaches his or her mid to late 20s, prophylactic gastrectomy should be considered along with aggressive breast cancer surveillance starting at the age of 30.[11] Diffuse GC families are one kindred subgroup to whom genetic testing can now be offered.

It is noteworthy that more than half to up to two-thirds of HDGC families reported have proven negative for the *E-cadherin* gene mutation.[14,27] Allele expression imbalance of *CDH1* was noted in a subset of these families[28]; however, most of these families likely have other molecular alterations underlying their cancer predisposition that are yet to be discovered.

Other hereditary cancer predisposition syndromes

Several other hereditary cancer predisposition syndromes exist that, in addition to other predominant cancers, also appear to have an increased risk of developing GC, as listed later in this article. The incidence of GC differs somewhat, but is generally low compared with other cancers in these syndromes and both intestinal and diffuse histologic subtypes of GC have been described. A subset of families with these syndromes; however, can exhibit a striking cluster of GC.

A now well-characterized inherited predisposition syndrome that may include GC development is Lynch syndrome.[29] GCs occurring in the setting of germline mismatch repair gene mutations underlying Lynch syndrome were diagnosed at a mean age of 56 years, were predominantly intestinal-type, tended to lack evidence of *H pylori* infection, and exhibited microsatellite instability in a Finnish Lynch syndrome registry study.[30]

Li-Fraumeni syndrome is a rare inherited cancer syndrome defined by a clustering of malignancies, including sarcoma, breast cancer, brain tumor, leukemia, adrenocortical, and GC, attributable to germline mutation of the tumor suppressor gene p53.[31] An extended family affected by this syndrome demonstrated strong evidence of linkage to p53, and 3 of 4 gastric tumors analyzed showed loss of the wild-type allele.[32] However, GCs account for fewer than 4% of all neoplasms in this rare syndrome.[33] GCs have also been associated with the hereditary breast and ovarian cancer syndrome.[34]

Polyposis syndromes The Peutz-Jeghers syndrome is a rare autosomal dominant disorder characterized by germline mutations of STK11, hamartomatous polyposis, and pigmentation of the lips, buccal mucosa, and digits that carries an increased risk of many types of cancer, including those of the gastrointestinal tract, with gastric carcinomas observed.[35] An increased risk of GC associated with familial adenomatous polyposis has been reported in high-risk regions, such as Asia, whereas no significant increased risk was exhibited in other populations.[29,36] Overall, GC is rare in this setting, and the exact contribution of the polyposis and underlying germline alterations of the APC and MYH genes is unclear. Inherited allelic defects of the *MYH* base excision repair gene have been linked to 2.1% of sporadic cases of GC, and even to as many as 9.9% of patients with a familial pattern of GC.[37]

GCs have been noted to occur in patients with other gastrointestinal polyposis disease entities, such as juvenile polyposis, who harbor germline mutations in SMAD4 or BMPR1A.[38] Up to 24% of those with generalized juvenile gastrointestinal polyposis developed GC, which was similar to a subset of patients who presented with predominantly gastric polyposis and was found to have neoplastic tissue arising in 25% of the resected gastric specimens.[39] Cowden syndrome is a gastrointestinal hamartosis polyposis syndrome that is associated with multiple cancers, including rare GC.[40,41]

Other inherited syndromes

Rare kindreds exhibiting site-specific GC predilection have been reported, occasionally associated with other inherited abnormalities.[42,43] Indeed, a constitutional deletion of 18p inherited from her mother, with somatic loss of the remaining long arm of this chromosome, was observed in the GC of a 14-year-old girl with associated mental and cardiac abnormalities, suggesting a predisposing condition.[44] A few patients with GC have been rarely found to harbor germline mutations in the ATM (ataxia-telangiectasia mutated) gene and the proto-oncogene MET.[45] Familial intestinal GC not attributed to the previously mentioned well-characterized inherited cancer susceptibility syndromes has been described as well, although the underlying defect(s) remain uncertain.[46] Moreover, a kindred manifesting the autosomal dominant inheritance of familial gastric hyperplastic polyposis and GC development was demonstrated not to have *E-cadherin* or other identifiable genetic alteration.[47]

GENETIC ALTERATIONS

Molecular analyses of sporadic GCs for acquired changes have described many somatic alterations, but the significance of these changes in gastric tumorigenesis remains to be established in most instances. A study by Wright and colleagues[48] demonstrated that the human gastric mucosa is composed of clonal units with several multipotent stem cells. Additionally, intestinal metaplasia crypts exhibited clonality containing multiple pluripotent stem cells that can spread by crypt fission. Taken together, these findings provide evidence for how genetic mutations spread clonally in human gastric mucosa.

Chromosomal Instability

Most GCs exhibit significant gross chromosomal aneuploidy. One study found that 72% of differentiated tumors and 43% of undifferentiated gastric tumors were aneuploid.[49] Variability in the classification of instability or histopathologic subtype and in the number of loci examined account for some of this variation in aneuploidy, with a trend toward more frequent occurrence in intestinal-type cancers at more advanced stages. Cytogenetic studies of GCs are few in number and have failed to identify any consistent chromosomal abnormalities. A variable number of numerical or structural aberrations have been reported in GC cells, such as those involving chromosomes 3 (rearrangements), 6 (deletion distal to 6q21), 8 (trisomy), 11 (11p13-p15 aberrations), and 13 (monosomy and translocations).[50,51]

Comparative genomic hybridization (CGH) analyses have revealed several regions of consensus change in DNA copy number, indicating the possible location of candidate gastric oncogenes or tumor suppressor genes involved in gastric tumorigenesis.[52] A knowledge of these alterations is important, as GCs of different histopathologic features have been shown to be associated with distinct patterns of genetic alterations, supporting the notion that these cancers evolve via distinct genetic pathways. Chromosomal arms 4q, 5q, 9p, 17p, and 18q exhibited frequent decreases in DNA copy number, whereas chromosomes 8q, 17q, and 20q showed frequent increases in DNA copy number.[53] CGH analysis showed an increased frequency of 20q gains and 18q losses in tumors that metastasized to lymph nodes.[54] As described later in this article, several known or candidate tumor suppressor genes have been isolated within some of these frequently lost regions.

Comprehensive loss of heterozygosity (LOH) analysis of these tumors has identified 3p, 4p, 4q, 5p, 8q, 13p, 17p, and 18q to be frequently lost.[55] In LOH analysis of more than 100 archived GCs, allelic loss was most frequently noted on chromosome 3p.[56] Moreover, 3 distinct regions of chromosome 4q were found to be frequently lost in gastroesophageal junctional adenocarcinomas, indicating the potential for multiple tumor suppressor genes to be located on this chromosomal arm.[57]

Microsatellite Instability

Microsatellite instability (MSI) has been found in approximately 14% to 44% of sporadic GCs.[58] The degree of genome-wide instability also varies, with more significant instability (eg, with MSI-high [MSI-H] tumors exhibiting instability in >33% of loci tested) occurring in only 10% to 16% of GCs.[59]

Abnormal loss of protein expression of either MLH1 or MSH2 was demonstrated in all cases exhibiting MSI-H.[60] Altered expression of MLH1 was associated with increased methylation of the promoter region of MLH1 in MSI-H cases, suggesting a silencing role of hypermethylation.[61] Interestingly, no difference in the frequency of hMLH1 hypermethylation and MSI phenotype was noted between familial (non-Lynch and non-HDGC) and sporadic cases of GC, indicating epigenetic regulation in both these settings.[58]

MSI-H gastric tumors exhibit distinct clinicopathologic characteristics and a unique set of genetic alterations. Consistent associations of the MSI-H phenotype with intestinal subtype, distal location (eg, antral), and more favorable prognosis have been observed.[62] Several tumor suppressor genes have been shown to be critical targets of defective mismatch repair (MMR) in MSI-H tumors. At least one important target of MSI appears to be the transforming growth factor beta (TGF-β) type II receptor (*TGFβR2*) at a polyadenine tract within its gene.[63] Another gene involved in this signaling pathway, ACVR2, was found to be similarly mutated, even in a biallelic fashion, in gastric tumors exhibiting MSI.[64] Thus, alteration of TGF-β receptors and other members of this signaling path appears to be a critical event in the development of at least a subset of GCs, allowing escape from the growth control signal of TGF-β.

The proapoptotic BAX gene and additional MMR genes have also been demonstrated to be altered in MSI-H GCs. Somatic nonframeshift mutations have been reported in *BAX*.[65] Moreover, the relatively frequent missense mutations at codon 169 of *BAX* was shown to impair its proapoptotic activity.[66] These same genes are observed to be infrequently mutated or altered in MSI-low or MSS tumors.[62] Additional genes with simple tandem repeat sequences within their coding regions found to be specifically altered in GCs displaying MSI include *IGFRII*, *hMSH3*, *hMSH6*, and *E2F-4*, which are known to be involved in regulation of cell-cycle progression and apoptotic signaling.[67]

ACQUIRED SOMATIC GENETIC/MOLECULAR ALTERATIONS
TFF-1 Loss

Loss of the trefoil peptide TFF1(pS2), a stable 3-loop molecule synthesized in mucus-secreting cells, has been described in approximately 50% of GCs.[68] The biologic significance of this loss was reported in a knockout mouse model of gastric antral neoplasia.[69] Additionally, expression of TFF1 was observed to be lower in some gastric intestinal metaplasia and gastric adenomatous lesions compared with adjacent normal or hyperplastic mucosa.[70] *TFF1* resides on chromosome 21q22, a region noted to be deleted in some GCs in LOH studies.[71] Overexpression of TFF1 in the GC cell line, AGS, inhibited its growth.[72] Furthermore, the overwhelming majority of GCs studied had absent to minimal transcript levels compared with normal gastric mucosa.[73] Moreover, C/EBP-β was found to be overexpressed in most GCs in a corresponding manner and bind to the promoter of TFF1, suggesting a regulatory factor role.[74] Finally, cytokine signaling through the coreceptor gp130, with increased STAT-3 expression, has also been observed to decrease TFF1 and lead to gastric lesions in mice.[75] Additionally, characterization of gastrokine (GKN) 2, a stomach-specific tumor suppressor protein, was found to be structurally and physically related to TFF1.[76] Noteworthy, loss of GKN1 and GKN2 expression was found to occur in gastric adenocarcinoma and portend an overall shorter survival.[77]

E-Cadherin Alteration

In addition to germline mutations leading to HDGC described previously, several sporadic diffuse GCs have displayed altered *E-cadherin*. E-cadherin is a transmembrane, calcium ion–dependent adhesion molecule important in epithelial cell homotypic interactions, which, when decreased in expression, is associated with invasive properties.[78] Reduced *E-cadherin* expression determined by immunohistochemical analysis was noted in most GCs, 92% of 60 cases, when compared with their adjacent normal tissue.[79] Genetic abnormalities of the *E-cadherin* gene and transcripts were demonstrated in a third to one-half of diffuse GCs.[23,80] *E-cadherin* splice site alterations producing exon deletion and skipping, large deletions including allelic loss, and point mutations mostly of the missense nature have been demonstrated in diffuse-type cancers, some even exhibiting alterations in both alleles.[81] Methylation of the *E-cadherin* promoter region was found in 16 (26%) of 61 GCs studied.[61]

Kinases/Phosphatases

Activation of protein kinases by tyrosine kinases and phosphatases has been shown to affect many cellular activities, including cell growth, differentiation, and survival.[82] Noteworthy, a novel KGF-R2 phosphorylation inhibitor, Ki23057, decreased proliferation of 2 scirrhous GC cell lines with K-sam amplification.[83] Phosphatidylinositol 3-kinases (PI3K) are lipid kinases that regulate pathways for neoplastic proliferation, adhesion, survival and motility.[84] Mutations in *PIC3A,* which encodes a catalytic subunit of PI3K, have been characterized in several cancers including gliobastoma, colon, and up to 25% of GCs analyzed.[85] Further attempts at identifying mutations in *PIC3A* have reported a lower prevalence of 4.3% in GCs; however, this study also reported increased expression of this gene product in gastric tumors and a specific expression profile associated with this upregulation.[86] Moreover, increased PI3K/AKT signaling from nuclear factor kappaB (NF-kB) has been shown to activate transcription of HuR, which has proliferative and antiapoptotic effects on GC cells.[87] Furthermore, a kinase involved in chromosome segregation and stability, STK15 (BTAK, Aurora2), was found to be amplified and overexpressed in GCs.[88]

Wang and colleagues[89] identified 83 somatic mutations in human protein tyrosine phosphatases (PTPs), most affecting colon cancer, but also found them in 17% of GCs analyzed. The most commonly altered PTP, protein-tyrosinase phosphatase-receptor type (PTPRT) was found to decrease its activity, suggesting a role as a tumor suppressor gene. However, an additional polymerase chain reaction–based study suggests a much smaller role for alterations in PTPRT in gastric tumorigenesis, being found in only 1% of cases.[90] Overexpression of DARP32 and a novel truncated isoform was found in most GCs.[91] Moreover, an antiapoptotic effect of this overexpression of DARP32 and t-DARP was observed in vitro.[92]

Overexpression of the *MET* gene, which encodes a tyrosine kinase receptor for the hepatocyte growth factor, has been reported to have prognostic value to indicate poorer survival in multivariate analysis.[93] There have been numerous reports in the literature indicating that the *MET* gene is amplified in approximately 15% and its expression elevated in up to 50% of GCs.[94]

Methylation Silencing Alterations (Epigenetic Alteration)

A significant number (41%) of GCs exhibited CpG island methylation in a study of the promoter region of p16.[61] Many of these cases with hypermethylation of promoter regions displayed the MSI-H phenotype with multiple sites of methylation, including the *MLH1* promoter region.[95]

RUNX3, a tumor suppressor gene, appears to suppress gastric epithelial cell growth by inducing p21 (WAF1/Cip1) expression in cooperation with TGF-β–activated SMAD.[96] RUNX3 was found to be altered in 82% of GCs through either gene silencing or protein mislocalization to the cytoplasm.[97] Multiple other tumor suppressor genes and candidates, including protocadherin 10 (PCDH10), CDKN2A, GSTP1, APC, MGMT, DAKP, XAF1, THBS-1, RUNX1, and CDH1, have been shown to be methylated in GCs.[98]

Apoptosis Signaling Alterations

Mutations of the BAX gene, believed to be a promoter of apoptosis, have been identified in up to 33% of GCs, as well as in colorectal and endometrial cancers.[99] Another study supporting the role of the BAX gene in tumor suppression linked low expression levels of the protein Bax-interacting factor-1 (Bif-1) in GCs, suggesting another breakdown in the pathway of regulating apoptosis.[100] The bcl-2 homolog BAK, another promoter of apoptosis, was found to have missense mutations in 12.5% of GCs analyzed.[101] Defects in cell surface receptors of the apoptosis pathway have also been observed in gastric tumors, such as in the death receptors DR4 and DR5.[102]

Other Alterations

The *p53* gene has consistently been demonstrated to be altered in GCs, both by allelic loss in more than 60% of cases and mutations identified in approximately 30% to 50% of cases.[103] The spectrum of mutations in this gene is similar to other cancers, with a predominance of base transitions, especially at CpG dinucleotides.

The human epidermal growth factor receptor 2 (HER2/neu/ERBB2) has been demonstrated to be overexpressed in many types of cancer, including GC; and to be associated with metastasis. HER2 was shown to interact with CD44 and upregulated CXCR4 through epigenetic silencing of microRNA (miRNA)-139 in GC cells.[104] Several of the vascular endothelial growth factor (VEGF) gene polymorphisms were found to be independent prognostic markers for patients with GC and the analysis of VEGF gene polymorphisms may help identify patients at greatest risk for poor outcomes.[105]

Evidence of tumor suppressor loci on chromosome 3p has accumulated from a variety of studies, including allelic loss in primary GCs (46%) and homozygous deletion in a GC cell line (KATO III), as well as xenografted tumors.[106] The *FHIT* gene was isolated from the common fragile site FRA3B region at 3p14.2 and found to have abnormal transcripts with deleted exons in 5 of 9 GCs.[107] Furthermore, loss of FHIT protein expression was demonstrated immunohistochemically in most GCs.[108] One somatic missense mutation was identified in exon 6 of the *FHIT* gene during a coding region analysis of 40 GCs.[109] Additional studies are needed to determine the role that breakpoints in this region of 3p have in GC development.

Somatic mutations in the chromatin remodeling gene, ARIDIA, occurred in several GCs as well as other tumors.[110] Only 1 of 35 GCs contained an intragenic mutation of SMAD4 along with allelic loss, suggesting this gene is infrequently altered in sporadic gastric tumorigenesis.[96,111] Additionally, only one missense change of uncertain functional significance in the *LKB1* (STK11) gene was noted in a study of 28 sporadic GCs.[112]

Members of the Wnt signaling pathway, *APC* and *β-Catenin*, have had several somatic alterations noted in a few cases of GC.[113] Missense somatic mutations in *β-Catenin*, which also has connections with the cell adhesion complex involving E-cadherin, as well as Lcf/LEF transcription regulation, were identified in a few cases of intestinal-type GC.[114] Elevated expressions of the hedgehog target genes, human patched gene 1 (PTCH1) or Glil, were reported in 63 of 99 primary GCs. Interestingly, treatment of GC cells with KAAD-cyclopamine, a hedgehog signaling inhibitor, decreased expression of Glil and PTCH1, resulting in cell growth inhibition and apoptosis.[115] Additionally, cyclopamine decreased the growth of GC cell lines that expressed high levels of spermine oxidase.[116]

GLOBAL MOLECULAR PROFILING

Deregulation of canonical pathways, such as TFF1, HER2, p53, and Wnt/B-catenin, are known to occur with varying frequency in GC; however, studies have typically focused on single pathways measuring only one or a few targets. Recent evidence indicates that most cancers are products of complex interactions between multiple pathways. More global analyses are beginning to provide better definition of higher-order relationships between distinct oncogenic pathways. Elucidating these relationships may help to bridge the gap to clinical utility. Moreover, the advancement in our molecular understanding of tumorigenesis as a whole with these global profiling studies may result in specific targeted chemotherapy with dramatic effects in controlling tumor growth and survival.

Genomics

High-throughput analyses, such as microarrays and next-generation sequencing that comprehensively determine gene sequences or DNA copy number patterns, are being explored in various diseases, including GC. Genome-wide association studies have led to identification of multigene markers that correlate with prognostic significance in GCs. One study analyzed 47,296 transcripts from GC and, through microarray analysis, identified a 10-gene panel that correlated with overall prognosis from 39 cancer samples.[117] The panel consisted of 6 ribosomal proteins (RPLP2, RPS12, RPS8, RPS19, RPS12, and RPS15P4) and EIF3S6, GLTSCR2, TMSB10, and SEC61G, thought to be targets of tumor suppressor and oncogenes. The panel was then validated in an independent data set containing 33 cancer samples. Furthermore, a genome-wide association study in 3279 individuals identified noncardia GC susceptibility loci at 5p13.1, which contains the PTGER gene responsible for regulation of cell migration and immune response and thought to induce growth inhibition of human GC cell lines.[118] The same study identified cancer susceptibility loci at 3q13.31, which contains the ZBtB20 gene that encodes zinc finger protein homologous to bcl6 that is involved in the immune response, hematopoiesis, and oncogenesis. Moreover, the investigators validated several other loci, including rs2294008 and rs2976392 on 8q24, rs4072037 on 1q22, and rs13042395 on 20p13 being associated with noncardia GC in a further 6897 subjects.

Using genome-wide promoter methylation analysis, ADAMTS9 was identified as a functional tumor suppressor in GC by blocking AKT/mTOR signaling.[119] Indeed epigenetic silencing through hypermethylation was identified in 29.2% of primary GC tumors.[119] Additionally, multivariate analysis showed that patients with ADAMTS9 methylation had a poorer overall survival.

Genome copy number aberrations (CNAs) have been extensively characterized by comparative genomic hybridization in GC, as stated previously. A more global study, by Kuroda and colleagues,[120] demonstrated no significant association between number of genomic CNAs and GC submucosal invasion or lymph node metastasis. They did, however, demonstrate that subclones that acquire gain of 11q13, 11q14, 11q22, 14q32, or amplification of 17q21 were more frequent in submucosal-invasive GCs.

Transcriptomes

Although genomics has identified numerous genes/pathways involved in GC, transcriptome analysis elaborates on this technique, specifically identifying those genes that are silenced or upregulated. Regulation of genes, through CNAs, methylation, and other epigenetic mechanisms, ultimately affects their expression. Comprehensive serial analysis of gene expression has identified novel genetic alterations, including overexpression of calcium-binding proteins.[121]

Noncoding RNA sequences, miRNAs, have demonstrated considerable association with tumorigenesis, including GC. Mechanisms that dysregulate miRNAs include aberrant miRNA biogenesis and transcription, DNA methylation, epigenetic alteration, and amplification or loss of genomic regions that encode miRNAs. This dysregulation can promote progression of the GC cell cycle by altering translation of mRNAs that encode cyclin-dependent kinase inhibitors (CKIs), such as p21 and p16.[122]

Furthermore, this altered expression of CKI mRNAs reduces apoptotic signaling through regulation of Bcl-2, which has previously been described as a prognostic factor associated with the stage of GC.[123] Genome-wide studies have also shown that miRNAs are frequently found at genomic regions where LOH and amplification occur. For instance, miR-486, which has a role as a tumor suppressor, was found to be downregulated via loss of its locus in 25% to 30% of 106 gastric tissue samples.[124] Several miRNAs expressed aberrantly in GCs affect important signaling pathways, such as TGF-β.[125] Expression profiles of miRNAs have revealed 21 individual miRNA and 6 miRNA clusters that are consistently upregulated in GCs.[122]

It was postulated that PRKAA2 was a target gene for miR-19a when an inverse correlation was observed.[126] PRKAA2 is involved in the AMPK pathway, which inhibits the mTOR pathway, a major cancer growth-promoting signaling that regulates hypoxia-inducible factor-1a (HIF-1a). Furthermore, hepatocyte-NF-4a (HNF4a) and HIF-1a expression levels were demonstrated to be significantly higher in stage I-II GC explants compared with stage III-IV or normal tissue, suggesting a role as a biomarker of early GC.[126] Interestingly, studies to amplify the AMPK pathway, and thereby increase the concentration of PRKAA2 mRNA levels using metformin, resulted in decreased expression of HNF4a and an inhibition of the expression and transactivating activity of HIF-1a.[126]

Although NF-kB has been shown to be activated by *H pylori*, a known GC carcinogen, and altered NF-kB is known to play a role in multiple inflammation-based cancers, studies to date have not demonstrated overt differences in NF-kB activation, perhaps because of the limitations of older technologies. However, pathway profiling analysis of multiple components, including posttranslational modification of gene transcripts, has demonstrated NF-kB to be constitutively activated in GC.[127] Thus, targeted NF-kB inhibitors are currently being developed. Indeed, Sohma and colleagues[128] demonstrated NF-kB phosphorylation to be downregulated by the inhibitor parthenolide. Furthermore, they demonstrated that the inhibitory action of parthenolide on NF-kB signaling was associated with enhanced chemosensitivity to paclitaxel, thereby providing evidence of a promising potential therapeutic target against GC.

Proteomics

Multiple and multidimensional proteomic techniques, including 2-DE (dimensional electrophoresis), iTRAQ (isobaric tags for relative and absolute quantitation), ICAT (isotope-coded affinity tag), protein chip array and liquid chromatography, have become more advanced and are now being applied to analyzing quantitative differences in proteins present in various specimens. A proteomic analysis identified 9 proteins with increased expression and 13 proteins with decreased expression in GCs, which included those involved in mitotic check points, such as MAD1L1 and EB1, as well as others, including HSP27, CYR61, and CLPP.[129] Proteomic analysis using 2-DE profiles has revealed differential expression of annexins in *H pylori*–associated GCs.[130] Additionally, protein chip array and surface-enhanced laser desorption/ionization time-of-flight mass spectrometry (SELDI-TOF-MS) analyses have demonstrated upregulation of pepsinogen C and pepsin A, as well as downregulation of alpha-defensins in patients with GC.[131] Fibroblast growth factor–inducible factor 14 (Fn14), a type 1 transmembrane protein that belongs to the tumor necrosis factor (TNF) superfamily that functions through the NF-kB pathway, was found to be overexpressed in GC compared with normal tissue.[132] Moreover Fn14 expression levels were inversely correlated with patient survival in 87 patients with late-stage GC.

Although proteomic analysis in GCs has previously been focused on surgical specimens, one study using matrix-assisted laser desorption/ionizations (MALDI) mass spectrometry on endoscopic biopsies identified a signature protein profile consisting of 73 signals that included alpha-defensins that distinguished cancer samples from normal tissue.[133] In a validation set, this panel exhibited 93.8% sensitivity and 95.5% specificity. Furthermore, the investigators were also able to identify a protein signal that distinguished stage 1a GCs from more advanced lesions.

Novel splicing variants of ALDOC were identified by combined analysis with proteomics and transcriptome analysis. Specifically, the variant 4b was found to be highly expressed in most metastasis-related GC cell lines and poorly differentiated GC tumors with overexpression of ERB2/HER2/neu.[134] A total of 151 differentially expressed proteins, including galectin-2 and other proteins linked to TNF and p53, were upregulated in lymph node metastasis–negative GCs, providing candidate markers related to progression of tumor malignancy.[135] Twenty-two proteins involved in signal transduction controlling cancer cell proliferation/invasion/metastasis were found to be differentially expressed between the gastric tumor and the normal tissue, including Notch4, Akt, and B-catenin, which were upregulated, and cyclin E, p27, E-cadherin, HIF-3a, and NF-kB, which were downregulated.[136] Furthermore, changes in HIF-3a and NF-kB were associated with more invasive/metastatic tumors.

The most extensively studied biomarker of poor prognosis in GC is the HER2 protein.[137] This relationship was first described in 1986 and validated by numerous subsequent studies; however, the association was equivocal until Allgayer and colleagues[138] used directed antibodies against HER2 to demonstrate very high rates of membranous and cytoplasmic HER2 expression in a prospective series of 203 patients with GC. More recently, it has become evident that HER2 overexpression correlates more strongly with gastro-esophageal junction (GEJ) cancers than gastric tumors.[137] The demonstration that HER2-negative GCs correlated with a median survival twice as long as those of HER2-positive cancers (12.9 months vs 6.6 months)[139] highlights the fact that proteomic identification of biomarkers is critical to prognostication and directed future therapies.

BIOMARKERS: DIAGNOSTIC, PROGNOSTIC, TREATMENT GUIDANCE

The high mortality rate from GC is due to delayed detection and surgical resection at advanced stages of the disease. Currently, detection of early tumors is limited, as a reliable biomarker profile has not been elucidated. Diagnostic serum biomarkers in GC, such as carcinoembryonic antigen (CEA) and CA 10-9, have not proven to be sensitive or specific. Major efforts are being made to develop molecular signature-based methods complementing histopathological diagnosis and prognosis in GCs, as described previously. Some additional markers are expounded on in the following sections.

Potential biomarkers, such as phospholipase A2, signature profiles of gene expression, or copy number alterations identified may ultimately provide useful prognostic as well as diagnostic information about GC.[98,140,141] Elevated tissue levels of certain proteins have been shown to be associated with increased invasiveness of tumor cells, and some even associated with poorer survival, including urokinase-type plasminogen activator (uPA), VEGF, MET, MYC, tie-1 protein tyrosine kinase, CD44v6, PDGF-A, TGF-β1, and cyclin D2.[67] On the other hand, decreased levels of other proteins have been noted to be associated with more invasiveness and poorer survival, including loss of p27 (Kip1), p21 (CIP1), plasminogen activator inhibitor type-1 (PAI-1), and tissue-type plasminogen activator (tPA).[67] Nishigaki and colleagues[142] identified 9 proteins with increased expression and 13 proteins with decreased expression in GCs, notables include mitotic checkpoint (MAD1L1 and EB1) and mitochondrial functions (CLPP, COX5A, and ECH1). Thus, some of these molecules could potentially provide diagnostic and/or prognostic markers that may have clinical utilities.

Chemosensitization Markers

Measuring molecular markers in tumor cells may be able to predict how they will respond to specific treatment agents. The feasibility of this kind of testing was demonstrated in a small study of 30 patients in which overexpression of p53 by immunohistochemistry of locally advanced GCs was found to indicate a lower response rate to neoadjuvant cytotoxic therapy.[143] Furthermore, the expression of thymidine phosphorylase or even thymidine synthase in gastric tumors may help predict their response to fluorouracil agents.[144] In another small study of 23 patients with GC, those tumors with positive staining for BAX and Bcl-2 were more chemoresistant and had worse prognosis than those negative for Bcl-2 staining.[145,146] Kim and colleagues[147] demonstrated a shorter time to progression of HER2-positive GC in patients treated with FOLFOX-based (leucovorin, fluorouracil, oxaliplatin) chemotherapy.

The ToGA (Trastuzumab for Gastric Cancer) trial has provided evidence of the most efficacious target for GC to date. In the trial, trastuzumab, a monoclonal antibody to the HER2/neu receptor, resulted in a median overall survival of 13.8 months in those assigned to trastuzumab plus chemotherapy compared with 11.1 months in those assigned to chemotherapy alone ($P = .0046$).[148] Although results have been encouraging from the ToGA trial, it has been postulated that GCs are composed of genetically heterogeneous subpopulations and this tumor heterogeneity makes the development of effective drugs difficult, as tumors may differ in both biologic behavior and response to anticancer drugs, including molecular targeting agents.[120] Further biomarker/target elucidation may allow for improved outcomes in a larger subset of patients with GC.

Serum Markers

Additional diagnostic and prognostic markers for patients with GC have been sought in peripheral blood samples. High concentrations of tissue inhibitor of metalloproteinase (TIMP)-1, interleukin-10, hepatocyte growth factor, soluble receptor for interleukin-2, and soluble fragment of E-cadherin in the serum or plasma of patients with GC have been observed to be associated with more invasiveness and poorer survival.[144,149–152] Elevated plasma levels of osteopontin were an independent risk factor of poor survival in patients with GC.[153]

A proteomic evaluation of serum from patients with GC before and after surgical treatment and compared with controls suggested a panel of 5 protein markers had diagnostic potential, with a sensitivity of 83% and specificity of 95%.[154] Serum analysis of miRNAs, which are stable in blood as exosomal miRNAs, or most predominantly as Argonaute2 (Ago2) protein-bound miRNAs, found increased levels of miR-187, miR-371-5p, and miR-378 in patients with advanced-stage GC.[155] These studies, however, involved small sample sets and were mostly retrospective and case-control in nature; therefore, validation in larger independent prospective cohorts is required before these assays can be used for clinical purposes. The ultimate goal would be to identify a marker or panel that could be used to screen a population to make the diagnosis of GC early on, before symptoms appear.

REFERENCES

1. Goldgar DE, Easton DF, Cannon-Albright LA, et al. Systematic population-based assessment of cancer risk in first-degree relatives of cancer probands. J Natl Cancer Inst 1994;86:1600–8.

2. Lugli A, Zlobec I, Singer G, et al. Napoleon Bonaparte's gastric cancer: a clinicopathologic approach to staging, pathogenesis, and etiology. Nat Clin Pract Gastroenterol Hepatol 2007;4:52–7.

3. Antommarchi F. Les derniers moments de Napoleon, en compement du memorial de Sainte-Helene. 1st edition. Brusselles (Belgium): H Tarlier; 1825.

4. Hemminki K, Jiang Y. Familial and second gastric carcinomas: a nationwide epidemiologic study from Sweden. Cancer 2002;94:1157–65.

5. Zanghieri G, Di Gregorio C, Sacchetti C, et al. Familial occurrence of gastric cancer in the 2-year experience of a population-based registry. Cancer 1990; 66:2047–51.

6. Palli D, Galli M, Caporaso NE, et al. Family history and risk of stomach cancer in Italy. Cancer Epidemiol Biomarkers Prev 1994;3:15–8.

7. Lee FI. Carcinoma of the gastric antrum in identical twins. Postgrad Med J 1971; 47:622–4.

8. Aoki M, Yamamoto K, Noshiro H, et al. A full genome scan for gastric cancer. J Med Genet 2005;42:83–7.

9. Fitzgerald RC, Hardwick R, Huntsman D, et al. Hereditary diffuse gastric cancer: updated consensus guidelines for clinical management and directions for future research. J Med Genet 2010;47:436–44.

10. Guilford P, Hopkins J, Harraway J, et al. E-cadherin germline mutations in familial gastric cancer. Nature 1998;392:402–5.

11. Blair VR. Familial gastric cancer: genetics, diagnosis, and management. Surg Oncol Clin N Am 2012;21:35–56.

12. Barber M, Murrell A, Ito Y, et al. Mechanisms and sequelae of E-cadherin silencing in hereditary diffuse gastric cancer. J Pathol 2008;216:295–306.

13. Schrader K, Huntsman D. Hereditary diffuse gastric cancer. Cancer Treat Res 2010;155:33–63.

14. Oliveira C, Senz J, Kaurah P, et al. Germline CDH1 deletions in hereditary diffuse gastric cancer families. Hum Mol Genet 2009;18:1545–55.

15. Guilford PJ, Hopkins JB, Grady WM, et al. E-cadherin germline mutations define an inherited cancer syndrome dominated by diffuse gastric cancer. Hum Mutat 1999;14:249–55.

16. Pharoah PD, Guilford P, Caldas C. Incidence of gastric cancer and breast cancer in CDH1 (E-cadherin) mutation carriers from hereditary diffuse gastric cancer families. Gastroenterology 2001;121:1348–53.

17. Kluijt I, Siemerink EJ, Ausems MG, et al. CDH1-related hereditary diffuse gastric cancer syndrome: clinical variations and implications for counseling. Int J Cancer 2012;131:367–76.

18. Kaurah P, MacMillan A, Boyd N, et al. Founder and recurrent CDH1 mutations in families with hereditary diffuse gastric cancer. JAMA 2007;297:2360–72.

19. Humar B, Blair V, Charlton A, et al. E-cadherin deficiency initiates gastric signet-ring cell carcinoma in mice and man. Cancer Res 2009;69:2050–6.

20. Oliveira C, Sousa S, Pinheiro H, et al. Quantification of epigenetic and genetic 2nd hits in CDH1 during hereditary diffuse gastric cancer syndrome progression. Gastroenterology 2009;136:2137–48.

21. Norton JA, Ham CM, Van Dam J, et al. CDH1 truncating mutations in the E-cadherin gene: an indication for total gastrectomy to treat hereditary diffuse gastric cancer. Ann Surg 2007;245:873–9.

22. Brooks-Wilson AR, Kaurah P, Suriano G, et al. Germline E-cadherin mutations in hereditary diffuse gastric cancer: assessment of 42 new families and review of genetic screening criteria. J Med Genet 2004;41:508–17.

23. Ascano JJ, Frierson H Jr, Moskaluk CA, et al. Inactivation of the E-cadherin gene in sporadic diffuse-type gastric cancer. Mod Pathol 2001;14:942–9.

24. Corso G, Pedrazzani C, Pinheiro H, et al. E-cadherin genetic screening and clinico-pathologic characteristics of early onset gastric cancer. Eur J Cancer 2011;47:631–9.

25. Stone J, Bevan S, Cunningham D, et al. Low frequency of germline E-cadherin mutations in familial and nonfamilial gastric cancer. Br J Cancer 1999;79: 1935–7.

26. Caldas C, Carneiro F, Lynch HT, et al. Familial gastric cancer: overview and guidelines for management. J Med Genet 1999;36:873–80.

27. Lynch HT, Grady W, Suriano G, et al. Gastric cancer: new genetic developments. J Surg Oncol 2005;90:114–33 [discussion: 33].

28. Pinheiro H, Bordeira-Carrico R, Seixas S, et al. Allele-specific CDH1 downregulation and hereditary diffuse gastric cancer. Hum Mol Genet 2010;19:943–52.

29. Capelle LG, Van Grieken NC, Lingsma HF, et al. Risk and epidemiological time trends of gastric cancer in Lynch syndrome carriers in the Netherlands. Gastroenterology 2010;138:487–92.

30. Aarnio M, Salovaara R, Aaltonen LA, et al. Features of gastric cancer in hereditary non-polyposis colorectal cancer syndrome. Int J Cancer 1997;74:551–5.

31. Masciari S, Dewanwala A, Stoffel EM, et al. Gastric cancer in individuals with Li-Fraumeni syndrome. Genet Med 2011;13:651–7.

32. Varley JM, McGown G, Thorncroft M, et al. An extended Li-Fraumeni kindred with gastric carcinoma and a codon 175 mutation in TP53. J Med Genet 1995;32:942–5.

33. Kleihues P, Schauble B, zur Hausen A, et al. Tumors associated with p53 germline mutations: a synopsis of 91 families. Am J Pathol 1997;150:1–13.

34. Friedenson B. BRCA1 and BRCA2 pathways and the risk of cancers other than breast or ovarian. MedGenMed 2005;7:60.

35. van Lier MG, Westerman AM, Wagner A, et al. High cancer risk and increased mortality in patients with Peutz-Jeghers syndrome. Gut 2011;60:141–7.

36. Offerhaus GJ, Giardiello FM, Krush AJ, et al. The risk of upper gastrointestinal cancer in familial adenomatous polyposis. Gastroenterology 1992;102: 1980–2.

37. Win AK, Hopper JL, Jenkins MA. Association between monoallelic MUTYH mutation and colorectal cancer risk: a meta-regression analysis. Fam Cancer 2011;10:1–9.

38. Pollock J, Welsh JS. Clinical cancer genetics: part I: gastrointestinal. Am J Clin Oncol 2011;34:332–6.

39. Hizawa K, Iida M, Yao T, et al. Juvenile polyposis of the stomach: clinicopathological features and its malignant potential. J Clin Pathol 1997;50:771–4.

40. Heald B, Mester J, Rybicki L, et al. Frequent gastrointestinal polyps and colorectal adenocarcinomas in a prospective series of PTEN mutation carriers. Gastroenterology 2010;139:1927–33.

41. Stanich PP, Francis DL, Sweetser S. The spectrum of findings in Cowden syndrome. Clin Gastroenterol Hepatol 2011;9:e2–3.

42. Maimon SN, Zinninger MM. Familial gastric cancer. Gastroenterology 1953;25: 139–52 [discussion: 53–5].

43. Woolf CM, Isaacson EA. An analysis of 5 "stomach cancer families" in the state of Utah. Cancer 1961;14:1005–16.

44. Dellavecchia C, Guala A, Olivieri C, et al. Early onset of gastric carcinoma and constitutional deletion of 18p. Cancer Genet Cytogenet 1999;113:96–9.

45. Lee JH, Han SU, Cho H, et al. A novel germ line juxtamembrane Met mutation in human gastric cancer. Oncogene 2000;19:4947–53.
46. Oliveira C, Seruca R, Carneiro F. Genetics, pathology, and clinics of familial gastric cancer. Int J Surg Pathol 2006;14:21–33.
47. Gayther SA, Gorringe KL, Ramus SJ, et al. Identification of germ-line E-cadherin mutations in gastric cancer families of European origin. Cancer Res 1998;58:4086–9.
48. McDonald SA, Greaves LC, Gutierrez-Gonzalez L, et al. Mechanisms of field cancerization in the human stomach: the expansion and spread of mutated gastric stem cells. Gastroenterology 2008;134:500–10.
49. Sasaki O, Soejima K, Korenaga D, et al. Comparison of the intratumor DNA ploidy distribution pattern between differentiated and undifferentiated gastric carcinoma. Anal Quant Cytol Histol 1999;21:161–5.
50. Seruca R, Castedo S, Correia C, et al. Cytogenetic findings in eleven gastric carcinomas. Cancer Genet Cytogenet 1993;68:42–8.
51. Panani AD, Ferti A, Malliaros S, et al. Cytogenetic study of 11 gastric adenocarcinomas. Cancer Genet Cytogenet 1995;81:169–72.
52. El-Rifai W, Harper JC, Cummings OW, et al. Consistent genetic alterations in xenografts of proximal stomach and gastro-esophageal junction adenocarcinomas. Cancer Res 1998;58:34–7.
53. Kimura Y, Noguchi T, Kawahara K, et al. Genetic alterations in 102 primary gastric cancers by comparative genomic hybridization: gain of 20q and loss of 18q are associated with tumor progression. Mod Pathol 2004;17:1328–37.
54. Hidaka S, Yasutake T, Kondo M, et al. Frequent gains of 20q and losses of 18q are associated with lymph node metastasis in intestinal-type gastric cancer. Anticancer Res 2003;23:3353–7.
55. Yustein AS, Harper JC, Petroni GR, et al. Allelotype of gastric adenocarcinoma. Cancer Res 1999;59:1437–41.
56. Schneider BG, Pulitzer DR, Brown RD, et al. Allelic imbalance in gastric cancer: an affected site on chromosome arm 3p. Genes Chromosomes Cancer 1995;13:263–71.
57. Rumpel CA, Powell SM, Moskaluk CA. Mapping of genetic deletions on the long arm of chromosome 4 in human esophageal adenocarcinomas. Am J Pathol 1999;154:1329–34.
58. Leite M, Corso G, Sousa S, et al. MSI phenotype and MMR alterations in familial and sporadic gastric cancer. Int J Cancer 2011;128:1606–13.
59. dos Santos NR, Seruca R, Constancia M, et al. Microsatellite instability at multiple loci in gastric carcinoma: clinicopathologic implications and prognosis. Gastroenterology 1996;110:38–44.
60. Halling KC, Harper J, Moskaluk CA, et al. Origin of microsatellite instability in gastric cancer. Am J Pathol 1999;155:205–11.
61. Suzuki H, Itoh F, Toyota M, et al. Distinct methylation pattern and microsatellite instability in sporadic gastric cancer. Int J Cancer 1999;83:309–13.
62. Yamamoto H, Perez-Piteira J, Yoshida T, et al. Gastric cancers of the microsatellite mutator phenotype display characteristic genetic and clinical features. Gastroenterology 1999;116:1348–57.
63. Myeroff LL, Parsons R, Kim SJ, et al. A transforming growth factor beta receptor type II gene mutation common in colon and gastric but rare in endometrial cancers with microsatellite instability. Cancer Res 1995;55:5545–7.
64. Mori Y, Sato F, Selaru FM, et al. Instabilotyping reveals unique mutational spectra in microsatellite-unstable gastric cancers. Cancer Res 2002;62:3641–5.

65. Yamamoto H, Sawai H, Perucho M. Frameshift somatic mutations in gastrointestinal cancer of the microsatellite mutator phenotype. Cancer Res 1997;57: 4420–6.

66. Gil J, Yamamoto H, Zapata JM, et al. Impairment of the proapoptotic activity of Bax by missense mutations found in gastrointestinal cancers. Cancer Res 1999; 59:2034–7.

67. Powell SM. Stomach cancer. In: Childs B, Kinzler KW, Vogelstein B, editors. Metabolic and molecular basis of inherited diseases. 8th edition. New York: McGraw-Hill Companies, Inc; 2001. p. 1119–24.

68. Wu MS, Shun CT, Wang HP, et al. Loss of pS2 protein expression is an early event of intestinal-type gastric cancer. Jpn J Cancer Res 1998;89:278–82.

69. Lefebvre O, Chenard MP, Masson R, et al. Gastric mucosa abnormalities and tumorigenesis in mice lacking the pS2 trefoil protein. Science 1996;274: 259–62.

70. Nogueira AM, Machado JC, Carneiro F, et al. Patterns of expression of trefoil peptides and mucins in gastric polyps with and without malignant transformation. J Pathol 1999;187:541–8.

71. Nishizuka S, Tamura G, Terashima M, et al. Loss of heterozygosity during the development and progression of differentiated adenocarcinoma of the stomach. J Pathol 1998;185:38–43.

72. Calnan DP, Westley BR, May FE, et al. The trefoil peptide TFF1 inhibits the growth of the human gastric adenocarcinoma cell line AGS. J Pathol 1999; 188:312–7.

73. Beckler AD, Roche JK, Harper JC, et al. Decreased abundance of trefoil factor 1 transcript in the majority of gastric carcinomas. Cancer 2003;98: 2184–91.

74. Sankpal NV, Moskaluk CA, Hampton GM, et al. Overexpression of CEBPbeta correlates with decreased TFF1 in gastric cancer. Oncogene 2006;25:643–9.

75. Howlett M, Judd LM, Jenkins B, et al. Differential regulation of gastric tumor growth by cytokines that signal exclusively through the coreceptor gp130. Gastroenterology 2005;129:1005–18.

76. May FE, Griffin SM, Westley BR. The trefoil factor interacting protein TFIZ1 binds the trefoil protein TFF1 preferentially in normal gastric mucosal cells but the co-expression of these proteins is deregulated in gastric cancer. Int J Biochem Cell Biol 2009;41:632–40.

77. Moss SF, Lee JW, Sabo E, et al. Decreased expression of gastrokine 1 and the trefoil factor interacting protein TFIZ1/GKN2 in gastric cancer: influence of tumor histology and relationship to prognosis. Clin Cancer Res 2008;14: 4161–7.

78. Birchmeier W, Behrens J. Cadherin expression in carcinomas: role in the formation of cell junctions and the prevention of invasiveness. Biochim Biophys Acta 1994;1198:11–26.

79. Mayer B, Johnson JP, Leitl F, et al. E-cadherin expression in primary and metastatic gastric cancer: down-regulation correlates with cellular dedifferentiation and glandular disintegration. Cancer Res 1993;53:1690–5.

80. Becker KF, Atkinson MJ, Reich U, et al. E-cadherin gene mutations provide clues to diffuse type gastric carcinomas. Cancer Res 1994;54:3845–52.

81. Berx G, Becker KF, Hofler H, et al. Mutations of the human E-cadherin (CDH1) gene. Hum Mutat 1998;12:226–37.

82. Gschwind A, Fischer OM, Ullrich A. The discovery of receptor tyrosine kinases: targets for cancer therapy. Nat Rev Cancer 2004;4:361–70.

83. Nakamura K, Yashiro M, Matsuoka T, et al. A novel molecular targeting compound as K-samII/FGF-R2 phosphorylation inhibitor, Ki23057, for Scirrhous gastric cancer. Gastroenterology 2006;131:1530–41.
84. Vivanco I, Sawyers CL. The phosphatidylinositol 3-Kinase AKT pathway in human cancer. Nat Rev Cancer 2002;2:489–501.
85. Samuels Y, Wang Z, Bardelli A, et al. High frequency of mutations of the PIK3CA gene in human cancers. Science 2004;304:554.
86. Li VS, Wong CW, Chan TL, et al. Mutations of PIK3CA in gastric adenocarcinoma. BMC Cancer 2005;5:29.
87. Kang MJ, Ryu BK, Lee MG, et al. NF-kappaB activates transcription of the RNA-binding factor HuR, via PI3K-AKT signaling, to promote gastric tumorigenesis. Gastroenterology 2008;135:2030–42, 2042.e1–3.
88. Sakakura C, Hagiwara A, Yasuoka R, et al. Tumour-amplified kinase BTAK is amplified and overexpressed in gastric cancers with possible involvement in aneuploid formation. Br J Cancer 2001;84:824–31.
89. Wang Z, Shen D, Parsons DW, et al. Mutational analysis of the tyrosine phosphatome in colorectal cancers. Science 2004;304:1164–6.
90. Lee JW, Jeong EG, Lee SH, et al. Mutational analysis of PTPRT phosphatase domains in common human cancers. APMIS 2007;115:47–51.
91. El-Rifai W, Smith MF Jr, Li G, et al. Gastric cancers overexpress DARPP-32 and a novel isoform, t-DARPP. Cancer Res 2002;62:4061–4.
92. Belkhiri A, Zaika A, Pidkovka N, et al. Darpp-32: a novel antiapoptotic gene in upper gastrointestinal carcinomas. Cancer Res 2005;65:6583–92.
93. Nakajima M, Sawada H, Yamada Y, et al. The prognostic significance of amplification and overexpression of c-met and c-erb B-2 in human gastric carcinomas. Cancer 1999;85:1894–902.
94. Tsugawa K, Yonemura Y, Hirono Y, et al. Amplification of the c-met, c-erbB-2 and epidermal growth factor receptor gene in human gastric cancers: correlation to clinical features. Oncology 1998;55:475–81.
95. Toyota M, Ahuja N, Suzuki H, et al. Aberrant methylation in gastric cancer associated with the CpG island methylator phenotype. Cancer Res 1999;59:5438–42.
96. Chi XZ, Yang JO, Lee KY, et al. RUNX3 suppresses gastric epithelial cell growth by inducing p21(WAF1/Cip1) expression in cooperation with transforming growth factor {beta}-activated SMAD. Mol Cell Biol 2005;25:8097–107.
97. Ito K, Liu Q, Salto-Tellez M, et al. RUNX3, a novel tumor suppressor, is frequently inactivated in gastric cancer by protein mislocalization. Cancer Res 2005;65:7743–50.
98. Mishra R, Powell SM. Gastric cancer: molecular biology. In: Kelsen DP, Daly JM, Kern SE, et al, editors. Gastrointestinal oncology: principles and practice. Philadelphia: Lippincott, Williams & Wilkins; 2008. p. 245–55.
99. Ouyang H, Furukawa T, Abe T, et al. The BAX gene, the promoter of apoptosis, is mutated in genetically unstable cancers of the colorectum, stomach, and endometrium. Clin Cancer Res 1998;4:1071–4.
100. Lee JW, Jeong EG, Soung YH, et al. Decreased expression of tumour suppressor Bax-interacting factor-1 (Bif-1), a Bax activator, in gastric carcinomas. Pathology 2006;38:312–5.
101. Kondo S, Shinomura Y, Miyazaki Y, et al. Mutations of the bak gene in human gastric and colorectal cancers. Cancer Res 2000;60:4328–30.
102. Kuraoka K, Matsumura S, Sanada Y, et al. A single nucleotide polymorphism in the extracellular domain of TRAIL receptor DR4 at nucleotide 626 in gastric cancer patients in Japan. Oncol Rep 2005;14:465–70.

103. Hollstein M, Shomer B, Greenblatt M, et al. Somatic point mutations in the p53 gene of human tumors and cell lines: updated compilation. Nucleic Acids Res 1996;24:141–6.
104. Bao W, Fu HJ, Xie QS, et al. HER2 interacts with CD44 to up-regulate CXCR4 via epigenetic silencing of microRNA-139 in gastric cancer cells. Gastroenterology 2011;141:2076–2087.e6.
105. Kim J, Sohn S, Chae Y, et al. Vascular endothelial growth factor gene polymorphisms associated with prognosis for patients with gastric cancer. Ann Oncol 2007;18(6):1030–6.
106. Kastury K, Baffa R, Druck T, et al. Potential gastrointestinal tumor suppressor locus at the 3p14.2 FRA3B site identified by homozygous deletions in tumor cell lines. Cancer Res 1996;56:978–83.
107. Ohta M, Inoue H, Cotticelli MG, et al. The FHIT gene, spanning the chromosome 3p14.2 fragile site and renal carcinoma-associated t(3;8) breakpoint, is abnormal in digestive tract cancers. Cell 1996;84:587–97.
108. Baffa R, Veronese ML, Santoro R, et al. Loss of FHIT expression in gastric carcinoma. Cancer Res 1998;58:4708–14.
109. Gemma A, Hagiwara K, Ke Y, et al. FHIT mutations in human primary gastric cancer. Cancer Res 1997;57:1435–7.
110. Jones S, Li M, Parsons DW, et al. Somatic mutations in the chromatin remodeling gene ARID1A occur in several tumor types. Hum Mutat 2012; 33:100–3.
111. Powell SM, Harper JC, Hamilton SR, et al. Inactivation of Smad4 in gastric carcinomas. Cancer Res 1997;57:4221–4.
112. Park WS, Moon YW, Yang YM, et al. Mutations of the STK11 gene in sporadic gastric carcinoma. Int J Oncol 1998;13:601–4.
113. Nagase H, Nakamura Y. Mutations of the APC (adenomatous polyposis coli) gene. Hum Mutat 1993;2:425–34.
114. Park WS, Oh RR, Park JY, et al. Frequent somatic mutations of the beta-catenin gene in intestinal-type gastric cancer. Cancer Res 1999;59:4257–60.
115. Ma X, Chen K, Huang S, et al. Frequent activation of the hedgehog pathway in advanced gastric adenocarcinomas. Carcinogenesis 2005;26: 1698–705.
116. Fukaya M, Isohata N, Ohta H, et al. Hedgehog signal activation in gastric pit cell and in diffuse-type gastric cancer. Gastroenterology 2006;131:14–29.
117. Zhang YZ, Zhang LH, Gao Y, et al. Discovery and validation of prognostic markers in gastric cancer by genome-wide expression profiling. World J Gastroenterol 2011;17:1710–7.
118. Shi D, Wang S, Gu D, et al. The PSCA polymorphisms derived from genome-wide association study are associated with risk of gastric cancer: a meta-analysis. J Cancer Res Clin Oncol 2012;138:1339–45.
119. Du W, Wang S, Zhou Q, et al. ADAMTS9 is a functional tumor suppressor through inhibiting AKT/mTOR pathway and associated with poor survival in gastric cancer. Oncogene 2012. http://dx.doi.org/10.1038/onc.2012.359.
120. Kuroda A, Tsukamoto Y, Nguyen LT, et al. Genomic profiling of submucosal-invasive gastric cancer by array-based comparative genomic hybridization. PLoS One 2011;6:e22313.
121. El-Rifai W, Moskaluk CA, Abdrabbo MK, et al. Gastric cancers overexpress S100A calcium-binding proteins. Cancer Res 2002;62:6823–6.
122. Song JH, Meltzer SJ. MicroRNAs in pathogenesis, diagnosis, and treatment of gastroesophageal cancers. Gastroenterology 2012;143:35–47.e2.

123. Liu W, Liu B, Cai Q, et al. Proteomic identification of serum biomarkers for gastric cancer using multi-dimensional liquid chromatography and 2D differential gel electrophoresis. Clin Chim Acta 2012;413:1098–106.

124. Oh HK, Tan AL, Das K, et al. Genomic loss of miR-486 regulates tumor progression and the OLFM4 antiapoptotic factor in gastric cancer. Clin Cancer Res 2011;17:2657–67.

125. Petrocca F, Visone R, Onelli MR, et al. E2F1-regulated microRNAs impair TGFbeta-dependent cell-cycle arrest and apoptosis in gastric cancer. Cancer Cell 2008;13:272–86.

126. Kim YH, Liang H, Liu X, et al. AMPKalpha modulation in cancer progression: multilayer integrative analysis of the whole transcriptome in Asian gastric cancer. Cancer Res 2012;72:2512–21.

127. Lee BL, Lee HS, Jung J, et al. Nuclear factor-kappaB activation correlates with better prognosis and Akt activation in human gastric cancer. Clin Cancer Res 2005;11:2518–25.

128. Sohma I, Fujiwara Y, Sugita Y, et al. Parthenolide, an NF-kappaB inhibitor, suppresses tumor growth and enhances response to chemotherapy in gastric cancer. Cancer Genomics Proteomics 2011;8:39–47.

129. Boussioutas A, Li H, Liu J, et al. Distinctive patterns of gene expression in premalignant gastric mucosa and gastric cancer. Cancer Res 2003;63:2569–77.

130. Gerke V, Creutz CE, Moss SE. Annexins: linking Ca2+ signalling to membrane dynamics. Nat Rev Mol Cell Biol 2005;6:449–61.

131. Melle C, Ernst G, Schimmel B, et al. Characterization of pepsinogen C as a potential biomarker for gastric cancer using a histo-proteomic approach. J Proteome Res 2005;4:1799–804.

132. Kwon OH, Park SJ, Kang TW, et al. Elevated fibroblast growth factor-inducible 14 expression promotes gastric cancer growth via nuclear factor-kappaB and is associated with poor patient outcome. Cancer Lett 2012;314:73–81.

133. Kim HK, Reyzer ML, Choi IJ, et al. Gastric cancer-specific protein profile identified using endoscopic biopsy samples via MALDI mass spectrometry. J Proteome Res 2010;9:4123–30.

134. Hatakeyama K, Ohshima K, Fukuda Y, et al. Identification of a novel protein isoform derived from cancer-related splicing variants using combined analysis of transcriptome and proteome. Proteomics 2011;11:2275–82.

135. Jung JH, Kim HJ, Yeom J, et al. Lowered expression of galectin-2 is associated with lymph node metastasis in gastric cancer. J Gastroenterol 2012;47:37–48.

136. Wang D, Ye F, Sun Y, et al. Protein signatures for classification and prognosis of gastric cancer: a signaling pathway-based approach. Am J Pathol 2011;179:1657–66.

137. Gravalos C, Jimeno A. HER2 in gastric cancer: a new prognostic factor and a novel therapeutic target. Ann Oncol 2008;19:1523–9.

138. Allgayer H, Babic R, Gruetzner KU, et al. c-erbB-2 is of independent prognostic relevance in gastric cancer and is associated with the expression of tumor-associated protease systems. J Clin Oncol 2000;18:2201–9.

139. Tanner M, Hollmen M, Junttila TT, et al. Amplification of HER-2 in gastric carcinoma: association with Topoisomerase IIalpha gene amplification, intestinal type, poor prognosis and sensitivity to trastuzumab. Ann Oncol 2005;16:273–8.

140. Guan XY, Fu SB, Xia JC, et al. Recurrent chromosome changes in 62 primary gastric carcinomas detected by comparative genomic hybridization. Cancer Genet Cytogenet 2000;123:27–34.

141. Weiss MM, Kuipers EJ, Postma C, et al. Genomic alterations in primary gastric adenocarcinomas correlate with clinicopathological characteristics and survival. Cell Oncol 2004;26:307–17.
142. Nishigaki R, Osaki M, Hiratsuka M, et al. Proteomic identification of differentially-expressed genes in human gastric carcinomas. Proteomics 2005;5:3205–13.
143. Cascinu S, Graziano F, Del Ferro E, et al. Expression of p53 protein and resistance to preoperative chemotherapy in locally advanced gastric carcinoma. Cancer 1998;83:1917–22.
144. Saito H, Tsujitani S, Ikeguchi M, et al. Serum level of a soluble receptor for interleukin-2 as a prognostic factor in patients with gastric cancer. Oncology 1999;56:253–8.
145. Muguruma K, Nakata B, Hirakawa K, et al. p53 and Bax protein expression as predictor of chemotherapeutic effect in gastric carcinoma. Gan To Kagaku Ryoho 1998;25(Suppl 3):400–3 [in Japanese].
146. Nakata B, Muguruma K, Hirakawa K, et al. Predictive value of Bcl-2 and Bax protein expression for chemotherapeutic effect in gastric cancer. A pilot study. Oncology 1998;55:543–7.
147. Kim JW, Im SA, Kim M, et al. The prognostic significance of HER2 positivity for advanced gastric cancer patients undergoing first-line modified FOLFOX-6 regimen. Anticancer Res 2012;32:1547–53.
148. Bang YJ, Van Cutsem E, Feyereislova A, et al. Trastuzumab in combination with chemotherapy versus chemotherapy alone for treatment of HER2-positive advanced gastric or gastro-oesophageal junction cancer (ToGA): a phase 3, open-label, randomised controlled trial. Lancet 2010;376:687–97.
149. Gofuku J, Shiozaki H, Doki Y, et al. Characterization of soluble E-cadherin as a disease marker in gastric cancer patients. Br J Cancer 1998;78:1095–101.
150. De Vita F, Orditura M, Galizia G, et al. Serum interleukin-10 levels in patients with advanced gastrointestinal malignancies. Cancer 1999;86:1936–43.
151. Han SU, Lee JH, Kim WH, et al. Significant correlation between serum level of hepatocyte growth factor and progression of gastric carcinoma. World J Surg 1999;23:1176–80.
152. Yoshikawa T, Saitoh M, Tsuburaya A, et al. Tissue inhibitor of matrix metalloproteinase-1 in the plasma of patients with gastric carcinoma. A possible marker for serosal invasion and metastasis. Cancer 1999;86:1929–35.
153. Wu CY, Wu MS, Chiang EP, et al. Elevated plasma osteopontin associated with gastric cancer development, invasion and survival. Gut 2007;56:782–9.
154. Poon TC, Sung JJ, Chow SM, et al. Diagnosis of gastric cancer by serum proteomic fingerprinting. Gastroenterology 2006;130:1858–64.
155. Liu H, Zhu L, Liu B, et al. Genome-wide microRNA profiles identify miR-378 as a serum biomarker for early detection of gastric cancer. Cancer Lett 2012;316:196–203.

Pathology of Gastric Cancer and Its Precursor Lesions

Evgeny Yakirevich, MD, DSc, Murray B. Resnick, MD, PhD*

KEYWORDS

- Chronic gastritis • *Helicobacter pylori* • Atrophic gastritis • Intestinal metaplasia
- Spasmolytic polypeptide–expressing metaplasia • Intestinal-type adenocarcinoma
- Diffuse (signet ring) type adenocarcinoma • Proximal gastric cancer

KEY POINTS

- The intestinal and diffuse types of gastric adenocarcinoma have unique and overlapping epidemiologic, pathogenetic, molecular, and histologic features.
- The development of the intestinal type of gastric adenocarcinoma is a multistep process starting with chronic gastritis triggered by *Helicobacter pylori* and progressing through atrophy, intestinal metaplasia, and dysplasia to carcinoma (Correa model).
- In addition to intestinal metaplasia a distinct type of metaplasia, spasmolytic polypeptide–expressing metaplasia, has been recognized and has a strong association with the intestinal type of gastric adenocarcinoma.
- Loss of E-cadherin expression caused by *CDH1* gene alteration is the primary carcinogenic event in the Carneiro model of the hereditary diffuse gastric cancer.
- Proximal gastric adenocarcinoma results from either gastroesophageal reflux or *Helicobacter pylori* gastritis, each with distinct morphologic, immunohistochemical, and molecular features.

INTRODUCTION

Gastric cancer is the fourth most common malignancy and the second leading cause of cancer-related death worldwide.[1] Although the incidence of gastric cancer in North America is lower than other parts of the world, survival remains poor. It has been recognized that gastric carcinogenesis is a multistep process.[2] Precancerous conditions, including chronic *Helicobacter pylori*–associated gastritis, epithelial atrophy, intestinal and spasmolytic polypeptide–expressing metaplasia (SPEM), and precancerous lesions (dysplasia or intraepithelial neoplasia) precede the development of the intestinal type of gastric adenocarcinoma. Recent genetic advances have shed light on the molecular pathogenesis of hereditary diffuse gastric cancer (HDGC). A

Department of Pathology, Rhode Island Hospital, APC-12, 593 Eddy Street, Providence, RI 02903, USA
* Corresponding author.
E-mail address: mresnick@lifespan.org

Gastroenterol Clin N Am 42 (2013) 261–284
http://dx.doi.org/10.1016/j.gtc.2013.01.004
0889-8553/13/$ – see front matter © 2013 Elsevier Inc. All rights reserved.

better understanding and definition of gastric cancer and the molecular events preceding its development is critical in the prevention, diagnosis, and targeted therapy for this malignancy.

CLASSIFICATION OF GASTRIC CANCER

Gastric cancer is not a single disease, but a heterogeneous group of tumors with different morphologies, molecular backgrounds, and histogenesis. Most (95%) gastric malignancies originate from glandular epithelium and are designated as adenocarcinoma. Several systems have been proposed to aid in the classification of gastric adenocarcinoma based on macroscopic features (Borrmann)[3] or exclusively on the histologic tumor growth pattern (Ming, Carniero, Goseki).[4–6] The two most commonly used histologic classifications are the Lauren and World Health Organization (WHO) systems (**Table 1**).[7,8] More recently, molecular classifications based on gene expression profiles and proteomics have been proposed; however, these have not been routinely used.[9–11]

Lauren Classification: Intestinal and Diffuse Types of Gastric Cancer

A seminal classification system of gastric adenocarcinomas was introduced by Lauren[7] in the mid-1960s. The Lauren scheme separates gastric adenocarcinomas into two primary types: intestinal and diffuse. Tumors exhibiting features of both the intestinal and diffuse types are designated as mixed-type adenocarcinoma. **Table 2** summarizes the clinicopathologic features of the intestinal and diffuse types of gastric adenocarcinoma. In the past, intestinal-type tumors were considered more common, accounting for more than 50% of gastric adenocarcinomas; however, more recently the incidences of intestinal and diffuse cancers have been shown to be equal in the Western world.[12] The intestinal type is characterized by the formation of glands exhibiting various degrees of differentiation and extracellular mucin production (**Fig. 1**A). In contrast, the diffuse type of gastric adenocarcinoma is composed of poorly cohesive cells with no gland formation (see **Fig. 1**B). This type of tumor often contains cells with abundant intracytoplasmic mucin, known as "signet ring cells."

The Lauren classification is used by pathologists in routine practice, and by epidemiologists and clinicians for evaluating the natural history of gastric adenocarcinoma, especially with regard to incidence trends, and etiologic precursors,[13] although all

Table 1	
Lauren and World Health Organization classification systems of gastric cancer	
Lauren	**World Health Organization 2010**
Intestinal type	Papillary adenocarcinoma Tubular adenocarcinoma Mucinous adenocarcinoma
Diffuse type	Poorly cohesive carcinoma (including signet ring cell carcinoma and other variants)
Mixed type (equal intestinal and diffuse)	Mixed type, mixture of glandular (tubular/papillary) and poorly cohesive/signet ring
Indeterminate	Undifferentiated carcinoma
	Adenosquamous carcinoma Carcinoma with lymphoid stroma (medullary carcinoma) Hepatoid adenocarcinoma Squamous cell carcinoma

Table 2
Clinicopathologic features of intestinal and diffuse types of gastric adenocarcinoma

	Intestinal Type	Diffuse Type
Gender	Males > females (2:1)	Males = females
Age	Older age (>50 y)	Younger age (<50 y)
Areas	High-risk (Japan, China, Korea)	Uniform across the world
Incidence	Decreasing	Increasing
Inheritance	Hereditary nonpolyposis colorectal cancer, adenomatous polyposis coli	Hereditary diffuse gastric cancer
Location	Antrum (distal)	Corpus/body, but may arise anywhere in the stomach
Growth pattern	Usually exophytic	Flat, ulcerated, linitis plastica
Histology	Gland formation, extracellular mucin	Loss of cohesion, signet ring cells, no glands
Precursors	Correa pathway: chronic *Helicobacter pylori* gastritis, atrophy, metaplasia, dysplasia	Carneiro pathway: signet ring carcinoma in situ in hereditary diffuse gastric cancer

existing classifications of gastric adenocarcinoma, including that of Lauren, are of limited significance in terms of therapeutic decisions.[10]

WHO Classification of Gastric Cancer

In 2010 the WHO revised the classification of gastric adenocarcinoma according to the morphologic patterns commonly exhibited by tumors in other gastrointestinal sites, such as the small bowel, ampulla of Vater, and colon, resulting in a more uniform classification of gastrointestinal tumors as a whole.[8] The 2010 WHO classification recognizes five major types of gastric adenocarcinoma based on the predominant histologic growth pattern: (1) papillary; (2) tubular; (3) mucinous (tumors with mucinous pools exceeding 50% of the tumor); (4) poorly cohesive (including signet ring cell carcinoma and other variants); and (5) mixed adenocarcinomas.[8] Uncommon variants of gastric carcinomas include the squamous cell, adenosquamous, hepatoid, parietal cell, Paneth cell, micropapillary, and undifferentiated subtypes, and carcinoma with lymphoid stroma (medullary carcinoma).[8,14]

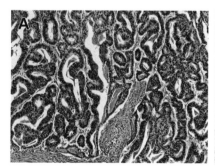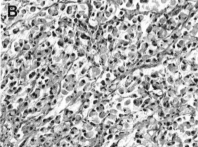

Fig. 1. (*A*) Intestinal type of gastric adenocarcinoma exhibiting gland formation (hematoxylin-eosin, original magnification ×100). (*B*) Diffuse type of gastric adenocarcinoma with signet ring cells containing abundant intracytoplasmic mucin (hematoxylin-eosin, original magnification ×200).

INTESTINAL TYPE OF GASTRIC ADENOCARCINOMA AND ITS PRECURSORS

The intestinal and diffuse subtypes of gastric adenocarcinoma are believed to result from two distinct pathogenetic pathways: the Correa pathway for the intestinal type[2] and the Carneiro model for the hereditary diffuse type of adenocarcinoma, discussed later.[15] Correa[2] postulated that the intestinal type of gastric adenocarcinoma is the consequence of progressive changes in the gastric mucosa with metamorphosis of normal gastric mucosa into carcinoma through the subsequent development of inflammation, atrophy, metaplasia, and dysplasia (**Fig. 2**).[16] This multistep process of carcinogenesis involves several genetic alterations, which may take years or even decades to develop.

Chronic Gastritis

Chronic gastritis is the most important and well-studied risk factor for the intestinal type of gastric cancer. *Helicobacter pylori*–associated and autoimmune gastritis are by far the two most common inflammatory conditions leading to the development of chronic gastritis and cancer. Although the etiologic agents are different, the end result of chronic inflammation in these two entities is atrophic gastritis. For routine histopathologic evaluation, the Sydney Classification System (later updated in Houston) was developed to provide information on the grade, topography (antrum, corpus, incisura), and origin of chronic gastritis.[17]

The morphologic attributes of chronic gastritis include inflammatory infiltrates containing mononuclear cells, predominantly lymphocytes, and plasma cells. Activity is determined by the presence of acute inflammatory cells (neutrophils) with a spectrum of grades from mild (neutrophils infiltrating the epithelium), to moderate (pit abscesses), to severe (erosions and ulcerations). To characterize the degree of chronicity, an international group of gastroenterologists and pathologists (Operative Link on Gastritis Assessment [OLGA]) developed a system for reporting the stage of gastritis, termed the OLGA Staging System.[18] The stage of gastritis is obtained by combining the extent of atrophy as scored histologically with the sites of atrophy identified by multiple biopsies from the antrum, incisura angularis (junctional area between

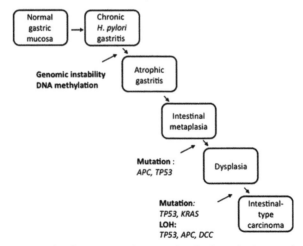

Fig. 2. The Correa cascade of gastric carcinogenesis. The intestinal type of gastric cancer is a multistep process with multiple genetic and epigenetic alterations that may take years or even decades to develop.

the anatomic antrum and body along the lesser curvature), and corpus according to the Sydney System protocol.[17,18]

Chronic Helicobacter pylori–associated gastritis

Helicobacter pylori is the most common chronic bacterial infectious agent in humans (>50% of the world population is infected) and is the only bacteria classified as a class I carcinogen by the WHO.[19] Numerous epidemiologic studies have confirmed the association of H pylori infection and gastric cancer, although only 1% to 3% of people infected with H pylori actually develop gastric cancer, suggesting that other factors, including those related to the host, may also play a role in carcinoma development.[20,21] In a combined analysis of 12 studies 81% of gastric cancers were associated with H pylori infection.[22] Although H pylori is strongly associated with the intestinal type and diffuse type of gastric cancer,[23] the underlying carcinogenic mechanisms may be different. Specifically, in intestinal-type cancers H pylori has been implicated in the multistep process from atrophic gastritis to intestinal metaplasia (IM) and dysplasia. In contrast, diffuse-type cancers have no recognizable precursor lesions besides chronic gastritis.

Helicobacter pylori infection results in a characteristic superficial chronic active gastritis with a dense lymphoplasmacytic lamina propria infiltrate often containing germinal centers (secondary lymphoid follicles) and active inflammation involving the epithelium (**Fig. 3**A). Because of the predominant anatomic location in the distal

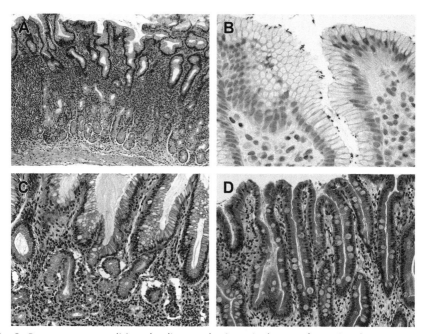

Fig. 3. Precancerous conditions leading to the intestinal type of gastric adenocarcinoma. (A) Chronic active Helicobacter pylori–associated gastritis (hematoxylin-eosin, original magnification ×100). (B) Immunostain highlights characteristic curved H pylori organisms (original magnification ×600). (C) Spasmolytic polypeptide–expressing metaplasia. Atrophic gastric body mucosa with oxyntic glands replaced by pseudopyloric metaplastic glands (hematoxylin-eosin, original magnification ×200). (D) Intestinal metaplasia, complete type, characterized by mature enterocytes with brush borders and goblet cells. Note normal gastric foveolar epithelium in the left upper corner (hematoxylin-eosin, original magnification ×200).

stomach *H pylori* gastritis has been also termed diffuse antral gastritis and chronic superficial gastritis. The presence of these typical histologic features is predictive of *H pylori* infection and in most cases routine hematoxylin-eosin staining is enough to detect the curved, sea-gull shaped microorganisms, although in some cases histochemical or immunohistochemical stains for *H pylori* organisms may be helpful (see **Fig. 3**B).[24,25]

Autoimmune gastritis

Autoimmune gastritis represents less than 5% of all chronic gastritis cases.[26] It is the consequence of an immune-mediated destruction of parietal cells, is restricted to the body and fundus, and is associated with characteristic neuroendocrine cell hyperplasia. The lack of parietal cells that secrete gastric intrinsic factor results in cobalamin deficiency and pernicious anemia, a late manifestation of autoimmune gastritis. In patients with pernicious anemia, the risk of gastric cancer increases threefold[27,28] and most adenocarcinomas are of the intestinal type.[29] Gastric type 1 neuroendocrine (carcinoid) tumors are associated with autoimmune atrophic gastritis; however, these usually are indolent in their behavior.

Atrophic Gastritis

Atrophy is defined as the loss of normal glandular epithelium. Two primary histologic variants of gastric atrophy include atrophy as the result of glandular destruction and subsequent replacement with lamina propria fibrosis, and glandular loss resulting from replacement of the native glands with metaplastic epithelium.[30] Atrophic gastritis occurs predominantly in the gastric antrum and incisura in *H pylori* gastritis, and is restricted to the oxyntic mucosa in corpus/fundus in autoimmune gastritis. Atrophy involves the antral and corpus mucosa in multifocal atrophic gastritis (formerly known as environmental atrophic gastritis) or in more advanced atrophic pangastritis. The relationship between antral atrophic gastritis and multifocal atrophic gastritis remains unclear, but they likely represent different stages of the same disease. In a long-term follow-up study invasive or intraepithelial gastric neoplasia was significantly associated with the degree of atrophy using the OLGA staging system.[31]

Metaplasia

Metaplasia is defined as a potentially reversible change in which one adult cell type is replaced by another adult cell type.[32] This alteration in phenotype is believed to help the mucosa to withstand a more adverse environment. In the stomach, three types of metaplasia are recognized: (1) SPEM; (2) intestinal; and (3) pancreatic (the latter is of no clinical significance and is more commonly seen in the proximal stomach).

Spasmolytic polypeptide–expressing metaplasia

SPEM is a metaplastic mucous cell lineage with morphologic features and the phenotype of deep antral glands, including strong expression of trefoil factor (TFF) 2 (previously designated as spasmolytic polypeptide) and MUC6; however, it lacks gastrin-producing G cells (see **Fig. 3**C).[33,34] This mucous lineage has been also termed pseudopyloric metaplasia, mucous metaplasia, or antralized oxyntic mucosa. These latter terms are recognized by pathologists and commonly used in pathology reports, as opposed to SPEM.

TFFs are a group of small secretory peptides that play a role in the protection and repair of the gastrointestinal mucosa.[35] TFF1 and TFF2 are specifically expressed in gastric epithelial cells, whereas TFF3, also termed intestinal trefoil factor, is expressed at high levels in the goblet cells of the small and large intestine in normal physiologic conditions and also in IM of the stomach and gastric carcinoma.[35]

SPEM was detected in 68% of patients with *H pylori* infection and is also seen in the setting of autoimmune atrophic gastritis targeting parietal cells in the corpus.[33] Recent studies have shown that SPEM is associated with 90% of gastric cancers and have suggested that SPEM may play a role in the preneoplastic process.[33,36,37] There is accumulating evidence that SPEM is the first metaplastic change preceding the development of IM.[34,38] SPEM may be present as a very localized phenomenon; however, extensive mapping of the stomach has revealed that in the intestinal type of gastric adenocarcinoma, atrophy in the corpus may exist as a continuous sheet of SPEM containing islands of IM (multifocal IM).[39] It is unclear whether SPEM or IM is a true precursor for intestinal-type cancer, or if they are merely associated with the carcinogenic process.[34,38]

Intestinal metaplasia

IM may arise in the background of SPEM or in the native mucous-secreting antral or cardia epithelium. Three types of IM have been recognized:

- Type I IM, also designated as the complete or small intestinal type, consists of mature enterocytes with brush borders, Paneth cells, and goblet cells, the latter secreting sialomucins (see **Fig. 3**D).[40] Complete IM is characterized by the expression of intestinal mucin MUC2, and markedly decreased levels of "gastric" mucins MUC1, MUC5AC, and MUC6.[41] Type I IM is the predominant subtype (73%) seen in biopsies with IM and is the most commonly seen in benign conditions, 70% in gastric ulcers and 76% in chronic gastritis.[42]
- Type II IM, or incomplete, immature, colonic type, is characterized by few or absent absorptive cells, and the presence of columnar "intermediate" cells in various stages of differentiation, secreting neutral and acid sialomucins, and goblet cells secreting sialomucins or occasionally sulfomucins (all cells contain mucin).[40,42]
- Type III IM, in which the predominant mucin secreted by the "intermediate" cells is acid sulfomucin rather than sialomucin as in type II IM.[42,43] Both type II and III incomplete IM maintain the expression of "gastric" mucins MUC1, MUC5AC, and MUC6.[41] On the molecular level all types of IM exhibit expression of the intestinal transcription factor CDX2, which is expressed in the normal bowel.[44] Type III IM has been identified in only 9.8% of all biopsies with IM and has a higher incidence in carcinoma (35%) than in benign conditions (7%).[42]

Although some studies have demonstrated that cancer risk is increased from type I to type III of IM,[42,43,45,46] currently the subtyping of IM is not recommended in routine practice because there is no conclusive evidence of the association between these subtypes and the risk of gastric cancer.

Recently, the modified OLGA system based on the assessment of IM, rather than atrophy (OLGIM) was introduced for the staging of chronic gastritis.[47] The OLGIM system provided a significantly higher agreement between pathologists compared with the OLGA system based on atrophy alone. The practical value of this system in predicting the development of dysplasia or cancer needs to be addressed.

At present, the reversibility of metaplasia involving the gastric mucosa is considered controversial. Although eradication of *H pylori* was associated with the reversibility of IM in some studies,[48–50] in other studies cancer risk decreased only after eradication in patients with nonatrophic mucosa.[51–53]

Gastric Dysplasia (Intraepithelial Neoplasia)

In tumor pathology, dysplasia is a term that literally means abnormal growth. The WHO defines dysplasia in the gastrointestinal system as the presence of histologic unequivocal neoplastic epithelium without evidence of tissue invasion.[54] Several classification systems of dysplasia, including the Padova, Vienna, and WHO (**Box 1**), were developed to standardize the definition of gastric dysplasia and neoplasia between pathologists of North America and Europe and those in Japan.[8,55,56] This standardization was necessary because gastric lesions diagnosed as high-grade dysplasia (HGD) by Western pathologists were invariably diagnosed as carcinoma by Japanese colleagues.[57] Noninvasive carcinoma (carcinoma in situ) was included in the category of high-grade noninvasive neoplasia (dysplasia) in the Vienna and Padova classifications, which corresponds to high-grade intraepithelial neoplasia (dysplasia) in the 2010 WHO classification.[8] The term "adenoma" is used for raised polypoid lesions, whereas nonadenomatous dysplasia is reserved for flat or depressed lesions. The latter group is not obvious with standard white light endoscopy; however, it may be visualized with chromoendoscopy or narrow-band imaging. Recently, a pit dysplasia limited to the gastric pit region without surface epithelial involvement characteristic of traditional dysplasia has been described.[58]

Two primary histologic types of gastric dysplasia have been described: the intestinal (adenomatous, type I) and the gastric (foveolar, type II).[8,59,60] The intestinal type is the most common; is similar to colonic adenomas; and may be recognized histologically by hyperchromatic pseudostratified, pencillate, columnar cell nuclei.[8] The intestinal phenotype expresses MUC2, CDX2, and CD10 by immunohistochemistry.[61,62] Characteristic features of foveolar dysplasia include glands lined by a single layer of cuboidal to columnar epithelium with pale or clear cytoplasm, and round to oval nuclei with variably prominent nucleoli.[8] Immunohistochemically, the foveolar type is characterized by the expression of gastric mucins; TFF1; and low expression of CDX2 and CD10 ($MUC5AC^+MUC6^+/CDX2^-/CD10^-$).[61,63] Several studies have attempted to better delineate the background mucosal pathology and assess the risk of malignant progression in these two types of gastric dysplasia[61,64]; however, phenotyping of dysplasia is not recommended because the significance of these subtypes remains controversial.

The prevalence of dysplasia varies from less than 4% in the Western world to up to 20% in high-risk areas for gastric adenocarcinoma, such as Colombia and China.[60] The natural history of gastric dysplasia depends on its grade, extent, and surface appearance (polypoid vs flat or depressed). Dysplasia is graded based on cytologic and architectural features as either low- or high-grade.[8] Low-grade dysplasia (LGD) is characterized by minimal architectural abnormalities and only mild-to-moderate cytologic atypia. The nuclei are hyperchromatic, elongated, or pseudostratified, and mitotic activity is low (**Fig. 4A**). HGD is distinguished by the presence of architectural

---

Box 1
WHO (2010) classification of gastric dysplasia (epithelial neoplasia)

1. Negative for intraepithelial neoplasia (dysplasia)

2. Indefinite for intraepithelial neoplasia (dysplasia)

3. Intraepitehlial neoplasia (dysplasia)

    a. Low-grade intraepithelial neoplasia (dysplasia)

    b. High-grade intraepithelial neoplasia (dysplasia)

4. Intramucosal invasive neoplasia/intramucosal carcinoma

5. Invasive neoplasia

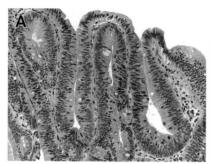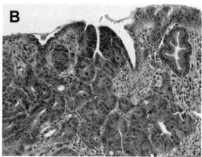

Fig. 4. Gastric dysplasia (intraepithelial neoplasia). (*A*) Low-grade dysplasia with limited architectural abnormalities and hyperchromatic, elongated, pseudostratified nuclei (hematoxylin-eosin, original magnification ×200). (*B*) High-grade dysplasia characterized by architectural abnormalities with glandular crowding and loss of polarity and severe cytologic atypia with rounded hyperchromatic nuclei, high nuclear/cytoplasmic ratio, prominent nucleoli, and high mitotic activity. Note normal gastric foveolar epithelium in the right upper corner (hematoxylin-eosin, original magnification ×200).

disarray with loss of nuclear polarity and marked cytologic atypia with rounded nuclei, high nuclear/cytoplasmic ratio, prominent nucleoli, and high mitotic activity including atypical mitotic figures (see **Fig. 4**B).

LGD diagnosed on endoscopic biopsies has been shown to regress in 38% to 75% of cases, to persist in 19% to 50%, and to progress to HGD in 0% to 9% of cases.[65] Several long-term follow-up studies have demonstrated that LGD lesions do not progress rapidly to HGD or carcinoma, thus some authors have advocated a management approach of scheduled endoscopic surveillance and rebiopsy.[66,67] However, other groups have suggested removal of LGD lesions because of the histologic discrepancies found between forceps biopsy specimens and resected specimens ranging from 19% to 35%.[68–70] The best independent predictors of progression of LGD to HGD or cancer are size greater than 2 cm and the presence of depression on endoscopic examination.[68,70]

HGD regresses in only 0% to 16% of cases, persists in 14% to 58%, and progresses in 10% to 100% of cases to invasive carcinoma.[65] In a cohort of patients with premalignant gastric lesions approximately 25% of patients with HGD progressed to carcinoma within 1 year of follow-up.[71] For these reasons, a lesion diagnosed as HGD by endoscopic forceps biopsy material should be considered for endoscopic mucosal resection.[67]

Gastric Polyps and Polyposis Syndromes

Gastric polyps are defined as lesions that project above the plain of the mucosal surface. Fundic gland polyps (FGP) are the most common and account for up to 77% of all gastric polyps, followed by hyperplastic polyps and adenomas.[72,73]

FGPs occur in two different clinical settings: sporadic and syndromic. Dysplasia in sporadic FGPs is extremely rare (<1%) and there is no association between sporadic FGPs and the development of gastric cancer.[74] FGPs may also be seen as a manifestation of familial adenomatous polyposis syndrome. In this setting patients present at a younger age and may have numerous FGPs. Although dysplasia is seen in up to 48% of these polyps, progression to carcinoma is rare in the North American population.[75] Recently, a new hereditary gastric cancer syndrome has been identified that is associated with a significant risk of gastric carcinoma: gastric adenocarcinoma and proximal polyposis syndrome.[76] This autosomal-dominant syndrome is characterized by the development of numerous FGPs, with areas of dysplasia or intestinal-type gastric cancer.[76]

Most hyperplastic polyps are associated with chronic gastritis and *H pylori* infection. Dysplasia may be found in 1% to 3% of hyperplastic polyps, and is usually associated with size larger than 2 cm and older age. Complete excision with entire histologic examination of large hyperplastic polyps is believed to be curative even if dysplasia or intramucosal carcinoma is present.[77]

Gastric adenomas are raised polypoid lesions that by definition exhibit low- or high-grade epithelial dysplasia and comprise 0.5% to 3.75% of all gastric polyps in the Western hemisphere, in contrast to 9% to 20% in areas of high-risk gastric cancer.[72] The prevalence of gastric adenoma in a large nationwide US population series was 0.69%.[73] Histologically, gastric adenomas may be classified as tubular, tubulovillous, or villous based on architecture. Gastric adenomas may be also subtyped based on the epithelial phenotype into intestinal and gastric types. The intestinal type of adenoma is more common and contains absorptive, goblet, and Paneth cells.[61,64] Paneth cell adenoma, a rare variant composed exclusively of Paneth cells, has also been described.[78] Gastric-type adenomas may be classified as foveolar or the pyloric type.[61,64,79,80] Recently, an oxyntic gland polyp or adenoma has also been proposed, which likely represents the previously described variant of gastric adenocarcinoma with chief cell differentiation.[81] The clinicopathologic characteristics of gastric adenomas are presented in **Table 3**. The risk of carcinoma progression of gastric adenomas is related to the size of the lesions and is increased in lesions larger than 2 cm in diameter.

Intramucosal Adenocarcinoma

Intramucosal adenocarcinoma is defined by Western pathologists as unequivocal invasion of neoplastic cells into the lamina propria or muscularis mucosa, but not into the submucosa. Histologic criteria for invasion include the presence of single cells or small cell clusters, irregular budding of the tumor cells into surrounding lamina propria, or marked architectural complexity with fused glands.[54] Differentiating an intramucosal adenocarcinoma from HGD may be challenging; however, because of the minimal risk of lymphatic involvement (0%–7%), in many circumstances the management of patients with intramucosal carcinoma is similar to those with HGD.[82,83] The prognosis of intramucosal gastric adenocarcinomas is excellent with 5-year survival close to 100%.[82,83]

Early Gastric Cancer

Early gastric cancer (EGC) is defined as intramucosal or submucosal tumor invasion independent of lymph node involvement.[9] Although EGC represents 15% to 21% of all gastric cancers in the Western world, it accounts for more than 50% of the gastric carcinomas in Japan.[8,82–84] These differences are likely related to endoscopic screening programs implemented in Japan, although differences in diagnostic criteria may also play a role. The Japanese Gastric Cancer Association has grouped the gross classification of early gastric carcinoma as protruded, elevated, flat, depressed, excavated, or combined forms; however, these subtypes correlate weakly with microscopic appearance and prognosis.[85] Histologically, most EGC are intestinal-type adenocarcinomas, whereas signet ring carcinoma represents 26% of the cases.[83] The prognosis of EGC is excellent with more than 90% 5-year survival.[83]

Table 3
Clinicopathologic characteristics of gastric adenomas according to histologic subtypes

Adenoma Type	Sex	Location	Histologic Features	Mucin	Association	Malignant Transformation
Intestinal	M > F	Antrum	Elongated hyperchromatic nuclei, focal goblet cells and Paneth cells	$MUC2^+, 5^-, 6^-$	Gastritis and IM	High
Foveolar	M = F	Body	Round to oval nuclei, pale or clear cytoplasm, apical mucin	$MUC2^-, 5^+, 6^-$	FAP	Controversial
Pyloric	F > M	Body	Round bland or atypical nuclei, ground glass cytoplasm	$MUC2^-, 5^+, 6^+$	Autoimmune gastritis and IM	High
Oxyntic	M ≈ F	Fundus/cardia	Chief cells, mucous neck cells	$MUC2^-, 5^-, 6^+$	Some with mild chronic gastritis	None

Abbreviations: FAP, familial adenomatous polyposis; IM, intestinal metaplasia.

Advanced Gastric Cancer

Intestinal-type adenocarcinomas are usually bulky tumors with a variety of gross appearances including polypoid, fungating, or ulcerated subtypes. The intestinal-type carcinomas are similar histologically to colorectal adenocarcinoma with formation of glands exhibiting various degrees of differentiation and extracellular mucin production. The tumors are graded into well-differentiated (>95% of tumor composed of glands); moderately differentiated (50%–95% of tumor composed of glands); and poorly differentiated (<50% composed of glands). The morphologic distinction between poorly differentiated intestinal-type tumors and diffuse-type tumors is often problematic. The immunohistochemical phenotype is similar for the intestinal and diffuse type carcinoma, both stain with low- and high-molecular-weight keratins, and may exhibit positivity for CDX2 and TFF3.[86] MUC2, MUC5AC, and MUC6 are frequently expressed in gastric adenocarcinomas; however, this cannot distinguish between the intestinal and diffuse types.[87] Although MUC1 expression was shown to be more frequent in the intestinal type, there is significant overlap with diffuse carcinoma.[87] Intestinal gastric cancer metastasizes primarily by lymphatics to the regional lymph nodes of the lesser and greater curvature, porta hepatis, and subpyloric region. Distant lymphatic metastases also occur, most commonly to the supraclavicular node, called Virchow node. The depth of invasion and the extent of nodal and distant metastasis at the time of presentation is the most powerful prognostic indicator for gastric cancer. In the United States most patients with gastric cancer present at advanced stage with metastatic disease at presentation, with an overall 5-year survival less than 30%.

The Molecular Pathology of Intestinal Gastric Adenocarcinoma and its Precursors

The genomic changes involved in the multistep process of carcinogenesis of intestinal-type cancer are the result of genetic and epigenetic abnormalities including (1) silencing of tumor-suppressor genes and activation of oncogenes; (2) genomic instability through two distinct pathways, microsatellite instability (MSI) and chromosomal instability; and (3) epigenetic alterations.

Tumor-suppressor genes

The tumor-suppressor gene *TP53* is a nuclear transcription factor involved in the regulation of the cell cycle. Alterations in *TP53* were found in at least 30% of regions of IM, and in 33% to 58% of gastric dysplasia and adenomas, indicating that *TP53* is an early event in gastric carcinogenesis.[88] TP53 nuclear immunoreactivity is seen in approximately one-third of cases of gastric dysplasia and adenoma, predominantly in areas with HGD.[89–91] Inactivation of *TP53* gene by loss of heterozygosity or mutation is observed in up to 40% of the intestinal subtype in contrast to 0% to 21% in diffuse cancer.[8,88]

APC is a tumor suppressor gene that is a susceptibility factor for familial polyposis coli and plays a crucial role in sporadic colorectal cancer. Somatic mutations in the *APC* gene are present in 6% of IM and in 20% to 40% of gastric adenomas and therefore are also considered as an early event in gastric carcinogenesis.[8,88] Between 20% and 40% of intestinal type gastric cancers harbor APC mutations, whereas the diffuse type gastric cancers have less than 2%.[8,88] Loss of heterozygosity at the *DCC* locus also is one of the characteristics of intestinal-type gastric cancer and is seen in 60% of tumors.[88]

Oncogenes

Among the oncogenes mutated or amplified in gastric cancer, several, such as *HER2* and *EGFR*, have been evaluated as possible candidates for targeted therapies.[92–96]

Amplification and overexpression of HER2, a member of the human tyrosine kinase receptor family, is detected in 7% to 34% of gastric adenocarcinomas and is most prevalent in the intestinal type of gastric cancer.[92,93,97] In contrast to HER2 expression in breast cancer, HER2 immunohistochemical expression in gastric cancer is more heterogeneous (focal staining) and may exhibit incomplete membrane staining. Therefore, an HER2 scoring system specific for gastric cancer has been developed with separate scores for endoscopic biopsies and surgical resection specimens.[98] In a multicenter phase III ToGA trial involving patients with gastric or gastroesophageal junction (GEJ) adenocarcinoma the addition of Trastuzumab (Herceptin, Genentech), a humanized monoclonal antibody targeting the HER2 receptor, to the chemotherapy protocol significantly improved the overall survival of patients with HER2-positive locally advanced, recurrent, or metastatic gastric cancer.[93] In the ToGA study the highest HER2 expression (33%) was observed in the gastric cardia.[93] In a more recent study, the rate of HER2 expression in the distal stomach (32%) was comparable with that in the gastric cardia of the ToGA study.[99] HER2 overexpression seems to be an early event in gastric carcinogenesis, because HER2 expression rises significantly from LGD to HGD to adenocarcinoma.[99]

EGFR is another member of the human tyrosine kinase receptor family. EGFR has been shown to be overexpressed by immunohistochemistry in 27% of gastric carcinomas, whereas gene amplification by fluorescence in situ hybridization was evident in less than 3% in one large series.[94] Several clinical trials adding a monoclonal anti-EGFR antibody to chemotherapy regimens in advanced gastric cancer have been undertaken; however, none have found EGFR expression to be predictive of overall survival or response to therapy.[95,96] EGFR activates a signaling cascade by several pathways, including RAS-activated protein kinase. Activating KRAS mutations result in RAS proteins that are constitutively active, leading to stimulation of downstream signaling pathway independent of EGFR signaling. KRAS mutations have been detected in 1% to 28% of intestinal carcinoma, but not in diffuse carcinoma.[8,88]

Genomic instability

MSI is caused by dysfunction of the DNA mismatch repair system. The mismatch repair system functions to recognize and repair nucleotide mismatches and consists of the MLH1, PMS2, MLH2, and MLH6 proteins. MSI has been detected in early stages of carcinogenesis including chronic gastritis, IM, dysplasia, and adenoma and in 15% to 49% of sporadic gastric cancers.[88] Gastric carcinomas with a high frequency of MSI are often seen in patients older than 73 years and characterized by an antral location, intestinal type, abundant lymphoid infiltrates, multiple tumors, and favorable prognosis as opposed to MSI-low tumors.[8,88]

Gastric carcinomas may occur in 11% of patients with the hereditary nonpolyposis colon cancer syndrome, also known as Lynch syndrome, arising in families with MLH1, MSH2, or MSH6 germline mutations.[100] Most of these cancers are of the intestinal type and have the same natural history as sporadic cancer.[100]

Chromosomal instability results in chromosomal gains or losses with an aneuploid DNA pattern and represents an early event in gastric carcinogenesis.

Epigenetic alterations

Methylation of gene promoters leads to gene silencing. An increasing frequency of promoter methylation involving multiple genes has been shown to occur in the progression from chronic gastritis to carcinoma.[101] CpG island methylator phenotype is characterized by simultaneous methylation of the CpG islands in multiple genes.

Recent studies revealed that CpG island methylator phenotype is more prevalent in the diffuse as opposed to the intestinal type of gastric cancer.[102,103]

DIFFUSE TYPE OF GASTRIC ADENOCARCINOMA

Diffuse gastric cancers characteristically present with a diffusely thickened gastric wall, classically known as "linitis plastica." Histologically, this type of cancer is best recognized by a dyscohesive diffuse growth pattern and the presence of signet ring cells, although plasmacytoid, histiocytic, anaplastic, and desmoplastic variants have also been described.[104] Most diffuse gastric cancers are sporadic; however, familial clustering is present in 10%, and 1% to 3% of gastric cancers arise as a hereditary syndrome.[105] Inherited gastric carcinomas are more often of the diffuse type and are generally referred to as HDGC. Hereditary and sporadic diffuse gastric cancers have similar histologic appearances.

Hereditary Diffuse Gastric Cancer and the Carneiro Model of Carcinogenesis

The diffuse type of gastric adenocarcinoma is characterized by alterations in molecules involved in cell-to-cell interaction and adhesion resulting in the invasion of single or small cell groups. Three main classes of epithelial junctional proteins have been shown to be dysregulated in gastric cancer: (1) E (epithelial)-cadherin, a calcium-dependent cell adhesion molecule; (2) tight junction proteins including the claudin family of proteins; and (3) gap junction proteins, including connexins.[106–108]

Germline mutations in the E-cadherin gene *CDH1* are the genetic basis of the HDGC autosomal-dominant syndrome, which is associated with the development of diffuse gastric cancer and lobular carcinoma of the breast.[109] Germline mutations in the E-cadherin tumor-suppressor gene *CDH1* are responsible for HDGC in 30% to 40% of cases.[110] To date, 122 mutations have been described in the *CDH1* gene.[111] A second *CDH1* hit is required to initiate diffuse gastric carcinoma in mutant carriers. Inactivation of a second allele occurs in most cases of hereditary and sporadic diffuse gastric cancers epigenetically by hypermethylation of the *CDH1* promoter.[111] The result of these genetic alterations is low or absent E-cadherin protein expression. Promoter methylation leads to downregulation but not always complete silencing of *CDH1*, and therefore may explain the conflicting results describing the immunohistochemical expression of E-cadherin in the diffuse type of adenocarcinoma (varying from 0%–68%).[112] Because 60% to 70% of patients with HDGC are negative for *CDH1* germline mutations, the search for additional genes involved in HDGC is of great importance. Catenins, proteins that are downstream molecules involved in E-cadherin signaling, were suggested as potential candidates involved in HDGC; however, a recent study did not find any common mutation in the catenin genes in non-*CDH1* HDGC families.[113] Novel next-generation sequencing technologies should provide whole genome and exome sequencing data, which will be invaluable in the identification of additional genetic alterations in hereditary and sporadic gastric cancers.

Despite the low frequency of HDGC, gastrectomies from *CDH1* mutation carriers are extremely helpful in understanding the pathogenesis of diffuse gastric cancer. The Carneiro model for the development of diffuse gastric cancer has been proposed based on the detailed histologic examination of the entire gastric mucosa from prophylactic gastrectomy specimens of *CDH1* germline mutation carriers (**Fig. 5**).[15] The precursor lesion of signet ring cell carcinoma has been identified as signet ring cell carcinoma in situ, which may show pagetoid spread of signet ring cells under normal foveolar epithelium similar to that seen in breast lobular carcinoma in situ.[15] Histologically, in situ carcinomas are characterized by foveolae and glands with intact

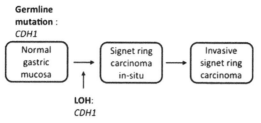

Fig. 5. The Carneiro model of hereditary diffuse gastric cancer. Germline mutations in the E-cadherin gene *CDH1* are responsible for 30% to 40% of hereditary diffuse gastric cancer syndrome. The second hit occurs in most cases by epigenetic silencing of *CDH1* promoter by hypermethylation.

basement membranes totally or partially lined by signet ring cells with excentric hyperchromatic nuclei and mucous vacuoles. Absent or low E-cadherin expression in in situ carcinoma suggests that E-cadherin inactivation is an early event in the development of diffuse gastric cancer.[15]

The distribution of tumor foci in the stomachs of patients with HDGC remains controversial. Although some studies described HDGC from the cardia to the pre-pyloric region, others have demonstrated a predilection to the distal stomach and the body-antral transitional zone.[15,114] Usually the foci are multiple, up to 487 in an individual case, and vary in size from 0.1 to 10 mm.[115] Currently, no genetic or epigenetic alterations have been shown to correlate with the histologic changes in the background gastric mucosa. These changes include a mild chronic *H pylori*–negative nonatrophic gastritis and foveolar hyperplasia with tufting of superficial epithelium and focal globoid change, described as increased retention of mucin in the supranuclear cytoplasm without nuclear atypia or disruption of epithelial structures.[116]

Sporadic Diffuse Gastric Cancer

Although HDGC is not associated with *H pylori*, there is a strong association of sporadic diffuse gastric cancer with *H pylori* infection.[22,23] A combined analysis of prospective studies did not find a risk difference between *H pylori* infection and the incidence of intestinal or diffuse-type noncardia gastric cancers.[22] It has been shown that *H pylori* infection induces promoter methylation and silencing of the E-cadherin gene in nonneoplastic gastric mucosa and in gastric cancer.[117] Methylation of nonneoplastic gastric mucosa may be reversed after successful *H pylori* eradication.[118]

Somatic mutations in E-cadherin were identified in 50% to 70% of the sporadic diffuse type of gastric adenocarcinoma, and were not observed or infrequently detected as harmless silent mutations not affecting the E-cadherin protein structure in the intestinal tumor type.[112] *CDH1* germline mutations presenting as de novo mutations have also been identified in 4% to 7% of sporadic early onset gastric cancer in patients younger than 35 years of age.[110]

The diffuse type of gastric adenocarcinomas has been considered more aggressive, irrespective of its histologic features.[119] However, a "desmoplastic" variant, characterized by prominent desmoplasia surrounding individual tumor cells, has been shown to have stage-independent improved survival.[104] It seems that the biologic behavior of signet ring cell carcinoma differs between early (mucosal and submucosal) and advanced stages of the disease. Patients with EGC with signet ring carcinoma seem to have a better prognosis compared with early non–signet ring carcinoma.[120,121] In contrast, patient survival may be worse in advanced signet ring cell carcinoma compared with the non–signet ring group.[122]

PROXIMAL GASTRIC CANCER: ESOPHAGEAL OR GASTRIC?

The incidence of adenocarcinoma of the GEJ has increased sixfold within the past 40 years in the United States and Western Europe.[123] Recent studies have demonstrated that adenocarcinomas anatomically located within the gastric cardia are a heterogeneous group with different molecular pathogenesis, biologic behavior, and clinical outcomes. This is confounded by the fact as to whether adenocarcinomas involving the GEJ region and gastric cardia originate in the esophagus or the stomach. This may be caused in part by different anatomic definitions of the gastric cardia. Although some pathologists recognize this short 5- to 15-mm normal segment of transition zone between the esophageal squamous and gastric oxyntic mucosa, others consider it a consequence of gastroesophageal reflux.[124,125] Adenocarcinomas of the distal third of the esophagus, the GEJ, and cardia are classified as gastric cardia adenocarcinomas according to the International Classification of Diseases.[126] In contrast, the most recent American Joint Commission on Cancer Staging System requires gastric cardia carcinomas (within the arbitrary proximal 5 cm of the stomach) involving the GEJ or esophagus to be staged as esophageal, rather than gastric cancer.[127]

Two primary pathways of gastric cardia and GEJ carcinogenesis have been recognized. One is the result of gastroesophageal reflux disease and obesity, and is associated with nonatrophic gastric mucosa; the other is associated with chronic atrophic H pylori gastritis with IM, resembling intestinal or diffuse noncardia cancer.[128,129]

In North America, where H pylori and gastric atrophy are relatively rare, most cancers arising at the GEJ are likely the result of gastroesophageal reflux. This is supported by a recent study in which most (86%) of gastric cardia and GEJ adenocarcinomas were not associated with chronic gastritis, H pylori infection, or IM in the distal stomach in North American patients.[130] Recent studies based on histologic features and immunophenotype have demonstrated that dysplasia and adenocarcinoma arising in the gastric cardia and GEJ are also heterogeneous including adenomatous (intestinal), foveolar (gastric), and mixed types.[131,132] The intestinal type arises in a background of intestinal (Barrett) metaplasia. The gene expression profile of cardiac IM in patients without pangastric IM is similar to Barrett, and differs markedly from distal gastric IM.[133] Histologically, the intestinal-type tumors are glandular tumors, and immunohistochemically show $CDX2^+/CD10^+/MUC2^+/MUC5AC^-/MUC6^-$ intestinal phenotype and better survival compared with the gastric type.[131] The intestinal type of cardia cancer expresses β-catenin and HER2.[131] The second, foveolar (gastric) type, expresses gastric markers, such as MUC5AC and MUC6, and is associated with EGFR expression.[131]

The association of H pylori with gastric cardia cancer is more evident in high-risk East Asian populations, including Japan, Korea, and China.[134,135] Although H pylori infection is a strong risk factor for noncardia gastric cancer, it seems to be inversely associated with the risk of gastric cardia cancer in Western countries.[135,136] This inverse association suggests that H pylori eradication may increase the risk of gastric cardia cancer in Western populations, although these two events may be coincidental.

SUMMARY

Recently, the pathways leading to the development of intestinal and diffuse type of gastric adenocarcinoma have been better elucidated; however, there are still many unanswered questions involving different steps of the carcinogenic cascade. Currently, it remains unclear whether SPEM or IM are true precursors of the intestinal type of adenocarcinoma. Although significant progress has been made in the understanding of HDGC, the pathways leading to the sporadic diffuse type remain less clear. Contemporary immunohistochemical and molecular techniques will likely identify novel biomarkers leading to better classification, prognostification, and prediction of chemotherapeutic responses in patients with gastric cancer.

REFERENCES

1. Ferlay J, Shin HR, Bray F, et al. Estimates of worldwide burden of cancer in 2008: GLOBOCAN 2008. Int J Cancer 2010;127:2893–917.
2. Correa P. A human model of gastric carcinogenesis. Cancer Res 1988;48: 3554–60.
3. Borrmann R. Geshwulste des Magens und Duodenums. In: Henke F, Lubrasch O, editors. Handbuch der Speziellen Pathologischen Anatomie und Histologie. Berlin: Springer-Verlag; 1926. p. 865.
4. Ming SC. Gastric carcinoma. A pathobiological classification. Cancer 1977;39: 2475–85.
5. Carneiro F. Classification of gastric carcinomas. Curr Diagn Pathol 1997;4:51–9.
6. Goseki N, Takizawa T, Koike M. Differences in the mode of the extension of gastric cancer classified by histological type: new histological classification of gastric carcinoma. Gut 1992;33:606–12.
7. Lauren P. The two histological main types of gastric carcinoma: diffuse and so-called intestinal-type carcinoma. An attempt at a histo-clinical classification. Acta Pathol Microbiol Scand 1965;64:31–49.
8. Lauwers GY, Carneiro F, Graham DY, et al. Gastric carcinoma. In: Bosman FT, Carneiro F, Hruban RH, et al, editors. WHO classification of tumours of the digestive system. 4th edition. Lyon (France): IARC Press; 2010. p. 48–58.
9. Tay ST, Leong SH, Yu K, et al. A combined comparative genomic hybridization and expression microarray analysis of gastric cancer reveals novel molecular subtypes. Cancer Res 2003;63:3309–16.
10. Tan IB, Ivanova T, Lim KH, et al. Intrinsic subtypes of gastric cancer, based on gene expression pattern, predict survival and respond differently to chemotherapy. Gastroenterology 2011;141:476–85.
11. Lee HS, Cho SB, Lee HE, et al. Protein expression profiling and molecular classification of gastric cancer by the tissue array method. Clin Cancer Res 2007;13: 4154–63.
12. Henson DE, Dittus C, Younes M, et al. Differential trends in the intestinal and diffuse types of gastric carcinoma in the United States, 1973-2000: increase in the signet ring cell type. Arch Pathol Lab Med 2004;128:765–70.
13. Fuchs CS, Mayer RJ. Gastric carcinoma. N Engl J Med 1995;333:32–41.
14. Eom DW, Kang GH, Han SH, et al. Gastric micropapillary carcinoma: a distinct subtype with a significantly worse prognosis in TNM stages I and II. Am J Surg Pathol 2011;35:84–91.
15. Carneiro F, Huntsman DG, Smyrk TC, et al. Model of the early development of diffuse gastric cancer in E-cadherin mutation carriers and its implications for patient screening. J Pathol 2004;203:681–7.
16. Correa P. Human gastric carcinogenesis: a multistep and multifactorial process – First American Cancer Society Award lecture on cancer epidemiology and prevention. Cancer Res 1992;52:6735–40.
17. Dixon MF, Genta RM, Yardley JH, et al. Classification and grading of gastritis. The updated Sydney System. International Workshop on the Histopathology of Gastritis, Houston 1994. Am J Surg Pathol 1996;20:1161–81.

18. Rugge M, Genta RM, OLGA Group. Staging gastritis: an international proposal. Gastroenterology 2005;129:1807–8.
19. Schistosomes, liver flukes and *Helicobacter pylori*. IARC Working Group on the Evaluation of Carcinogenic Risks to Humans. Lyon, 7–14 June 1994. IARC Monogr Eval Carcinog Risks Hum 1994;61:1–241.
20. Fox JG, Wang TC. Inflammation, atrophy, and gastric cancer. J Clin Invest 2007; 117:60–9.
21. Uemura N, Okamoto S, Yamamoto S, et al. *Helicobacter pylori* infection and the development of gastric cancer. N Engl J Med 2001;345:784–9.
22. Helicobacter and Cancer Collaborative Group. Gastric cancer and *Helicobacter pylori*: a combined analysis of 12 case control studies nested within prospective cohorts. Gut 2001;49:347–53.
23. Huang JQ, Sridhar S, Chen Y, et al. Meta-analysis of the relationship between *Helicobacter pylori* seropositivity and gastric cancer. Gastroenterology 1998; 114:1169–79.
24. Smith SB, Snow AN, Perry RL, et al. *Helicobacter pylori*: to stain or not to stain? Am J Clin Pathol 2012;137:733–8.
25. Hartman DJ, Owens SR. Are routine ancillary stains required to diagnose *Helicobacter* infection in gastric biopsy specimens? An institutional quality assurance review. Am J Clin Pathol 2012;137:255–60.
26. Strickland RG. The Sydney System: auto-immune gastritis. J Gastroenterol Hepatol 1991;6:238–43.
27. Brinton LA, Gridley G, Hrubec Z, et al. Cancer risk following pernicious anaemia. Br J Cancer 1989;59:810–3.
28. Hsing AW, Hansson LE, McLaughlin JK, et al. Pernicious anemia and subsequent cancer. A population-based cohort study. Cancer 1993;71:745–50.
29. Solcia E, Rindi G, Fiocca R, et al. Distinct patterns of chronic gastritis associated with carcinoid and cancer and their role in tumorigenesis. Yale J Biol Med 1992; 65:793–804.
30. Rugge M, Meggio A, Pennelli G, et al. Gastritis staging in clinical practice: the OLGA staging system. Gut 2007;56:631–6.
31. Rugge M, de Boni M, Pennelli G, et al. Gastritis OLGA-staging and gastric cancer risk: a twelve-year clinico-pathological follow-up study. Aliment Pharmacol Ther 2010;31:1104–11.
32. Kumar V, editor. Robbins and Cotran Pathologic basis of disease. 8th edition. Philadelphia: Saunders/Elsevier; 2010. p. 10.
33. Schmidt PH, Lee JR, Joshi V, et al. Identification of a metaplastic cell lineage associated with human gastric adenocarcinoma. Lab Invest 1999;79: 639–46.
34. Goldenring JR, Nam KT, Wang TC, et al. Spasmolytic polypeptide-expressing metaplasia and intestinal metaplasia: time for reevaluation of metaplasias and the origins of gastric cancer. Gastroenterology 2010;138:2207–10.
35. Wong WM, Poulsom R, Wright NA. Trefoil peptides. Gut 1999;44:890–5.
36. Halldórsdóttir AM, Sigurdardóttir M, Jónasson JG, et al. Spasmolytic polypeptide-expressing metaplasia (SPEM) associated with gastric cancer in Iceland. Dig Dis Sci 2003;48:431–41.
37. Yamaguchi H, Goldenring JR, Kaminishi M, et al. Identification of spasmolytic polypeptide expressing metaplasia (SPEM) in remnant gastric cancer and surveillance postgastrectomy biopsies. Dig Dis Sci 2002;47:573–8.
38. Goldenring JR, Nam KT. Oxyntic atrophy, metaplasia, and gastric cancer. Prog Mol Biol Transl Sci 2010;96:117–31.

39. El-Zimaity HM, Ota H, Graham DY, et al. Patterns of gastric atrophy in intestinal type gastric carcinoma. Cancer 2002;94:1428–36.
40. Jass JR, Filipe MI. The mucin profiles of normal gastric mucosa, intestinal metaplasia and its variants and gastric carcinoma. Histochem J 1981;13: 931–9.
41. Reis CA, David L, Correa P, et al. Intestinal metaplasia of human stomach displays distinct patterns of mucin (MUC1, MUC2, MUC5AC, and MUC6) expression. Cancer Res 1999;59:1003–7.
42. Filipe MI, Potet F, Bogomoletz WV, et al. Incomplete sulphomucin-secreting intestinal metaplasia for gastric cancer. Preliminary data from a prospective study from three centres. Gut 1985;26:1319–26.
43. Jass JR, Filipe MI. Sulphomucins and precancerous lesions of the human stomach. Histopathology 1980;4:271–9.
44. Barros R, Freund JN, David L, et al. Gastric intestinal metaplasia revisited: function and regulation of CDX2. Trends Mol Med 2012;18:555–63.
45. Pagnini CA, Bozzola L. Precancerous significance of colonic type intestinal metaplasia. Tumori 1981;67:113–6.
46. Filipe MI, Muñoz N, Matko I, et al. Intestinal metaplasia types and the risk of gastric cancer: a cohort study in Slovenia. Int J Cancer 1994;57:324–9.
47. Capelle LG, de Vries AC, Haringsma J, et al. The staging of gastritis with the OLGA system by using intestinal metaplasia as an accurate alternative for atrophic gastritis. Gastrointest Endosc 2010;71:1150–8.
48. Correa P, Fontham ET, Bravo JC, et al. Chemoprevention of gastric dysplasia: randomized trial of antioxidant supplements and anti-*Helicobacter pylori* therapy. J Natl Cancer Inst 2000;92:1881–8.
49. Ley C, Mohar A, Guarner J, et al. *Helicobacter pylori* eradication and gastric preneoplastic conditions: a randomized, double-blind, placebo-controlled trial. Cancer Epidemiol Biomarkers Prev 2004;13:4–10.
50. Zhou L, Sung JJ, Lin S, et al. A five-year follow-up study on the pathological changes of gastric mucosa after *H. pylori* eradication. Chin Med J (Engl) 2003;116:11–4.
51. Wong BC, Lam SK, Wong WM, et al, China Gastric Cancer Study Group. *Helicobacter pylori* eradication to prevent gastric cancer in a high-risk region of China: a randomized controlled trial. JAMA 2004;291:187–94.
52. Asfeldt AM, Steigen SE, Løchen ML, et al. The natural course of *Helicobacter pylori* infection on endoscopic findings in a population during 17 years of follow-up: the Sørreisa gastrointestinal disorder study. Eur J Epidemiol 2009; 24:649–58.
53. Barros R, Peleteiro B, Almeida R, et al. Relevance of high virulence *Helicobacter pylori* strains and futility of CDX2 expression for predicting intestinal metaplasia after eradication of infection. Scand J Gastroenterol 2010;45:828–34.
54. Odze RD, Riddell RH, Bosman FT, et al. Premalignant lesions of the digestive system. In: Bosman FT, editor. WHO Classification of tumours of the digestive system. 4th edition. Lyon (France): IARC Press; 2010. p. 10–2.
55. Rugge M, Correa P, Dixon MF, et al. Gastric dysplasia: the Padova international classification. Am J Surg Pathol 2000;24:167–76.
56. Schlemper RJ, Riddell RH, Kato Y, et al. The Vienna classification of gastrointestinal epithelial neoplasia. Gut 2000;47:251–5.
57. Lauwers GY, Shimizu M, Correa P, et al. Evaluation of gastric biopsies for neoplasia: differences between Japanese and Western pathologists. Am J Surg Pathol 1999;23:511–8.

58. Shin N, Jo HJ, Kim WK, et al. Gastric pit dysplasia in adjacent gastric mucosa in 414 gastric cancers: prevalence and characteristics. Am J Surg Pathol 2011;35: 1021–9.
59. Jass JR. A classification of gastric dysplasia. Histopathology 1983;7(2):181–93.
60. Lauwers GY, Riddell RH. Gastric epithelial dysplasia. Gut 1999;45:784–90.
61. Park do Y, Srivastava A, Kim GH, et al. Adenomatous and foveolar gastric dysplasia: distinct patterns of mucin expression and background intestinal metaplasia. Am J Surg Pathol 2008;32:524–33.
62. Park do Y, Srivastava A, Kim GH, et al. CDX2 expression in the intestinal-type gastri epithelial neoplasia: frequency and significance. Mod Pathol 2010;23: 54–61.
63. Nogueira AM, Machado JC, Carneiro F, et al. Patterns of expression of trefoil peptides and mucins in gastric polyps with and without malignant transformation. J Pathol 1999;187:541–8.
64. Abraham SC, Montgomery EA, Singh VK, et al. Gastric adenomas: intestinal-type and gastric-type adenomas differ in the risk of adenocarcinoma and presence of background mucosal pathology. Am J Surg Pathol 2002;26:1276–85.
65. Srivastava A, Lauwers GY. Gastric epithelial dysplasia: the Western perspective. Dig Liver Dis 2008;40(8):641–9.
66. Yamada H, Ikegami M, Shimoda T, et al. Long term follow-up study of gastric adenoma/dysplasia. Endoscopy 2004;36:390–6.
67. Dinis-Ribeiro M, Areia M, de Vries AC, et al, European Society of Gastrointestinal Endoscopy, European Helicobacter Study Group, European Society of Pathology, Sociedade Portuguesa de Endoscopia Digestiva. Management of precancerous conditions and lesions in the stomach (MAPS): guideline from the European Society of Gastrointestinal Endoscopy (ESGE), European *Helicobacter* Study Group (EHSG), European Society of Pathology (ESP), and the Sociedade Portuguesa de Endoscopia Digestiva (SPED). Endoscopy 2012;44:74–94.
68. Kim YJ, Park JC, Kim JH, et al. Histologic diagnosis based on forceps biopsy is not adequate for determining endoscopic treatment of gastric adenomatous lesions. Endoscopy 2010;42:620–6.
69. Won CS, Cho MY, Kim HS, et al. Upgrade of lesions initially diagnosed as low-grade gastric dysplasia upon forceps biopsy following endoscopic resection. Gut Liver 2011;5:187–93.
70. Kasuga A, Yamamoto Y, Fujisaki J, et al. Clinical characterization of gastric lesions initially diagnosed as low-grade adenomas on forceps biopsy. Dig Endosc 2012;24:331–8.
71. de Vries AC, van Grieken NC, Looman CW, et al. Gastric cancer risk in patients with premalignant gastric lesions: a nationwide cohort study in the Netherlands. Gastroenterology 2008;134:945–52.
72. Park do Y, Lauwers GY. Gastric polyps: classification and management. Arch Pathol Lab Med 2008;132:633–40.
73. Carmack SW, Genta RM, Schuler CM, et al. The current spectrum of gastric polyps: a 1-year national study of over 120,000 patients. Am J Gastroenterol 2009;104:1524–32.
74. Genta RM, Schuler CM, Robiou CI, et al. No association between gastric fundic gland polyps and gastrointestinal neoplasia in a study of over 100,000 patients. Clin Gastroenterol Hepatol 2009;7:849–54.
75. Zwick A, Munir M, Ryan CK, et al. Gastric adenocarcinoma and dysplasia in fundic gland polyps of a patient with attenuated adenomatous polyposis coli. Gastroenterology 1997;113:659–63.

76. Worthley DL, Phillips KD, Wayte N, et al. Gastric adenocarcinoma and proximal polyposis of the stomach (GAPPS): a new autosomal dominant syndrome. Gut 2012;61:774–9.

77. Carmack SW, Genta RM, Graham DY, et al. Management of gastric polyps: a pathology-based guide for gastroenterologists. Nat Rev Gastroenterol Hepatol 2009;6:331–41.

78. Rubio CA. Paneth cell adenoma of the stomach. Am J Surg Pathol 1989;13: 325–8.

79. Vieth M, Kushima R, Borchard F, et al. Pyloric gland adenoma: a clinico-pathological analysis of 90 cases. Virchows Arch 2003;442:317–21.

80. Chen ZM, Scudiere JR, Abraham SC, et al. Pyloric gland adenoma: an entity distinct from gastric foveolar type adenoma. Am J Surg Pathol 2009;33: 186–93.

81. Singhi AD, Lazenby AJ, Montgomery EA. Gastric adenocarcinoma with chief cell differentiation: a proposal for reclassification as oxyntic gland polyp/adenoma. Am J Surg Pathol 2012;36:1030–5.

82. Everett SM, Axon AT. Early gastric cancer in Europe. Gut 1997;41:142–50.

83. Alfaro EE, Lauwers GY. Early gastric neoplasia: diagnosis and implications. Adv Anat Pathol 2011;18:268–80.

84. Noguchi Y, Yoshikawa T, Tsuburaya A, et al. Is gastric carcinoma different between Japan and the United States? Cancer 2000;89:2237–46.

85. Japanese Gastric Cancer Association. Japanese classification of gastric carcinoma: 2nd English edition. Gastric Cancer 1998;1:10–24.

86. Krasinskas AM, Goldsmith JD. Immunohistology of the gastrointestinal tract. In: Dabbs DJ, editor. Diagnostic immunohistochemistry. 3rd edition. Philadelphia: WB Saunders; 2010. p. 505–11.

87. Gürbüz Y, Kahlke V, Klöppel G. How do gastric carcinoma classification systems relate to mucin expression patterns? An immunohistochemical analysis in a series of advanced gastric carcinomas. Virchows Arch 2002;440:505–11.

88. Tahara E. Genetic pathways of two types of gastric cancer. IARC Sci Publ 2004; 157:327–49.

89. Brito MJ, Williams GT, Thompson H, et al. Expression of p53 in early (T1) gastric carcinoma and precancerous adjacent mucosa. Gut 1994;35:1697–700.

90. Lauwers GY, Wahl SJ, Melamed J, et al. p53 expression in precancerous gastric lesions: an immunohistochemical study of PAb 1801 monoclonal antibody on adenomatous and hyperplastic gastric polyps. Am J Gastroenterol 1993;88: 1916–9.

91. Joypaul BV, Newman EL, Hopwood D, et al. Expression of p53 protein in normal, dysplastic, and malignant gastric mucosa: an immunohistochemical study. J Pathol 1993;170:279–83.

92. Hofmann M, Stoss O, Shi D, et al. Assessment of a HER2 scoring system for gastric cancer: results from a validation study. Histopathology 2008;52: 797–805.

93. Bang YJ, Van Cutsem E, Feyereislova A, et al. ToGA Trial Investigators Trastuzumab in combination with chemotherapy versus chemotherapy alone for treatment of HER2-positive advanced gastric or gastro-oesophageal junction cancer (ToGA): a phase 3, open-label, randomised controlled trial. Lancet 2010;376:687–97.

94. Kim MA, Lee HS, Lee HE, et al. EGFR in gastric carcinomas: prognostic significance of protein overexpression and high gene copy number. Histopathology 2008;52:738–46.

95. Pinto C, Di Fabio F, Siena S, et al. Phase II study of cetuximab in combination with FOLFIRI in patients with untreated advanced gastric or gastroesophageal junction adenocarcinoma (FOLCETUX study). Ann Oncol 2007;18:510–7.

96. Han SW, Oh DY, Im SA, et al. Phase II study and biomarker analysis of cetuximab combined with modified FOLFOX6 in advanced gastric cancer. Br J Cancer 2009;100:298–304.

97. Yoon HH, Shi Q, Sukov WR, et al. Association of HER2/ErbB2 expression and gene amplification with pathologic features and prognosis in esophageal adenocarcinomas. Clin Cancer Res 2012;18:546–54.

98. Rüschoff J, Hanna W, Bilous M, et al. HER2 testing in gastric cancer: a practical approach. Mod Pathol 2012;25:637–50.

99. Fassan M, Mastracci L, Grillo F, et al. Early HER2 dysregulation in gastric and oesophageal carcinogenesis. Histopathology 2012;61:769–76.

100. Aarnio M, Sankila R, Pukkala E, et al. Cancer risk in mutation carriers of DNA-mismatch-repair genes. Int J Cancer 1999;81:214–8.

101. Kang GH, Lee S, Kim JS, et al. Profile of aberrant CpG island methylation along the multistep pathway of gastric carcinogenesis. Lab Invest 2003;83:635–41.

102. Kang GH, Lee S, Cho NY, et al. DNA methylation profiles of gastric carcinoma characterized by quantitative DNA methylation analysis. Lab Invest 2008;88:161–70.

103. Park SY, Kook MC, Kim YW, et al. CpG island hypermethylator phenotype in gastric carcinoma and its clinicopathological features. Virchows Arch 2010;457:415–22.

104. Chiaravalli AM, Klersy C, Tava F, et al. Lower- and higher-grade subtypes of diffuse gastric cancer. Hum Pathol 2009;40:1591–9.

105. Carneiro F. Hereditary gastric cancer. Pathologe 2012;33(Suppl 2):231–4.

106. Guilford P, Hopkins J, Harraway J, et al. E-cadherin germline mutations in familial gastric cancer. Nature 1998;392:402–5.

107. Resnick MB, Gavilanez M, Newton E, et al. Claudin expression in gastric adenocarcinomas: a tissue microarray study with prognostic correlation. Hum Pathol 2005;36:886–92.

108. Jee H, Nam KT, Kwon HJ, et al. Altered expression and localization of connexin32 in human and murine gastric carcinogenesis. Dig Dis Sci 2011;56:1323–32.

109. Fitzgerald RC, Hardwick R, Huntsman D, et al, International Gastric Cancer Linkage Consortium. Hereditary diffuse gastric cancer: updated consensus guidelines for clinical management and directions for future research. J Med Genet 2010;47:436–44.

110. Corso G, Pedrazzani C, Pinheiro H, et al. E-cadherin genetic screening and clinico-pathologic characteristics of early onset gastric cancer. Eur J Cancer 2011;47:631–9.

111. Carneiro P, Fernandes MS, Figueiredo J, et al. E-cadherin dysfunction in gastric cancer-cellular consequences, clinical applications and open questions. FEBS Lett 2012;586:2981–9.

112. Becker KF, Atkinson MJ, Reich U, et al. E-cadherin gene mutations provide clues to diffuse type gastric carcinomas. Cancer Res 1994;54:3845–52.

113. Schuetz JM, Leach S, Kaurah P, et al. Catenin family genes are not commonly mutated in hereditary diffuse gastric cancer. Cancer Epidemiol Biomarkers Prev 2012;21(12):2272–4.

114. Charlton A, Blair V, Shaw D, et al. Hereditary diffuse gastric cancer: predominance of multiple foci of signet ring cell carcinoma in distal stomach and transitional zone. Gut 2004;53:814–20.

115. Guilford P, Humar B, Blair V. Hereditary diffuse gastric cancer: translation of CDH1 germline mutations into clinical practice. Gastric Cancer 2010;13:1–10.
116. Solcia E, Fiocca R, Cornaggia M, et al. Precancerous lesions of the stomach. In: Dobrilla G, Bertaccini G, Langman MJ, et al, editors. Problems and controversies in gastroenterology. New York: Raven Press; 1985. p. 241–8.
117. Chan AO, Lam SK, Wong BC, et al. Promoter methylation of E-cadherin gene in gastric mucosa associated with *Helicobacter pylori* infection and in gastric cancer. Gut 2003;52:502–6.
118. Chan AO, Huang C, Hui WM, et al. Stability of E-cadherin methylation status in gastric mucosa associated with histology changes. Aliment Pharmacol Ther 2006;24:831–6.
119. Kubo T. Histologic appearance of gastric carcinoma in high and low mortality countries: comparison between Kyushu, Japan and Minnesota, USA. Cancer 1971;28:726–34.
120. Hyung WJ, Noh SH, Lee JH, et al. Early gastric carcinoma with signet ring cell histology. Cancer 2002;94:78–83.
121. Chiu CT, Kuo CJ, Yeh TS, et al. Early signet ring cell gastric cancer. Dig Dis Sci 2011;56:1749–56.
122. Li C, Kim S, Lai JF, et al. Advanced gastric carcinoma with signet ring cell histology. Oncology 2007;72:64–8.
123. Devesa SS, Blot WJ, Fraumeni JF Jr. Changing patterns in the incidence of esophageal and gastric carcinoma in the United States. Cancer 1998;83: 2049–53.
124. Glickman JN, Fox V, Antonioli DA, et al. Morphology of the cardia and significance of carditis in pediatric patients. Am J Surg Pathol 2002;26:1032–9.
125. Chandrasoma PT, Der R, Ma Y, et al. Histology of the gastroesophageal junction: an autopsy study. Am J Surg Pathol 2000;24:402–9.
126. International classification of diseases. 9th revision, clinical modification (ICD-9-CM). 6th edition. Hyattsville (MD): National Center for Health Statistics; 2008.
127. Edge SB, editor. AJCC cancer staging manual. 7th edition. New York: Springer-Verlag; 2010. p. 103–15.
128. Carneiro F, Chaves P. Pathologic risk factors of adenocarcinoma of the gastric cardia and gastroesophageal junction. Surg Oncol Clin N Am 2006;15: 697–714.
129. Derakhshan MH, Malekzadeh R, Watabe H, et al. Combination of gastric atrophy, reflux symptoms and histological subtype indicates two distinct aetiologies of gastric cardia cancer. Gut 2008;57(3):298–305.
130. Wijetunge S, Ma Y, DeMeester S, et al. Association of adenocarcinomas of the distal esophagus, "gastroesophageal junction," and "gastric cardia" with gastric pathology. Am J Surg Pathol 2010;34:1521–7.
131. Demicco EG, Farris AB III, Baba Y, et al. The dichotomy in carcinogenesis of the distal esophagus and esophagogastric junction: intestinal-type vs cardiac-type mucosa-associated adenocarcinoma. Mod Pathol 2011;24:1177–90.
132. Khor TS, Alfaro EE, Ooi EM, et al. Divergent expression of MUC5AC, MUC6, MUC2, CD10, and CDX-2 in dysplasia and intramucosal adenocarcinomas with intestinal and foveolar morphology: is this evidence of distinct gastric and intestinal pathways to carcinogenesis in Barrett Esophagus? Am J Surg Pathol 2012;36:331–42.
133. Oh DS, DeMeester SR, Tanaka K, et al. The gene expression profile of cardia intestinal metaplasia is similar to that of Barrett's esophagus, not gastric intestinal metaplasia. Dis Esophagus 2011;24:516–22.

134. Dawsey SM, Mark SD, Taylor PR, et al. Gastric cancer and *H. pylori*. Gut 2002; 51:457–8.

135. Cavaleiro-Pinto M, Peleteiro B, Lunet N, et al. *Helicobacter pylori* infection and gastric cardia cancer: systematic review and meta-analysis. Cancer Causes Control 2011;22(3):375–87.

136. Kamangar F, Dawsey SM, Blaser MJ, et al. Opposing risks of gastric cardia and noncardia gastric adenocarcinomas associated with *Helicobacter pylori* seropositivity. J Natl Cancer Inst 2006;98:1445–52.

Helicobacter pylori in Gastric Carcinogenesis: Mechanisms

Lydia E. Wroblewski, PhD[a], Richard M. Peek Jr, MD[a,b],*

KEYWORDS

- Helicobacter pylori • Gastric cancer • Virulence factors

KEY POINTS

- Infection with Helicobacter pylori plays a central role in the development of gastric cancer.
- The pathogenicity of H pylori infection is attributable to specific interactions between virulence components, variable host inflammatory responses, and environmental factors.
- Mechanisms for the carcinogenesis induced by H pylori include changes in host gene expression, alterations in proliferation and apoptosis, and disruption of apical-junctional complexes.

INTRODUCTION

Helicobacter pylori was definitively identified by culture in 1984 by Robin Warren and Barry Marshall,[1] and 10 years later this organism was recognized by the International Agency for Research on Cancer (WHO) as a type I carcinogen. H pylori infection is the strongest known risk factor for gastric cancer, and epidemiologic studies have estimated that, in the absence of H pylori infection, 75% of gastric cancers would not exist.[2] H pylori is considered to be the most common causative agent of infection-related cancers, and is estimated to be responsible for 5.5% of all cancers worldwide.[3] Although it is clear that H pylori is the strongest causative agent for gastric cancer, the precise mechanisms for gastric cancer development in response to H pylori infection are less well defined, and a complex interplay of strain-specific bacterial constituents, inflammatory responses governed by host genetic diversity, and/or environmental influences are involved in determining the fate of the host that is persistently colonized by H pylori.[4] This review focuses on the specific mechanisms used by H pylori to drive gastric carcinogenesis.

Grant Support: NIH P01 CA116087; R01 CA77955; R01 DK58587; DK-58404.

[a] Department of Medicine, Vanderbilt University, 1030 C MRB IV, 2215 Garland Avenue, Nashville, TN 37232, USA; [b] Department of Cancer Biology, Vanderbilt University, 1030 C MRB IV, 2215 Garland Avenue, Nashville, TN 37232, USA
* Corresponding author. Division of Gastroenterology, Hepatology and Nutrition, Vanderbilt University, 1030C MRB IV, 2215B Garland Avenue, Nashville, TN 37232-2279.
E-mail address: richard.peek@vanderbilt.edu

H PYLORI VIRULENCE FACTORS THAT MEDIATE CARCINOGENESIS
The H pylori Type IV cag Secretion System

The cag pathogenicity island (cag PAI) is a well-characterized and intensively studied H pylori virulence determinant, and strains that harbor the cag PAI increase the risk for distal gastric cancer compared with strains that lack the cag island.[5] Genes within the cag island encode proteins that form a bacterial type IV secretion system (T4SS) that translocates proteins across the bacterial membrane into host gastric epithelial cells.[6–8] The terminal gene product of the cag island is CagA, and this is one of the substrates that is translocated into host cells by the T4SS.[9] CagA translocation occurs through the interaction of the H pylori protein CagL, which is located on the distal tip of the T4SS pilus, with integrin $\alpha_5\beta_1$ on host epithelial cells.[10] CagI and CagY have also been shown to interact with β_1 integrin and mediate CagA translocation,[11] and CagL physically associates with CagI and CagH.[12] In addition, CagA facilitates its own translocation through specific binding to β_1 integrin.[11,13] CagA is also reported to be delivered into host epithelial cells by T4SS-induced externalization of phosphatidylserine from the inner leaflet of the cell membrane. The N-terminus of CagA then interacts with phosphatidylserine to gain entry into host epithelial cells.[14,15] Once inside host cells, CagA is tyrosine phosphorylated by Src and Abl kinases at glutamate-proline-isoleucine-tyrosine-alanine (EPIYA) motifs located within the carboxyl-terminus of CagA.

There are 4 distinct CagA EPIYA motifs (A, B, C, or D) and these are distinguished by different amino acid sequences surrounding the EPIYA motif.[16–18] In contrast to EPIYA-A and EPIYA-B motifs, which are present in strains throughout the world, EPIYA-C is typically found only in strains from Western countries (Europe, North America, and Australia), and in these strains, an increased number of CagA EPIYA-C sites confers a heightened risk for developing gastric cancer.[19,20] The EPIYA-D motif is almost exclusively found in East Asian strains.[21] Tyrosine phosphorylation of CagA is tightly regulated, and on injection into the host cell, CagA is immediately phosphorylated on EPIYA-C or EPIYA-D by Src kinase, followed later by phosphorylation on A, B, C, or D motifs by Abl.[22]

Once phosphorylated by members of the Abl and Src family kinases, phospho-CagA targets and interacts with numerous intracellular effectors to lower the threshold for carcinogenesis. Phospho-CagA activates a eukaryotic tyrosine phosphatase (SHP-2), leading to sustained activation of extracellular signal-regulated kinase 1 and 2 (ERK1/2), Crk adaptor, and C-terminal Src kinase, and induces morphologic transformations similar to the changes induced by growth factor stimulation.[23] Interaction of phospho-CagA with C-terminal Src kinase rapidly activates a negative feedback loop to downregulate Src signaling and subsequently the generation of phospho-CagA.[24]

The quantity of phospho-CagA is tightly self-regulated; however, nonphosphorylated CagA also exerts effects within the cell that contribute to pathogenesis. Nonphosphorylated CagA interacts with the cell adhesion protein E-cadherin, the hepatocyte growth factor receptor c-Met, the phospholipase PLC-γ, the adaptor protein Grb2, and the kinase PAR1b/MARK2, and activates β-catenin,[25–28] culminating in proinflammatory and mitogenic responses, disruption of cell-cell junctions, and loss of cell polarity, all of which promote neoplastic progression. Nonphosphorylated CagA also associates with the epithelial tight junction scaffolding protein ZO-1, and the transmembrane protein, junctional adhesion molecule (JAM)-A, leading to nascent but incomplete assembly of tight junctions at sites of bacterial attachment distant from sites of cell-cell contacts.[29] CagA also directly binds PAR1b/MARK2, a central regulator of cell polarity, inhibits its kinase activity, and promotes loss of cell polarity.[25,30,31] These events are discussed in more detail later (**Fig. 1**).

Another pathway through which *H pylori* CagA can increase the risk for gastric cancer is through manipulation of apoptosis, by increasing spermine oxidase production in gastric epithelial cells. This generates oxidative damage and selects for a subpopulation of DNA damaged cells that are resistant to apoptosis.[32] *H pylori* also targets the tumor suppressor p53 to regulate apoptosis in a CagA-dependent manner.[33,34] CagA interacts with the apoptosis-stimulating protein of p53 (ASPP2) and prevents ASPP2 from inducing apoptosis through activation of p53. This results in proteasomal degradation of p53 and resistance to apoptosis.[33] Recent findings suggest that *H pylori* induces specific p53 isoforms that inhibit p53 and p73 activities, induce nuclear factor kappa B (NF-κB) activity, and increase cell survival.[34]

CagA is not the only bacterial product delivered through the T4SS; components of *H pylori* peptidoglycan are also delivered into host cells and trigger signaling pathways that lower the threshold for carcinogenesis. Peptidoglycan interacts with the host intracellular pattern recognition molecule Nod1, which leads to activation of NF-κB-dependent proinflammatory responses such as secretion of IL-8[35] or β-defensin-2, as well as production of type I interferon (IFN).[36,37] Translocated peptidoglycan can also activate phosphatidylinositol 3-kinase (PI3K)/Akt signaling, leading to decreased apoptosis, increased proliferation, and increased cell migration.[38,39]

Vacuolating Cytotoxin A (VacA)

Vacuolating cytotoxin A (VacA), a toxin produced by *H pylori*, is associated with increased disease risk.[40] VacA exerts multiple effects on epithelial cells including vacuolation, induction of apoptosis, and suppression of T-cell responses, which may contribute to the longevity of infection.[41–43]

Most *H pylori* strains possess the *vacA* gene; however, there is considerable variation in *vacA* gene structures within the signal (s) region, the middle (m) region, and the intermediate (i) region.[44] The s-region and m-region are stratified into s1 or s2 and m1 or m2 alleles, respectively. *vacA* s1/m1 strains induce greater vacuolation than s1/m2 strains, and there is typically no vacuolating activity in s2/m2 strains.[44–47] The *vacA* s1/m1 allele is strongly associated with duodenal and gastric ulcer disease, and gastric cancer.[47–49] There are 2 i region subtypes, i1 and i2; and the i region plays a functional role in vacuolating activity.[44] Colonization with *vacA* i1 strains is strongly associated with the presence of CagA, *vacA* s1, and gastric cancer.[44,50]

Of great interest are recent reports suggesting that VacA and CagA are able to counterregulate the effects of each other on the host, representing an effective mechanism to promote persistent colonization of *H pylori*.[51,52] Phospho-CagA is able to inhibit trafficking of VacA and thus prevents VacA from reaching its intracellular targets and inducing vacuoles. Nonphosphorylated CagA is also able to oppose vacuolation by blocking VacA activity at the mitochondria.[51] Another example of the antagonistic effects of CagA and VacA is CagA activation of the NFAT (nuclear factor of activated T cells) family of transcription factors. CagA induces translocation of NFAT from the cytoplasm to the nucleus, whereas VacA prevents the translocation of NFAT.[53] VacA is also able to counteract the effects of CagA by inactivating epithelial growth factor receptor, suppressing activation of ERK1/2 mitogen-activated protein kinase, and preventing CagA-mediated cellular elongation.[52] Recent work has identified another mechanism for regulation of CagA by VacA, whereby VacA induces autophagy and degradation of CagA through specific binding of VacA m1 to low-density lipoprotein receptor-related preotein-1 (LRP1) on epithelial cells.[54] In cells expressing a marker of stem cells, CD44 variant 9 (CD44v9) VacA-induced degradation of CagA is circumvented as a result of resistance to reactive oxygen species.[54] These findings

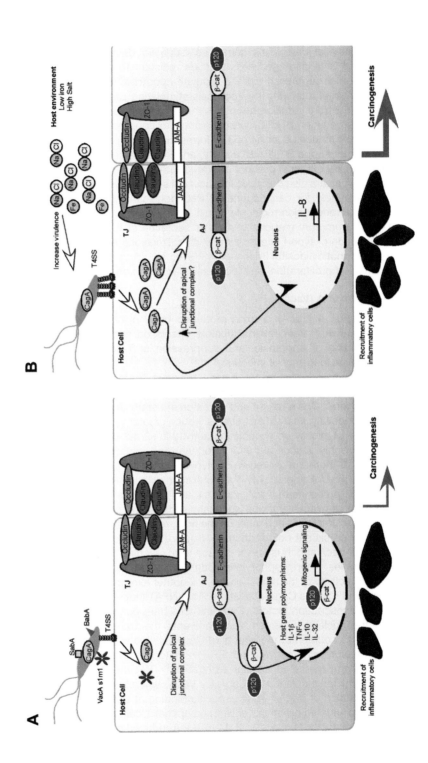

further highlight mechanisms through which *H pylori* can avoid the induction of excess cellular damage and maintain long-term persistence in the gastric niche.

Although CagA and VacA clearly counteract the effects of each other, an exception is facilitation of iron uptake from polarized host epithelial monolayers. In this situation, CagA and VacA act synergistically to create a replicative niche on the apical surface of host epithelial cells by inducing apical mislocalization of transferrin receptors to sites of bacterial attachment.[55]

Adhesins and Outer Membrane Proteins

For *H pylori* to colonize, deploy virulence factors, and persist within the gastric niche, adherence of *H pylori* to gastric epithelium is required. Sequence analyses have revealed that an unusually high proportion of the *H pylori* genome is predicted to encode outer membrane proteins (OMPs), and OMP expression is associated with gastroduodenal ulceration and may heighten the risk for developing gastric cancer (see **Fig. 1**).[56]

Blood group antigen-binding adhesin (BabA) is an OMP encoded by the *babA2* gene and binds to fucosylated Lewis[b] antigen (Le[b]) on the surface of gastric epithelial cells.[57–59] Le[b]-mediated colonization may increase the pathogenic potential of *H pylori*[60] and *H pylori babA2*[+] strains are associated with an increased risk of developing gastric cancer, especially when found in conjunction with *cagA* and *vacA* s1 alleles.[57]

Another *H pylori* adhesin is sialic acid-binding adhesin (SabA). SabA binds to the carbohydrate structure sialyl-Lewis[x] antigen expressed on gastric epithelium, and is associated with increased gastric cancer risk.[61] Sialyl-Lewis[x] expression is induced during chronic gastric inflammation, suggesting that *H pylori* modulates host cell glycosylation patterns to enhance attachment and colonization.[62]

Outer inflammatory protein (OipA) is an inflammation-related outer membrane protein,[63] and the presence of a functional *oipA* gene is associated with more severe disease outcome and gastric cancer.[61,64] OipA expression is linked to increased production of proinflammatory cytokines including IL-8, IL-1, IL-17, and tumor necrosis factor α (TNF-α),[65,66] as well as other host effector proteins such as upregulation of matrix metalloproteinase (MMP)-1, an MMP associated with gastric cancer, and induction of OipA can result in activation of β-catenin.[64,67]

EFFECTS OF *H PYLORI* ON THE HOST IMMUNE RESPONSE THAT MEDIATE CARCINOGENESIS

Infection with *H pylori* invariably results in chronic gastric inflammation, and this occurs through a variety of pathways.[68] As discussed earlier, bacterial factors play

---

Fig. 1. Gastric cancer is a result of a complex interplay between bacterial virulence factors, host inflammatory responses, and environmental influences. (A) *H pylori* virulence factors, including SabA, BabA, CagA, and VacA, influence the outcome of *H pylori* infection; CagA and VacAs1m1 types are associated with increased disease severity. *H pylori* disrupts the apical-junctional complex at the level of the tight junction (TJ) and adherens junction (AJ), and disrupts cell polarity. Disruption of the adherens junction results in translocation of β-catenin and p120 to the nucleus, altering transcription of genes that promote disease progression. Host genetic diversity also contributes to gastric cancer, including polymorphisms within IL-1β, TNFα, IL-10, and IL-32. (B) Host iron (Fe) levels and salt (NaCl) concentrations also affect the virulence of *H pylori*. High salt increases CagA production and low iron levels increase assembly of T4SS pili, CagA translocation, and IL-8 secretion.

an important role in determining the severity of disease outcome; however, these alone are not sufficient to dictate the outcome of *H pylori* infection. The immune response of the host is a key determinant of the development of gastric cancer. *H pylori* upregulates several inflammatory molecules including interleukin (IL)-1β, IL-32, IL-10, and TNF-α and this plays a key role in *H pylori*–induced disease progression.[5]

IL-1β is a Th1 cytokine that inhibits acid secretion and is increased within the gastric mucosa of individuals infected with *H pylori*.[69] Polymorphisms in the IL-1β gene cluster, specifically *IL-1β*-31 and *IL-1β*-511, are associated with increased IL-1β production, and are associated with a significantly increased risk for hypochlorhydria, gastric atrophy, and distal gastric adenocarcinoma compared with persons with genotypes that limit IL-1β expression, but only among persons infected with *H pylori*.[70–72] Given that IL-1β is a potent inhibitor of acid secretion, is profoundly proinflammatory, and is upregulated by *H pylori*, colonized individuals harboring high-expression IL-1β polymorphisms are at increased risk for the development of gastric cancer.

Another cytokine that may increase the risk for gastric cancer is TNF-α. TNF-α is a proinflammatory, acid-suppressive cytokine that is increased within human gastric mucosa colonized by *H pylori*.[73] TNF-α polymorphisms that increase TNF-α production are associated with an increased risk of gastric cancer and its precursors.[72,74] TNF-α expression has been linked to increased β-catenin signaling through inhibition of glycogen synthase kinase (GSK)-3β through the use of transgenic mice that overexpress the β-catenin agonist Wnt1, and these mice develop gastric dysplasia. In vitro studies have revealed that supernatants from activated macrophages promote β-catenin signaling in gastric epithelial cells, which is attenuated by inhibition of binding of TNF-α to its receptor on gastric epithelial cells, providing a potential mechanism through which enhanced levels of TNF-α may increase the risk for gastric cancer.[75]

In contrast to IL-1β and TNF-α polymorphisms, which lead to increased cytokine production and are associated with increased risk for gastric cancer, polymorphisms that decrease the production of the antiinflammatory cytokine IL-10 reciprocally increase the risk for distal gastric cancer.[74] Investigations into the combinatorial effects of IL-1β, TNF-α, and IL-10 polymorphisms on the development of cancer have revealed that the risk of cancer increases progressively with an increasing number of proinflammatory polymorphisms and 3 high-risk polymorphisms increased the risk of cancer 27-fold over baseline.[74]

The role of IL-32, a recently described proinflammatory cytokine that is overexpressed in various inflammatory diseases and cancer, has also been investigated in *H pylori* infection.[76] Expression of IL-32 parallels the severity of gastric pathology, with increased expression in gastritis and gastric cancer compared with uninfected gastric mucosa. IL-32 expression induced by *H pylori* is *cag*PAI-dependent and requires activation of NF-κB. Within the context of *H pylori* infection, IL-32 expression is linked to expression of the cytokines CXCL1, CXCL2, and IL-8, suggesting that IL-32 may function as a master regulatory protein that controls cytokine expression in *H pylori* infection.[76]

MANIPULATION OF THE APICAL-JUNCTIONAL COMPLEX BY *H PYLORI*

Gastric mucosal barrier function is controlled by the apical-junctional complex and is essential for preventing potentially immunogenic elements present in the gastric lumen from gaining access to the gastric mucosa.[77] The apical-junctional complex is composed of tight junctions and adherens junctions, and studies have revealed that *H pylori* targets many of the host molecules that form apical-junctional complexes, which lowers the threshold for carcinogenesis (see **Fig. 1**).

Studies focused on tight junction proteins have revealed that *H pylori* recruits the tight junction proteins ZO-1 and JAM-A to the site of bacterial attachment,[29] and disrupts occludin localization at the tight junction.[78–80] *H pylori* also induces redistribution of claudin-4 and claudin-5 and disrupts barrier function.[80]

One mechanism through which *H pylori* can disrupt the tight junction is via the interaction of CagA with partitioning-defective 1b (PAR1b)/microtubule affinity-regulating kinase 2 (MARK2). PAR1b is a member of the PAR1 family of kinases, and has an essential role in maintaining epithelial cell polarity.[25,81–83] The PAR1b-binding region of CagA is a sequence of 16 amino acids known as the CagA-multimerization (CM) sequence, which is involved in CagA dimerization.[84] The CM motif binds to the MARK2 kinase substrate binding site and mimics a host cell substrate that inactivates the kinase activity of PAR1, leading to defects in epithelial cell polarity and disruption of tight junctions.[25,85] Dysregulation of tight junctions also permits *H pylori* to gain access into sites previously deemed sanctuary sites, such as intercellular spaces and the lamina propria.

H pylori also targets specific components that comprise the adherens junction to promote progression toward gastric carcinogenesis (see **Fig. 1**). Adherens junctions are required for maintenance of adhesive cell-cell contacts, cell polarity, and for signal transduction to the nucleus to regulate transcription. E-cadherin is 1 adherens junction protein that *H pylori* dysregulates via methylating the E-cadherin gene promoter, thereby reducing E-cadherin expression.[86–88] Loss of E-cadherin function is associated with gastric cancer,[86–88] and hypermethylation of the E-cadherin promoter can be reversed by eradication of *H pylori*.[87–89]

H pylori infection also disrupts the adherens junction by inducing translocation of membranous E-cadherin, β-catenin, and p120 to the cytoplasm of epithelial cells.[90–93] Specifically, nonphosphorylated CagA interacts with E-cadherin,[26,94] leading to destabilization of the E-cadherin/β-catenin complex, and accumulation of cytoplasmic and nuclear β-catenin, which subsequently transactivates β-catenin–dependent genes that may promote carcinogenesis.[26,95] Through activation of PI3K/Akt signaling by nonphosphorylated CagA, *H pylori* inactivates GSK-3β, which results in increased cytoplasmic expression of β-catenin.[96,97] *H pylori* closely regulates β-catenin activation within host cells through an inhibitory domain within the N-terminus of CagA.[98] The N-terminus of CagA counteracts the effects exerted by the C-terminus of CagA to reduce host cell responses by strengthening cell-cell contacts and decreasing CagA-induced β-catenin activity.[98]

H pylori can also cleave E-cadherin through the actions of the secreted virulence factor high-temperature requirement A (HtrA).[99] Loss of E-cadherin from the adherens junction is associated with dissociation and movement of β-catenin and p120 from the adherens junction into the cytosol. Under normal physiologic conditions, nuclear expression of p120 is low; however, in transformed cells, expression of p120 is increased.[100–102] *H pylori* is associated with mislocalization of p120 to the nucleus in human gastric epithelia and in infected murine primary gastric epithelial cells.[93,103] Further analysis of downstream signaling pathways has determined that p120 mislocalized to the nucleus in response to *H pylori* acts to relieve transcriptional repression of *mmp-7*, an MMP implicated in gastric tumorigenesis, by an interaction with Kaiso.[93] Nagy and colleagues[38] have also reported that a p120 and β-catenin target gene, PPARδ, regulates gastric epithelial proliferation via activation of cyclin E, representing another important mechanism through which *H pylori* may lower the threshold for the development of gastric cancer.

THE ROLE OF ENVIRONMENTAL INFLUENCES

There are many ways in which H pylori manipulates the host to lower the threshold for carcinogenesis and, conversely, the host can also signal to and alter the bacterium. Recent work has demonstrated that CagA expression is significantly upregulated when certain strains of H pylori are cultured in a medium containing high salt concentrations, an epidemiologically defined risk factor for gastric cancer (see **Fig. 1**).[104] Using sequence analysis and site-directed mutagenesis, it was determined that salt-responsive strains of H pylori are more likely to contain 2 copies of a TAATGA motif within the cagA promoter, whereas strains containing only a single copy of this motif are less likely to possess properties of salt-responsive CagA expression.[105]

Host iron levels have also been found to manipulate the virulence potential of H pylori. H pylori harvested from gerbils with low iron levels were found to assemble more T4SS pili per bacterium, translocate increased amounts of CagA, and increase IL-8 secretion compared with H pylori strains isolated from gerbils with normal iron levels (see **Fig. 1**). Furthermore, strains isolated from patients with low ferritin levels induced significantly higher levels of IL-8 compared with strains isolated from patients with the highest ferritin levels, suggesting that iron deficiency in the host increases the virulence of H pylori and the risk for developing gastric cancer.[106]

SUMMARY

H pylori infection induces chronic inflammation and is the strongest known risk factor for gastric cancer. The genomes of H pylori are highly diverse and therefore bacterial virulence factors play an important role in determining the outcome of H pylori infection, in combination with host responses that are augmented by environmental and dietary risk factors. It is important to gain further understanding of the pathogenesis of H pylori infection to develop more effective treatments for this common but deadly malignancy.

REFERENCES

1. Marshall BJ, Warren JR. Unidentified curved bacilli in the stomach of patients with gastritis and peptic ulceration. Lancet 1984;1(8390):1311–5.
2. Herrera V, Parsonnet J. Helicobacter pylori and gastric adenocarcinoma. Clin Microbiol Infect 2009;15(11):971–6.
3. Parkin DM, Bray F, Ferlay J, et al. Global cancer statistics, 2002. CA Cancer J Clin 2005;55(2):74–108.
4. Blaser MJ, Berg DE. Helicobacter pylori genetic diversity and risk of human disease. J Clin Invest 2001;107(7):767–73.
5. Wroblewski LE, Peek RM Jr, Wilson KT. Helicobacter pylori and gastric cancer: factors that modulate disease risk. Clin Microbiol Rev 2010;23(4):713–39.
6. Covacci A, Rappuoli R. Tyrosine-phosphorylated bacterial proteins: Trojan horses for the host cell. J Exp Med 2000;191(4):587–92.
7. Censini S, Lange C, Xiang Z, et al. cag, a pathogenicity island of Helicobacter pylori, encodes type I-specific and disease-associated virulence factors. Proc Natl Acad Sci U S A 1996;93(25):14648–53.
8. Akopyants NS, Clifton SW, Kersulyte D, et al. Analyses of the cag pathogenicity island of Helicobacter pylori. Mol Microbiol 1998;28(1):37–53.

9. Odenbreit S, Puls J, Sedlmaier B, et al. Translocation of *Helicobacter pylori* CagA into gastric epithelial cells by type IV secretion. Science 2000; 287(5457):1497–500.

10. Kwok T, Zabler D, Urman S, et al. *Helicobacter* exploits integrin for type IV secretion and kinase activation. Nature 2007;449(7164):862–6.

11. Jimenez-Soto LF, Kutter S, Sewald X, et al. *Helicobacter pylori* type IV secretion apparatus exploits beta1 integrin in a novel RGD-independent manner. PLoS Pathog 2009;5(12):e1000684.

12. Shaffer CL, Gaddy JA, Loh JT, et al. *Helicobacter pylori* exploits a unique repertoire of type IV secretion system components for pilus assembly at the bacteria-host cell interface. PLoS Pathog 2011;7(9):e1002237.

13. Kaplan-Turkoz B, Jimenez-Soto LF, Dian C, et al. Structural insights into *Helicobacter pylori* oncoprotein CagA interaction with beta1 integrin. Proc Natl Acad Sci U S A 2012;109(36):14640–5.

14. Murata-Kamiya N, Kikuchi K, Hayashi T, et al. *Helicobacter pylori* exploits host membrane phosphatidylserine for delivery, localization, and pathophysiological action of the CagA oncoprotein. Cell Host Microbe 2010;7(5): 399–411.

15. Hayashi T, Senda M, Morohashi H, et al. Tertiary structure-function analysis reveals the pathogenic signaling potentiation mechanism of *Helicobacter pylori* oncogenic effector CagA. Cell Host Microbe 2012;12(1):20–33.

16. Hatakeyama M. Oncogenic mechanisms of the *Helicobacter pylori* CagA protein. Nat Rev Cancer 2004;4(9):688–94.

17. Higashi H, Yokoyama K, Fujii Y, et al. EPIYA motif is a membrane-targeting signal of *Helicobacter pylori* virulence factor CagA in mammalian cells. J Biol Chem 2005;280(24):23130–7.

18. Naito M, Yamazaki T, Tsutsumi R, et al. Influence of EPIYA-repeat polymorphism on the phosphorylation-dependent biological activity of *Helicobacter pylori* CagA. Gastroenterology 2006;130(4):1181–90.

19. Basso D, Zambon CF, Letley DP, et al. Clinical relevance of *Helicobacter pylori* cagA and vacA gene polymorphisms. Gastroenterology 2008;135(1):91–9.

20. Ferreira RM, Machado JC, Leite M, et al. The number of *Helicobacter pylori* CagA EPIYA C tyrosine phosphorylation motifs influences the pattern of gastritis and the development of gastric carcinoma. Histopathology 2012; 60(6):992–8.

21. Argent RH, Hale JL, El-Omar EM, et al. Differences in *Helicobacter pylori* CagA tyrosine phosphorylation motif patterns between western and East Asian strains, and influences on interleukin-8 secretion. J Med Microbiol 2008;57(Pt 9): 1062–7.

22. Mueller D, Tegtmeyer N, Brandt S, et al. c-Src and c-Abl kinases control hierarchic phosphorylation and function of the CagA effector protein in Western and East Asian *Helicobacter pylori* strains. J Clin Invest 2012;122(4): 1553–66.

23. Higashi H, Tsutsumi R, Muto S, et al. SHP-2 tyrosine phosphatase as an intracellular target of *Helicobacter pylori* CagA protein. Science 2002;295(5555): 683–6.

24. Tsutsumi R, Higashi H, Higuchi M, et al. Attenuation of *Helicobacter pylori* CagA x SHP-2 signaling by interaction between CagA and C-terminal Src kinase. J Biol Chem 2003;278(6):3664–70.

25. Saadat I, Higashi H, Obuse C, et al. *Helicobacter pylori* CagA targets PAR1/MARK kinase to disrupt epithelial cell polarity. Nature 2007;447(7142):330–3.

26. Murata-Kamiya N, Kurashima Y, Teishikata Y, et al. *Helicobacter pylori* CagA interacts with E-cadherin and deregulates the beta-catenin signal that promotes intestinal transdifferentiation in gastric epithelial cells. Oncogene 2007;26(32): 4617–26.

27. Churin Y, Al-Ghoul L, Kepp O, et al. *Helicobacter pylori* CagA protein targets the c-Met receptor and enhances the motogenic response. J Cell Biol 2003;161(2): 249–55.

28. Franco AT, Israel DA, Washington MK, et al. Activation of beta-catenin by carcinogenic *Helicobacter pylori*. Proc Natl Acad Sci U S A 2005;102(30):10646–51.

29. Amieva MR, Vogelmann R, Covacci A, et al. Disruption of the epithelial apical-junctional complex by *Helicobacter pylori* CagA. Science 2003;300(5624): 1430–4.

30. Lu HS, Saito Y, Umeda M, et al. Structural and functional diversity in the PAR1b/MARK2-binding region of *Helicobacter pylori* CagA. Cancer Sci 2008;99(10): 2004–11.

31. Umeda M, Murata-Kamiya N, Saito Y, et al. *Helicobacter pylori* CagA causes mitotic impairment and induces chromosomal instability. J Biol Chem 2009; 284(33):22166–72.

32. Chaturvedi R, Asim M, Romero-Gallo J, et al. Spermine oxidase mediates the gastric cancer risk associated with *Helicobacter pylori* CagA. Gastroenterology 2011;141(5):1696–1708.e1–2.

33. Buti L, Spooner E, Van der Veen AG, et al. *Helicobacter pylori* cytotoxin-associated gene A (CagA) subverts the apoptosis-stimulating protein of p53 (ASPP2) tumor suppressor pathway of the host. Proc Natl Acad Sci U S A 2011;108(22):9238–43.

34. Wei J, Noto J, Zaika E, et al. Pathogenic bacterium *Helicobacter pylori* alters the expression profile of p53 protein isoforms and p53 response to cellular stresses. Proc Natl Acad Sci U S A 2012;109(38):E2543–50.

35. Viala J, Chaput C, Boneca IG, et al. Nod1 responds to peptidoglycan delivered by the *Helicobacter pylori cag* pathogenicity island. Nat Immunol 2004;5(11): 1166–74.

36. Boughan PK, Argent RH, Body-Malapel M, et al. Nucleotide-binding oligomerization domain-1 and epidermal growth factor receptor: critical regulators of beta-defensins during *Helicobacter pylori* infection. J Biol Chem 2006; 281(17):11637–48.

37. Watanabe T, Asano N, Fichtner-Feigl S, et al. NOD1 contributes to mouse host defense against *Helicobacter pylori* via induction of type I IFN and activation of the ISGF3 signaling pathway. J Clin Invest 2010;120(5):1645–62.

38. Nagy TA, Wroblewski LE, Wang D, et al. β-Catenin and p120 mediate PPARdelta-dependent proliferation induced by *Helicobacter pylori* in human and rodent epithelia. Gastroenterology 2011;141(2):553–64.

39. Nagy TA, Frey MR, Yan F, et al. *Helicobacter pylori* regulates cellular migration and apoptosis by activation of phosphatidylinositol 3-kinase signaling. J Infect Dis 2009;199(5):641–51.

40. Cover TL, Blanke SR. *Helicobacter pylori* VacA, a paradigm for toxin multifunctionality. Nat Rev Microbiol 2005;3(4):320–32.

41. Boncristiano M, Paccani SR, Barone S, et al. The *Helicobacter pylori* vacuolating toxin inhibits T cell activation by two independent mechanisms. J Exp Med 2003; 198(12):1887–97.

42. Gebert B, Fischer W, Weiss E, et al. *Helicobacter pylori* vacuolating cytotoxin inhibits T lymphocyte activation. Science 2003;301(5636):1099–102.

43. Sundrud MS, Torres VJ, Unutmaz D, et al. Inhibition of primary human T cell proliferation by *Helicobacter pylori* vacuolating toxin (VacA) is independent of VacA effects on IL-2 secretion. Proc Natl Acad Sci U S A 2004;101(20): 7727–32.

44. Rhead JL, Letley DP, Mohammadi M, et al. A new *Helicobacter pylori* vacuolating cytotoxin determinant, the intermediate region, is associated with gastric cancer. Gastroenterology 2007;133(3):926–36.

45. Van Doorn LJ, Figueiredo C, Megraud F, et al. Geographic distribution of *vacA* allelic types of *Helicobacter pylori*. Gastroenterology 1999;116(4):823–30.

46. Cover TL, Blaser MJ. Purification and characterization of the vacuolating toxin from *Helicobacter pylori*. J Biol Chem 1992;267(15):10570–5.

47. Atherton JC, Cao P, Peek RM Jr, et al. Mosaicism in vacuolating cytotoxin alleles of *Helicobacter pylori*. Association of specific *vacA* types with cytotoxin production and peptic ulceration. J Biol Chem 1995;270(30):17771–7.

48. Atherton JC, Peek RM Jr, Tham KT, et al. Clinical and pathological importance of heterogeneity in *vacA*, the vacuolating cytotoxin gene of *Helicobacter pylori*. Gastroenterology 1997;112(1):92–9.

49. Miehlke S, Kirsch C, Agha-Amiri K, et al. The *Helicobacter pylori vacA* s1, m1 genotype and *cagA* is associated with gastric carcinoma in Germany. Int J Cancer 2000;87(3):322–7.

50. Chung C, Olivares A, Torres E, et al. Diversity of VacA intermediate region among *Helicobacter pylori* strains from several regions of the world. J Clin Microbiol 2010;48(3):690–6.

51. Oldani A, Cormont M, Hofman V, et al. *Helicobacter pylori* counteracts the apoptotic action of its VacA toxin by injecting the CagA protein into gastric epithelial cells. PLoS Pathog 2009;5(10):e1000603.

52. Tegtmeyer N, Zabler D, Schmidt D, et al. Importance of EGF receptor, HER2/Neu and Erk1/2 kinase signalling for host cell elongation and scattering induced by the *Helicobacter pylori* CagA protein: antagonistic effects of the vacuolating cytotoxin VacA. Cell Microbiol 2009;11(3):488–505.

53. Yokoyama K, Higashi H, Ishikawa S, et al. Functional antagonism between *Helicobacter pylori* CagA and vacuolating toxin VacA in control of the NFAT signaling pathway in gastric epithelial cells. Proc Natl Acad Sci U S A 2005; 102(27):9661–6.

54. Tsugawa H, Suzuki H, Saya H, et al. Reactive oxygen species-induced autophagic degradation of *Helicobacter pylori* CagA is specifically suppressed in cancer stem-like cells. Cell Host Microbe 2012;12:764–77.

55. Tan S, Noto JM, Romero-Gallo J, et al. *Helicobacter pylori* perturbs iron trafficking in the epithelium to grow on the cell surface. PLoS Pathog 2011;7(5): e1002050.

56. Dossumbekova A, Prinz C, Gerhard M, et al. *Helicobacter pylori* outer membrane proteins and gastric inflammation. Gut 2006;55(9):1360–1.

57. Gerhard M, Lehn N, Neumayer N, et al. Clinical relevance of the *Helicobacter pylori* gene for blood-group antigen-binding adhesin. Proc Natl Acad Sci U S A 1999;96(22):12778–83.

58. Ilver D, Arnqvist A, Ogren J, et al. *Helicobacter pylori* adhesin binding fucosylated histo-blood group antigens revealed by retagging. Science 1998; 279(5349):373–7.

59. Boren T, Falk P, Roth KA, et al. Attachment of *Helicobacter pylori* to human gastric epithelium mediated by blood group antigens. Science 1993; 262(5141):1892–5.

60. Guruge JL, Falk PG, Lorenz RG, et al. Epithelial attachment alters the outcome of *Helicobacter pylori* infection. Proc Natl Acad Sci U S A 1998;95(7): 3925–30.

61. Yamaoka Y, Ojo O, Fujimoto S, et al. *Helicobacter pylori* outer membrane proteins and gastroduodenal disease. Gut 2006;55(6):775–81.

62. Mahdavi J, Sonden B, Hurtig M, et al. *Helicobacter pylori* SabA adhesin in persistent infection and chronic inflammation. Science 2002;297(5581):573–8.

63. Yamaoka Y, Kwon DH, Graham DY. A M(r) 34,000 proinflammatory outer membrane protein (*oipA*) of *Helicobacter pylori*. Proc Natl Acad Sci U S A 2000;97(13):7533–8.

64. Franco AT, Johnston E, Krishna U, et al. Regulation of gastric carcinogenesis by *Helicobacter pylori* virulence factors. Cancer Res 2008;68(2):379–87.

65. Yamaoka Y, Kudo T, Lu H, et al. Role of interferon-stimulated responsive element-like element in interleukin-8 promoter in *Helicobacter pylori* infection. Gastroenterology 2004;126(4):1030–43.

66. Sugimoto M, Ohno T, Graham DY, et al. Gastric mucosal interleukin-17 and -18 mRNA expression in *Helicobacter pylori*-induced Mongolian gerbils. Cancer Sci 2009;100(11):2152–9.

67. Wu JY, Lu H, Sun Y, et al. Balance between polyoma enhancing activator 3 and activator protein 1 regulates *Helicobacter pylori*-stimulated matrix metalloproteinase 1 expression. Cancer Res 2006;66(10):5111–20.

68. El-Omar EM. The importance of interleukin 1beta in *Helicobacter pylori* associated disease. Gut 2001;48(6):743–7.

69. Noach LA, Bosma NB, Jansen J, et al. Mucosal tumor necrosis factor-alpha, interleukin-1 beta, and interleukin-8 production in patients with *Helicobacter pylori* infection. Scand J Gastroenterol 1994;29(5):425–9.

70. El-Omar EM, Carrington M, Chow WH, et al. Interleukin-1 polymorphisms associated with increased risk of gastric cancer. Nature 2000;404(6776):398–402.

71. Figueiredo C, Machado JC, Pharoah P, et al. *Helicobacter pylori* and interleukin 1 genotyping: an opportunity to identify high-risk individuals for gastric carcinoma. J Natl Cancer Inst 2002;94(22):1680–7.

72. Santos JC, Ladeira MS, Pedrazzoli J Jr, et al. Relationship of IL-1 and TNF-alpha polymorphisms with *Helicobacter pylori* in gastric diseases in a Brazilian population. Braz J Med Biol Res 2012;45(9):811–7.

73. Crabtree JE, Shallcross TM, Heatley RV, et al. Mucosal tumour necrosis factor alpha and interleukin-6 in patients with *Helicobacter pylori* associated gastritis. Gut 1991;32(12):1473–7.

74. El-Omar EM, Rabkin CS, Gammon MD, et al. Increased risk of noncardia gastric cancer associated with proinflammatory cytokine gene polymorphisms. Gastroenterology 2003;124(5):1193–201.

75. Oguma K, Oshima H, Aoki M, et al. Activated macrophages promote Wnt signalling through tumour necrosis factor-alpha in gastric tumour cells. EMBO J 2008; 27(12):1671–81.

76. Sakitani K, Hirata Y, Hayakawa Y, et al. Role of interleukin-32 in *Helicobacter pylori*-induced gastric inflammation. Infect Immun 2012;80(11):3795–803.

77. Sun YQ, Soderholm JD, Petersson F, et al. Long-standing gastric mucosal barrier dysfunction in *Helicobacter pylori*-induced gastritis in mongolian gerbils. Helicobacter 2004;9(3):217–27.

78. Wroblewski LE, Shen L, Ogden S, et al. *Helicobacter pylori* dysregulation of gastric epithelial tight junctions by urease-mediated myosin II activation. Gastroenterology 2009;136(1):236–46.

79. Suzuki K, Kokai Y, Sawada N, et al. SS1 *Helicobacter pylori* disrupts the paracellular barrier of the gastric mucosa and leads to neutrophilic gastritis in mice. Virchows Arch 2002;440(3):318–24.

80. Fedwick JP, Lapointe TK, Meddings JB, et al. *Helicobacter pylori* activates myosin light-chain kinase to disrupt claudin-4 and claudin-5 and increase epithelial permeability. Infect Immun 2005;73(12):7844–52.

81. Cohen D, Brennwald PJ, Rodriguez-Boulan E, et al. Mammalian PAR-1 determines epithelial lumen polarity by organizing the microtubule cytoskeleton. J Cell Biol 2004;164(5):717–27.

82. Zeaiter Z, Cohen D, Musch A, et al. Analysis of detergent-resistant membranes of *Helicobacter pylori* infected gastric adenocarcinoma cells reveals a role for MARK2/Par1b in CagA-mediated disruption of cellular polarity. Cell Microbiol 2008;10(3):781–94.

83. Drewes G, Ebneth A, Preuss U, et al. MARK, a novel family of protein kinases that phosphorylate microtubule-associated proteins and trigger microtubule disruption. Cell 1997;89(2):297–308.

84. Ren S, Higashi H, Lu H, et al. Structural basis and functional consequence of *Helicobacter pylori* CagA multimerization in cells. J Biol Chem 2006;281(43): 32344–52.

85. Nesić D, Miller MC, Quinkert ZT, et al. *Helicobacter pylori* CagA inhibits PAR1-MARK family kinases by mimicking host substrates. Nat Struct Mol Biol 2010;17: 130–2.

86. Chan AO, Lam SK, Wong BC, et al. Promoter methylation of E-cadherin gene in gastric mucosa associated with *Helicobacter pylori* infection and in gastric cancer. Gut 2003;52(4):502–6.

87. Leung WK, Man EP, Yu J, et al. Effects of *Helicobacter pylori* eradication on methylation status of E-cadherin gene in noncancerous stomach. Clin Cancer Res 2006;12(10):3216–21.

88. Perri F, Cotugno R, Piepoli A, et al. Aberrant DNA methylation in non-neoplastic gastric mucosa of *H. Pylori* infected patients and effect of eradication. Am J Gastroenterol 2007;102(7):1361–71.

89. Chan AO, Peng JZ, Lam SK, et al. Eradication of *Helicobacter pylori* infection reverses E-cadherin promoter hypermethylation. Gut 2006;55(4):463–8.

90. Conlin VS, Curtis SB, Zhao Y, et al. *Helicobacter pylori* infection targets adherens junction regulatory proteins and results in increased rates of migration in human gastric epithelial cells. Infect Immun 2004;72(9):5181–92.

91. Suzuki M, Mimuro H, Suzuki T, et al. Interaction of CagA with Crk plays an important role in *Helicobacter pylori*-induced loss of gastric epithelial cell adhesion. J Exp Med 2005;202(9):1235–47.

92. Weydig C, Starzinski-Powitz A, Carra G, et al. CagA-independent disruption of adherence junction complexes involves E-cadherin shedding and implies multiple steps in *Helicobacter pylori* pathogenicity. Exp Cell Res 2007; 313(16):3459–71.

93. Ogden SR, Wroblewski LE, Weydig C, et al. p120 and Kaiso regulate *Helicobacter pylori*-induced expression of matrix metalloproteinase-7. Mol Biol Cell 2008;19(10):4110–21.

94. Kurashima Y, Murata-Kamiya N, Kikuchi K, et al. Deregulation of beta-catenin signal by *Helicobacter pylori* CagA requires the CagA-multimerization sequence. Int J Cancer 2008;122(4):823–31.

95. Oliveira MJ, Costa AM, Costa AC, et al. CagA associates with c-Met, E-cadherin, and p120-catenin in a multiproteic complex that suppresses

Helicobacter pylori-induced cell-invasive phenotype. J Infect Dis 2009;200(5): 745–55.

96. Nakayama M, Hisatsune J, Yamasaki E, et al. *Helicobacter pylori* VacA-induced inhibition of GSK3 through the PI3K/Akt signaling pathway. J Biol Chem 2009; 284(3):1612–9.

97. Suzuki M, Mimuro H, Kiga K, et al. *Helicobacter pylori* CagA phosphorylation-independent function in epithelial proliferation and inflammation. Cell Host Microbe 2009;5(1):23–34.

98. Pelz C, Steininger S, Weiss C, et al. A novel inhibitory domain of *Helicobacter pylori* protein CagA reduces CagA effects on host cell biology. J Biol Chem 2011;286(11):8999–9008.

99. Hoy B, Lower M, Weydig C, et al. *Helicobacter pylori* HtrA is a new secreted virulence factor that cleaves E-cadherin to disrupt intercellular adhesion. EMBO Rep 2010;11(10):798–804.

100. Mayerle J, Friess H, Buchler MW, et al. Up-regulation, nuclear import, and tumor growth stimulation of the adhesion protein p120 in pancreatic cancer. Gastroenterology 2003;124(4):949–60.

101. Wijnhoven BP, Pignatelli M, Dinjens WN, et al. Reduced p120ctn expression correlates with poor survival in patients with adenocarcinoma of the gastroesophageal junction. J Surg Oncol 2005;92(2):116–23.

102. Sarrio D, Moreno-Bueno G, Sanchez-Estevez C, et al. Expression of cadherins and catenins correlates with distinct histologic types of ovarian carcinomas. Hum Pathol 2006;37(8):1042–9.

103. Krueger S, Hundertmark T, Kuester D, et al. *Helicobacter pylori* alters the distribution of ZO-1 and p120ctn in primary human gastric epithelial cells. Pathol Res Pract 2007;203(6):433–44.

104. Loh JT, Torres V, Cover TL. Regulation of *Helicobacter pylori cagA* expression in response to salt. Cancer Res 2007;67(10):4709.

105. Loh JT, Friedman DB, Piazuelo MB, et al. Analysis of *Helicobacter pylori cagA* promoter elements required for salt-induced upregulation of CagA expression. Infect Immun 2012;80(9):3094–106.

106. Noto JM, Gaddy JA, Lee JY, et al. Iron deficiency accelerates *Helicobacter pylori*-induced carcinogenesis in rodents and humans. J Clin Invest 2013;123: 479–92.

Gastric Cancer Chemoprevention
The Current Evidence

Victoria P.Y. Tan*, Benjamin C.Y. Wong

KEYWORDS

- Gastric Cancer • Chemoprevention • NSAIDs • *Helicobacter pylori* eradication

KEY POINTS

- Chemoprevention may form the cornerstone in the management of gastric adenocarcinoma (GC) in the future.
- *Helicobacter pylori* (HP) eradication and aspirin and/or nonsteroidal anti-inflammatory drugs (NSAIDs) therapy have emerged as front-runner preventive strategies due to the putative pathogenic mechanisms that they address.
- Before a population-based chemopreventive strategy can be recommended on a large scale, randomized controlled trials (RCTs) with follow-up of more than 10 years of these 2 agents in populations at high GC risk are urgently awaited.

GC is the fourth most common cancer worldwide but the second leading cause of cancer deaths.[1] GC is a major public health burden internationally, especially in parts of the Asia-Pacific region, where this burden varies due to the heterogeneity of the ethnic populations that reside in this region. The risk of GC varies from high-risk areas in East Asia, including China, Japan, and Korea, where the age-standardized incidence rate (ASR) is greater than 20 per 100,000, to low-risk areas, such as Australia, India, and Thailand, where the ASR is less than half that.[2] This pattern of risk explains the types of clinical GC studies undertaken in the Asia-Pacific region, which have been focused on preventive strategies, early GC screening strategies, and endoscopic management of early GC.

The particular interest in GC-chemopreventive strategies in this region is driven by several factors. First, as discussed previously, some of the highest ASRs of GC internationally are in the Asia-Pacific region. Second, in the absence of screening programs to detect early GC, GC tends to present in an advanced stage because early GC is usually silent and symptoms are nonspecific. Third, treatment outcomes for patients with advanced GC are poor with the currently available chemotherapy regimens and even the newer biologics, with 5-year survival rates between 0% and 30%.[3–6] Finally, although population screening for occult GC in asymptomatic subjects may seem an

Department of Medicine, University of Hong Kong, Hong Kong
* Corresponding author.
E-mail address: vpytan@hku.hk

Gastroenterol Clin N Am 42 (2013) 299–316
http://dx.doi.org/10.1016/j.gtc.2013.02.001
0889-8553/13/$ – see front matter © 2013 Elsevier Inc. All rights reserved.

gastro.theclinics.com

appealing strategy, the costs associated with the program, suggested as high as $83,000 to detect 1 occult malignant lesion, may prove unsustainable.[7] By comparison, modeling on the chemoprevention of GC through therapy, such as HP eradication, suggests that the costs compare favorably to other well-established screening programs.[8] Although population-based chemoprevention seems an attractive option as a primary prevention for GC, for the strategy to be successful there needs to be an identifiable therapy that is low cost, easily implementable, and well tolerated by the target population. Two such agents have been identified, and this review examines the evidence for HP eradication and NSAIDs as chemoprophylactic agents. Other chemopreventive agents in GC also are discussed briefly.

HELICOBACTER PYLORI
Justification for Use of HP Eradication in the Prevention of GC

The most accepted model of gastric carcinogenesis is that GC, like colonic cancers, progresses through a cancer cascade.[9] This is particularly true for intestinal-type GC, where evidence shows there is a multistep progression from gastritis to glandular atrophy, intestinal metaplasia (IM), dysplasia, and ultimately cancer.[10] In early observational studies of the natural history of GC, it seemed that an unknown inciting agent triggered the start of this carcinogenesis cascade, which ultimately resulted in cancer.[11] Since 1982, when Marshall and Warren[12] identified HP and causally linked the bacterium with chronic gastritis and peptic ulcer disease, it has become evident that the putative pathogenic agent causing chronic gastritis in the majority of cases is HP. The hypothesis that prevention of GC may be achieved through HP eradication is based on the results of large-scale epidemiologic studies, experimental models, and meta-analysis of case-control studies.

In 1991, 3 seminal prospective case-control studies involving 324 GC subjects with matched controls were published, which demonstrated that the odds ratio (OR) for HP in subjects with GC was between 2.77 and 6.0, with the pooled analysis of the 3 prospective epidemiologic studies demonstrating a relative risk (RR) of 3.8, which was significant.[13,14] This led to the 1994 classification by the International Agency for Research on Cancer/World Health Organization of HP as a definite carcinogen based on the inference that HP causes histologic gastritis, which, when prolonged, may induce atrophic gastritis, considered the first step in the gastritis-metaplasia-carcinoma sequence of the stomach.[15] Unfortunately, subsequent studies found conflicting results, which prompted several meta-analyses to try to resolve the issue.[16,17] Of these, 2 meta-analyses used more rigorous entry criteria, including only prospective case-control studies, and both demonstrated pooled ORs for gastric cancer in HP-positive individuals of between 2 and 3.[18,19] So, in summary, several meta-analyses have found that HP infection is moderately to strongly associated with the risk of GC development. Coupled with the long lead times presumed involved in the transition between stages in the GC cascade, observational studies showing that non-atrophic gastritis progresses to glandular atrophy and IM over a period of 12 years, make HP eradication a natural choice for chemopreventive strategies, with a large window of opportunity during which to institute therapy. However, not all individuals infected with HP develop GC and the reason why certain individuals have a greater propensity to develop GC is most certainly a multi factorial process. So, although it may seem biologically plausible that HP eradication would result in a reduction in GC incidence, given these complex interactions between host factors, HP infection, and environmental factors, such as diet, it is critical that the evidence for the efficacy of HP eradication in GC prevention is examined.

Evidence for Effectiveness of HP Eradication on Gastric Cancer Incidence

Interventional studies of HP eradication would confirm whether eradication of this infection could prevent GC. Large population-based studies have not been performed, however, and are difficult to undertake for the following reasons. First, the incidence of GC is low, and second, the natural history of GC development is long, so that some investigators have projected that more than 35,000 subjects need to be enrolled and followed for more than 10 years to demonstrate a 50% reduction in the GC incidence after HP eradication.[20] This represents a possibly insurmountable issue in the design, execution, and financing of any proposed study, and these problems are demonstrated in the RCTs performed to examine this issue (discussed later). Finally, there are ethical issues involved in randomizing subjects from a high-risk GC region to placebo when there is strong evidence of HP's putative pathologic role in the development of GC. For these reasons, the authors believe both major cohort studies as well as all RCTs examining the efficacy of HP eradication on GC incidence warrant discussion. **Table 1** details the 6 major cohort studies examining the efficacy of HP eradication on GC incidence. Three of the studies are retrospective studies, which included more than 80,000 subjects and found that HP eradication was consistently and significantly associated with reduced GC incidence. The largest of these studies was conducted in Taiwan and demonstrated that in patients with peptic ulcer disease, HP eradication within an arbitrarily defined time frame (defined by the investigators as within a year of hospitalization for peptic ulcer disease) was associated with GC incidence rates similar to those of the general population. Moreover, this effect seemed time dependent, so that as the years posteradication of HP increased, this had the effect of decreasing the GC standardized incidence ratios (SIRs).[21] The remaining 3 cohort studies were prospective interventional studies, which again found benefit for HP eradication in reducing GC incidence. A study by Uemura and colleagues[22] is important because it was one of the first prospective studies to demonstrate that HP eradication caused a reduction in GC incidence and the subjects with duodenal ulcers seemed protected from GC development. The study's major flaws, however, are the significantly reduced follow-up time in the HP-eradicated cohort (mean 4.8 vs 8.5 years, respectively; P<.001) compared with the untreated cohort, meaning that GC developing later may have been missed in the HP-eradicated/negative group. Moreover, this study was never intended as an interventional study. The study by Yanaoka and colleagues[23] used pepsinogen levels as a surrogate marker of gastric atrophy, which probably would be more cost effective and less invasive if used in a GC chemoprevention program. The investigators suggest that there seems to be a point of no return in the stomach carcinogenesis cascade when HP eradication is of limited benefit. Similarly, the study by Take and colleagues[24] suggests HP eradication was most efficacious before the onset of significant atrophy. They noted, however, that HP eradication even in patients with mild gastric atrophy did not completely prevent GC.

The most robust evidence for the efficacy of HP eradication on GC incidence is derived from RCTs. To date, 5 population-based RCTs have been conducted investigating the effect (**Table 2**) after excluding earlier publications reporting outcomes from the same populations. A further study from Japan of a similar design examined the risk of GC post–HP eradication in subjects with treated early GC is also included.[25] A recent metanalysis was performed to answer the question of whether HP eradication reduced the GC incidence and included the 6 RCTs listed in **Table 2**, although the investigators used some of the data from earlier publications of the same trials due to some changes in methodology in the latest iterations.[26] The

Table 1
Cohort studies on efficacy of HP eradication on reducing GC incidence

Uemura et al,[22] 2001	Aims: to determine the relationship between HP infection and the development of GC Design: prospective, observational single-center study in Japan (N = 1526; 1246 with HP and 280 without HP) recruiting subjects with upper gastrointestinal disorders. HP status determined by positive histology, urease test, and/or serology. Subgroup of N = 253 who received HP eradication. Endoscopy performed at 1 y and 3 y post enrollment. Results: no cancers developed in HP-negative cohort; 36 cancers in the HP-positive cohort. Risk of GC by Kaplan-Meier analysis was 5% at 10 y. No cancers developed in the 253 patients who received HP eradication, although there were 36 cases of GC among 993 untreated patients (mean duration of follow-up 4.8 vs 8.5 y, respectively; P<.001); 63.9% of GC intestinal type and 36.1% diffuse type. Conclusions: HP-negative patients did not develop GC. HP infection is associated with development of both intestinal and diffuse GC, particularly when IM and/or corpus predominant gastritis is in conjunction with severe atrophy. By contrast, patients with HP infection and duodenal ulcer seemed protected from the development of GC. Limitations: nonrandomized. Not placebo controlled. Different follow-up between case and control groups.
Takenaka et al,[61] 2007	Aims: to determine the effect of HP eradication on GC incidence. Design: retrospective, multicenter, cohort study of 1807 subjects with HP positivity who received HP eradication (1519 HP eradicated; the rest had persistent infection). Subjects drawn from 11 hospitals in Japan. No uniform endoscopy at enrollment or post–HP eradication treatment. HP status posteradication determined by urea breath test or endoscopically. Median follow-up of patients was 3 y. Results: 11 subjects developed GC (6 in HP eradicated group and 5 in persistent infection group; P<.01). 3 Cases of diffuse and 8 cases of intestinal-type GC noted. On multivariate analysis, age >60 y (OR 5.5; 95% CI, 1.4–21) and successful HP eradication (OR 0.20; 95% CI, 0.061–0.66) were significant independent factors in the development of GC. Conclusions: HP eradication prevents, in particular, the development of the intestinal-type gastric cancer. Limitations: retrospective design and lack of control cohort. Short follow-up period. Histology at time of HP eradication unknown. 3% of patients lost to follow-up.
Ogura et al,[62] 2008	Aims: to determine the effect of HP eradication on GC incidence. Design: retrospective, open-label, interventional study of HP eradication. 1476 Subjects had a history of gastroduodenal disease, were HP positive, and were drawn from a single center in Japan with a high incidence of GC. Subjects were given HP eradication as an opt-in option (n = 853); subjects declining HP eradication were followed as the persistent HP infection cohort. HP eradication confirmed by urea breath test. 222 Subjects were withdrawn from the HP eradication cohort after a refusal or failure to eradicate HP on a second course of HP eradication. Subjects followed with yearly endoscopies, for a mean of 3 y. Results: a total of 19 cases of GC was reported during follow-up, 6 in the treatment group and 13 in the persistent HP infection group (P = .019). HR of GC development was 0.335 (95% CI, 0.114–0.985). Female gender and older age group also had significant associations with GC development. Conclusions: GC prevention through HP eradication is of benefit. Limitations: retrospective, open-label study. Small cohort study and short follow-up time may miss gastric cancer diagnoses.

Wu et al,[21] 2009	**Aims:** to determine GC risk in patients with peptic ulcer diseases who received early HP eradication (defined as within 1 y of hospitalization for peptic ulcer disease). **Design:** retrospective study of 80,255 subjects who were hospitalized with peptic ulcer disease and received HP eradication therapy. Data drawn from a Taiwanese database that covers 99% of the country's population. Follow-up for a mean of 5.92–7.22 y. **Results:** early HP eradication was associated with GC incidence rates similar to the general public (SIR 1.05; 95% CI, 0.96–1.14), but late eradication resulted in increased risk (SIR 1.36; 95% CI, 1.24–1.49). Early eradication in subjects with gastric ulcers demonstrated decreasing GC SIRs (1.60–1.05, 3–4 y vs 7–10 y, respectively) with increasing accumulated years post–HP treatment. Late eradication demonstrated a similar trend (SIRs decreased from 2.14 to 1.32, 3–4 y vs 7–10 y, respectively). Frequent aspirin or NSAID use (HR 0.65) was an independent protective factor for gastric cancer. **Conclusions:** early HP eradication before the onset of significant gastric atrophy decreases risk of gastric cancer in patients with known peptic ulcer disease, with incidence rates comparable to the general population. **Limitations:** retrospective study with varied follow-up, between 2 y and 10 y. No confirmation of outcome of HP eradication. Baseline HP status of cohort that received no HP eradication unknown (presumed HP negative). Finally, GC diagnosis abstracted from the database and uncertain of accuracy.
Yanaoka et al,[23] 2009	**Aims:** to determine the effect of HP eradication on chronic atrophic gastritis monitored by serum pepsinogen levels. **Design:** prospective, open-label cohort study of 4129 HP-positive male subjects. Follow-up for 9.3 y. Subjects were healthy factory workers recruited from a single province in Japan with high GC incidence. Subjects opted in for HP eradication and 473 successfully eradicated the HP infection. GC diagnosed through barium meal and/or pepsinogen levels, and confirmed with endoscopy. **Results:** 60 GC developed during the follow-up period, 5 in the HP-eradicated group, with no significant difference in GC incidence between HP eradication and persistent infection cohorts. Significant reduction in cancer incidence after HP eradication was observed only in pepsinogen test–negative subjects (P<.05). Pepsinogen test–positive subjects possibly represent the point of no return in stomach carcinogenesis for most GC development and HP eradication will have little impact on the incidence of GC development within 10 y of treatment. **Conclusions:** HP eradication is of most benefit in subjects with mild chronic atrophic gastritis as measured by pepsinogen levels. **Limitations:** GC incidence as secondary outcome measure. Surrogate measures of chronic atrophic gastritis used. Unblinded and no placebo control. Predominantly male subjects. Screening for GC with barium meal and/or pepsinogen level could miss some early GCs.
Take et al,[24] 2011	**Aims:** to determine the GC incidence over up to 14.1 y of follow-up in subjects with peptic ulcer disease who have had their HP eradicated. **Design:** prospective, uncontrolled, interventional study of 1674 subjects who were HP positive. HP eradication was given to every subject and eradication confirmed on a urea breath test within 2 mo of treatment. Yearly endoscopy followed thereafter to assess the histology. 96.7% Had peptic ulcer disease, because the original subjects studied by this group were patients with peptic ulcer disease and HP infection. Japanese single-center study. Subjects followed up for up to 14.1 y (mean 5.6 y). **Results:** 28 GC developed during the follow-up period; 16 were intestinal type and 12 were diffuse type. The risk of GC post–HP eradication was 0.30% per year. All GCs developed in the absence of histologic inflammation. Baseline mucosal atrophy (HR 14.4; 95% CI, 1.9–110.2; P = .01) was an independent risk factor on multivariate analysis for development of GC. **Conclusions:** HP eradication reduced GC incidence to 1/3 in patients with peptic ulcer disease (with no GC on enrollment endoscopy) and was most efficacious before significant gastric atrophy had developed, but HP eradication did not completely prevent GC even in patients with mild mucosal atrophy at time of treatment. The risk of intestinal and diffuse type GC was identical in subjects with HP eradication in this cohort. GC also developed in 2 subjects who initially presented with duodenal ulcers. Periodic follow-up of patients post–HP eradication should be for 10 y or more. **Limitations:** single-center study recruiting predominantly male factory workers. The majority of the cohort had peptic ulcer disease, with 61.4% had gastric ulcers with or without concomitant duodenal ulcers.

Table 2
Helicobacter pylori randomized controlled trials

Wong et al,[34] 2004	**Aims:** to determine whether treatment of HP infection reduces the incidence of GC. The secondary outcome was to determine the GC incidence in subjects with and without precancerous lesions between treatment groups.
	Design: prospective, placebo-controlled, population-based primary prevention study of 1630 healthy carriers of HP from Fujian province in China were randomized to receive HP eradication or placebo. Patients followed from 1994 to 2002.
	Results: there were 18 new cases of GC (HP eradication vs no HP eradication, 7 vs 11, respectively; *P* = .33). In subjects with no precancerous lesions on enrollment, no patient developed GC after HP eradication vs 6 subjects who developed GC after HP eradication but had precancerous lesions at enrollment (*P* = .02). Smoking (HR 6.2; 95% CI, 2.3–16.5; *P*<.001) and older age (HR 1.10; 95% CI, 1.05–1.15; *P*<.001) were independent risk factors for the development of GC.
	Conclusions: in patients with no precancerous lesions on enrollment, HP eradication prevented the development of GC during a 7.5-y follow-up period.
	Limitations: unblinded. Follow-up period of 7.5 y may not be sufficient to demonstrate a risk reduction in subjects with precancerous lesions after HP eradication.
Mera et al,[32] 2005	**Aims:** to determine the long-term effect on HP eradication on histology over a 12-y period.
	Design: prospective, randomized study of 609 subjects with precancerous lesions were randomized to receive HP eradication therapy and/or antioxidants. Patients followed for 12 y. Subjects recruited from a single high GC risk area in Nariño, Colombia.
	Results: HP-negative had 14.8% more regression and 13.7% less progression than patients who were positive at 12 y (*P* = .001). The rate of healing of gastric lesions was more evident in less-advanced lesions and seemed to correlate exponentially with the years free of infection accumulated. There were 9 cases of GC in the follow-up period, 5 in the HP eradication group (4 dysplasia and 1 IM at baseline) and 4 in the nontreated group (1 dysplasia and 3 IM at baseline).
	Conclusions: GC chemoprevention with HP eradication is a viable option; however, the effects may not be seen for the first 3–6 y of follow-up, due to the long lead times required for complete healing of the precancerous lesions.
	Limitations: not double blinded or placebo controlled. GC incidence as secondary outcome measure. Length of time between follow-ups does not allow insight into HP status during these periods and external confounders, including antibiotic treatment, which can influence HP status is unknown. Baseline lesions of average subjects were moderate to severe multifocal atrophic gastritis.
Saito et al,[30] 2005	**Aims:** to determine the regression/progression of gastric atrophy post–HP eradication
	Design: interventional, randomized, multicenter study involving 692 subjects randomized to HP eradication (n = 379) vs control. Subjects were healthy carriers of HP recruited from 145 institutions in Japan. Subjects were followed-up for more than 4 y.
	Results: a total of 5 subjects developed GC (n = 2 in HP eradicated group; *P*<.1). Overall, the endoscopic regression was 13% in both groups. Patients with gastric atrophy were observed to have lack of progression and regression during the subgroup analysis.
	Conclusions: mass eradication of HP is not recommended as a cost-effective method to reduce the incidence of GC. Eradication of HP seems to reduce the grade of atrophy in subjects with gastric atrophy.
	Limitations: published in abstract form only. GC incidence as secondary outcome measure. Uncertain if the control group was placebo controlled. Short follow-up period.

Zhou,[29] 2008	Aims: to determine the GC incidence post–HP eradication and the relationship between HP infection and gastric mucosa histopathology.
	Design: prospective, randomized, double-blinded, placebo-controlled study involving 552 subjects randomized to HP eradication (N ¼ 276) vs control. Subjects were healthy carriers of HP from Shandong county, China, with high incidence of GC. HP status determined 1 mo posteradication with urea breath test and followed for 10 y.
	Results: at 10 y, 9 cases of GC were detected (n = 2 in HP eradication group; $P = .13$). HP treatment group resulted in a significant reduction of the mean gastric body atrophy score ($P = .01$), there was also observed decreased mean polymorphonuclear infiltration and lymphocytic infiltration scores, which reached statistical significance.
	Conclusions: HP eradication shows a trend toward reducing the incidence of GC and HP eradication delays the progression of atrophy in the corpus.
	Limitations: published in abstract form only. GC incidence as secondary outcome measure. Baseline information about GC cases not known.
Fukase et al,[25] 2008	Aims: to determine the effect of HP eradication of the development of metachronous GC post–endoscopic resection for early GC
	Design: prospective, open-label, randomized, controlled trial involving 544 subjects (n = 272 randomized to HP eradication). Subjects had treated or soon-to-be treated early GC and HP positivity determined by rapid urease test or histologically. Subjects recruited from 51 centers in Japan. Patients were examined endoscopically at 6, 12, 24, and 36 mo after randomization. Median follow-up in both groups was 2.95 vs 2.85, HP eradication vs control, respectively.
	Results: a total of 31 GC were detected at the 3 y follow-up. OR for metachronous GC was 3.53 (95% CI, 0.161–0.775; $P = .09$) in the intention-to-treat analysis. In the eradication group, 7% of patients had diarrhea and 12% had soft stools.
	Conclusions: prophylactic eradication of HP should be used to prevent the development of metachronous GC.
	Limitations: no placebo control. Unblinded study. Short follow-up time. Examines patients at very high risk of GC.
Ma et al,[31] 2012	Aims: to determine the incidence of GC and cause-specific mortality post–HP eradication.
	Design: prospective, randomized, double-blinded, placebo-controlled study of HP eradication as part of a factorial design trial also studying the effect of other antioxidants enrolled 3365 subjects. Study participants were healthy subjects recruited randomly from Shandong county in China with high GC incidence. HP status at enrollment was determined by serology and subjects were followed-up for 14.7 y. HP eradication determined by urea breath test post–HP eradication. Endoscopy was performed at 3.3 y and 7.3 y after treatment.
	Results: there were 106 cases of GC during follow-up. GC was diagnosed in 3.0% of HP treatment and in 4.6% of HP treatment-naïve subjects (OR 0.61; 95% CI, 0.38 to 0.96; $P = .032$). GC deaths occurred among 1.5% of subjects assigned HP treatment vs 2.1% of subjects who received placebo (HR of death 0.67; 95% CI, 0.36–1.28).
	Conclusions: HP eradication reduced GC incidence by 39% 14.7 y after treatment and there was a trend toward GC deaths reduction.
	Limitations: no routine endoscopies performed after 7.3 y after enrollment, potentially missing early gastric cancers only able to be diagnosed on endoscopy. No information on long-term HP status after 7.3 y.

meta-analysis found that there was no reduction in the incidence of GC in subjects allocated to HP eradication (RR 0.65; 95% CI, 0.42–1.01) versus placebo (RR 0.70; 95% CI, 0.46–1.08).[27] Unfortunately, there were some serious questions raised about 1 of the data sets included in the meta-analyses due to a reduction in the numbers of GC reported at the 10-year follow-up compared with the 5-year follow-up.[28] Furthermore, 2 of the studies were published in abstract form only, limiting the rigorous assessment of the study methods, analyses, and results, although for the RCT by Zhou and colleagues,[29] information could be obtained from earlier reports of the same data set.[30] In light of the questions raised by the inclusion of these studies in this meta-analysis, in depth examination of the individual studies is warranted.

Only 2 studies have followed patients up for longer than 10 years,[31,32] although both did not design their studies to detect a difference in GC incidence as a primary outcome and both studies demonstrated a protocol change during the follow-up period. The study by Mera and colleagues[32] followed HP-positive patients for 12 years and did not find a difference in the GC incidence between HP-eradicated and HP-uneradicated cohorts but did find that successful and long-term HP eradication induced more regression and less progression on precancerous lesions. Moreover, this study found that HP eradication was more efficacious on less-advanced lesions and correlated exponentially with the number of years free of HP infection. The investigators postulated that the effects of HP eradication on GC incidence may not be evident in the first 3 to 6 years of follow-up due to the prolonged time required for healing of precancerous lesions. The study by Ma and colleagues[31] was a factorial design study that was originally designed to detect the effect of HP eradication and/or supplementation with garlic extract/vitamins. This study did find a reduction in the incidence of GC at 14.7 years' follow-up (OR 0.61; 95% CI, 0.38–0.96), which was not seen at the 7.3 years' follow-up.[33] The findings of this study seem to support the observation that HP eradication's effects may not be seen in the first 3 to 6 years of follow-up and may explain the results of the only meta-analyses performed to address this issue because half of the included RCTs had follow-up shorter than 10 years. These studies also demonstrate the difficulty with the logistics of executing a RCT to examine this issue. In the two studies with more than 10 year's follow up, there was a protocol change, including un-blinding and relaxation of endoscopic follow up, which may impact the findings of the study.[31,32]

The publication by Wong and colleagues[34] remains to date the only population-based RCT where the presented primary outcome is GC incidence post–HP eradication. This study found no difference in GC incidence at 7.5 years. The post hoc analyses found that HP eradication prevented GC development in the cohort without precancerous lesions at time of treatment. This finding again suggests that there is a point of no return, whereby HP eradication fails to reduce GC development, which carries significant biologic plausibility. Finally, the study by Fukase and colleagues,[25] although included in the meta-analysis by Fuccio and colleagues,[26] studied a completely different population from the other RCTs. This study examined patients with early GC who were HP positive and were randomized to HP eradication or to a control group and found that the OR for developing a metachronous GC was 3.53 (95% CI, 0.161–0.775; $P = .009$). This study raises several issues. First, the population studied already had GC, albeit cured endoscopically, and the findings should not be extrapolated to subjects with high GC risk and HP positivity. Second, from what is known about HP's role in the development of GC, randomization of patients with GC to a control arm raises ethical issues. Finally, the best available evidence from large cohort studies and RCTs suggests there is a point of no return in terms of GC prevention and HP eradication, when HP eradication seems less efficacious.

This study seems to suggest that even in patients who have developed early GC, HP eradication is still of significant benefit despite the gastric histology being past the point of no return. In summary, the Asia-Pacific region and South America have some of the highest rates of HP infection and GC prevalence rates, which explains why all the major cohort studies and RCTs on the effect of HP eradication on GC development have emerged from these regions. A meta-analysis has found that HP eradication does not prevent the development of GC, however questions about some of the studies included in the data set may impact on this conclusion. Examination of individual RCTs examining this issue suggest that HP eradication seems to prevent the development of GC in high-risk populations if instituted prior to the development of significant precancerous lesions. RCTs with GC incidence outcomes as the primary outcome and with longer-term follow-up are needed, however, before chemoprevention with HP eradication can be recommended in areas of high GC prevalence. In subjects with early gastric cancers, the evidence seems to suggest that HP eradication is still of significant benefit.

ASPIRIN, NSAIDS, AND COX-2 INHIBITORS
Justification for the Use of Aspirin, NSAIDs, and COX-2 Inhibitors in the Prevention of Gastric Cancer

Aspirin, other NSAIDs, and cyclooxygenase (COX)-2 inhibitors have effects on prostaglandin synthesis through inhibition of the COX enzymes. There are 2 isoforms of cyclooxygenase, COX-1 and COX-2. COX-1 is considered a housekeeping enzyme and is related to the cytoprotection of gastric mucosa. COX-2, conversely, is an inducible enzyme and has functions related to inflammation, pain, and carcinogenesis.[35] COX-2 mediates mitogenic growth factor signaling and down-regulates apoptosis, thus promoting tumor growth. Aspirin and NSAIDs nonselectively inhibit both COX-1 and COX-2 enzymes, whereas COX-2 inhibitors selectively inhibit the COX-2 enzyme. This raises the intriguing possibility of preventing tumorigenesis through the use of these agents. Initially first explored in rodent experiments in the late 1970s, these studies demonstrated that NSAIDs, including aspirin, inhibited chemically induced tumors of the gastrointestinal tract.[36] Moreover, it was also observed that tumor growth often resumed when NSAIDs were discontinued. Other investigators strengthened the hypothesis that aspirin and NSAIDs could possibly prevent cancer by demonstrating that these agents inhibited cell division, altered the cell cycle phase distribution, and caused apoptosis and tumor-induced angiogenesis.

Evidence on aspirin's role in the prevention of gastrointestinal cancers in humans came from an important retrospective case-control study in 1988 that found a 40% to 50% reduction in colon cancer incidence among regular users of aspirin, which was confirmed by subsequent case-control studies.[37] Current opinion is that some NSAIDs prevent tumor formation or induce regression of colorectal cancers in familial adenomatous polyposis syndrome patients and are recommended in this select cohort of patients.[38] A recent meta-analysis of RCTs found that aspirin use was associated with a significant reduction in both the absolute risk and RR of sporadic colonic neoplasia.[39]

The role of aspirin, NSAIDs, and COX-2 inhibitors in GC should be even more biologically convincing than that of colorectal cancers because HP infection induces COX-2 overexpression, and higher levels of COX-2 expression have been found in gastric carcinoma and premalignant lesions. It is, therefore, expected that intervention with aspirin, NSAIDs, and COX-2 inhibitors inhibit or reverse the process of HP related carcinogenesis and prevent the development of GC.

Evidence for Effectiveness of Aspirin, NSAIDS, and COX-2 Inhibitors on Gastric Cancer Incidence

Multiple retrospective case-control studies have been performed to examine the preventative effect of aspirin and NSAIDs on GC In contrast to the studies on HP and GC; however, these studies have ostensibly been performed in white populations with low GC ASRs. Most studies found a consistent association between aspirin and/or NSAIDs use and a reduction in the development of noncardia GC, by between 30% and 45%. This relationship seemed dose dependent.[40] One large UK study did not find an association between aspirin intake and a reduction in the odds for noncardia GC but did find a decrease in the odds for noncardia GC with NSAID ingestion.[41] Another study conducted in 5 Swedish countries found a reduction in the odds for noncardia GC and aspirin but not for NSAIDs.[42]

Because retrospective, case-control studies have many potential confounders that may not be adequately controlled for, and causation cannot be assumed, more robust evidence on the nature of the relationship between aspirin and NSAID ingestion is provided by cohort studies and RCTs. To date, there have been 4 prospective cohort studies and 1 RCT examining this issue (**Tables 3** and **4**). The duration of follow-up varies between 6 and 11 years. Thun and colleagues[43] and Ratnasinghe and colleagues[44] studied the relationship between aspirin and fatal GC, and although the study by Thun and colleagues found a reduced RR of fatal GC of 36% in aspirin users, the study by Ratsinghe and colleagues did not find a similar relationship. A study by Epplein and colleagues[45] examined both aspirin and NSAID use and found that aspirin but not NSAID use was associated with a reduced risk of the noncardia intestinal-type GC. By contrast, a study by Abnet and colleagues[46] found hazard ratio (HR) reductions of between 32% and 36% for aspirin and NSAID intake, respectively, for the development of noncardia GC. The final study is an RCT performed exclusively on women. This study, using alternate daily aspirin dosing, failed to find a reduction in GC deaths in subjects randomized to low-dose aspirin after an average follow-up of 10 years.[47] The studies performed thus far have had several design issues: first, the length of follow-up may not be sufficient to detect a difference in GC outcomes; second, the observational studies are subject to significant recall bias regarding aspirin and NSAID intake and, furthermore, doses taken are unknown; and, finally, most of the studies were not designed to detect GC incidence or GC death as a primary outcome.

To date, 3 meta-analyses and a pooled analysis of case-control or cohort studies have been performed to examine the relationship between aspirin and/or NSAID intake and GC development. A pooled analysis performed by Abnet and colleagues,[46] which included case-control or cohort studies, found a reduction in the odds of developing noncardia GC of 36% and 32% for aspirin and NSAIDs users, respectively. Three meta-analyses have been performed to resolve the issue of the association between aspirin and/or NSAIDs and GC development; the first meta-analysis to address this issue included 8 case-control studies and 1 cohort study and found that aspirin and NSAIDs use was associated with 27% and 22% reductions in the odds of developing GC, respectively, and that there was a significant dose-dependent relationship.[48] A later meta-analysis, which included 14 studies, 3 of which were cohort studies and 1 an RCT, found that there was 38% reduction in the odds of developing noncardia GC in subjects taking aspirin but there was no such association for cardia GC.[49] The final meta-analysis was published in 2011 and differed significantly from the prior 2 meta-analyses because the data used were individual patient data from RCTs of aspirin for primary or secondary prevention of vascular events

Table 3
Aspirin, NSAIDs, and COX-2 inhibitor studies for the prevention of gastric cancer

Thun et al,[43] 1993	Aims: to determine the relationship between aspirin use and fatal cancer risk
	Design: prospective cohort study of 635,031 aspirin users who were followed-up for 6 y (1982–1988). Study population was healthy relations of volunteers from the American Cancer Society, from 50 states in the United States. Aspirin use was determined by questionnaire administered at enrollment. Death determined by through personal enquiry from volunteer who recruited subject.
	Results: a total of 308 patients died of gastric cancer, of whom 152 were aspirin users. RR of death from GC was 0.64 (95% CI, 0.51–0.80) in aspirin compared with nonaspirin users. RRs of 0.73 (95% CI, 0.56–0.96) for occasional use (1–15 times per mo) and 0.49 (95% CI, 0.33–0.74) for use 16 or more times per month.
	Conclusions: aspirin use was inversely associated with fatal gastric cancers. The decrease risk of death was strongly correlated with more frequent and prolonged use of aspirin.
	Limitations: observational study. Short follow-up time. Recall bias for aspirin use. Aspirin dose unknown. Primary outcome is the effect of aspirin on all fatal cancers; GC death is a secondary outcome.
Cook et al,[47] 2005	Aims: to determine the effect of aspirin on the risk of cancer among healthy women.
	Design: prospective, randomized, placebo-controlled, double-blind study recruiting 39,876 healthy female health care workers from multiple centers in the United States and followed for a mean of 10 y. Subjects randomized to aspirin (100 mg every second d) or placebo.
	Results: there were 10 cases of GC death during follow-up (N = 10 for aspirin users). The RR of GC deaths was 1.00 (0.42–2.40, P>.99) in aspirin vs nonaspirin users.
	Conclusions: aspirin at a dose of 100 mg every other day is not effective in reducing the risk of GC in healthy women.
	Limitations: aspirin dose on every alternate day may be insufficient. 10 y follow-up may be insufficient. Primary outcome is the effect of aspirin on all cancers; GC death is a secondary outcome.
Ratnasinghe et al,[44] 2004	Aims: to determine the association between aspirin use and mortality from cancer, heart disease, and stroke.
	Design: prospective observational cohort study recruiting 22,843 subjects from a cross-sectional sample of the healthy population from multiple sites in the United States. Subjects followed for up to 10 y. Aspirin use was determined at face-to-face interview.
	Results: there were 48 cases of GC deaths during follow-up (N = 23 in aspirin users) and the RR for GC mortality was 0.82 (95% CI, 0.38–1.81) for aspirin vs nonaspirin users.
	Conclusions: aspirin use is not associated with a reduction in GC survival.
	Limitations: observational study. Unclear length of follow-up for subjects. Recall bias for aspirin use. Aspirin dose unknown. Primary outcome is the effect of aspirin on all cancer deaths; GC death is a secondary outcome.

(continued on next page)

Table 3
(continued)

Abnet et al,[46] 2009	Aims: to determine the association between NSAID (aspirin and nonaspirin) use and the development of cardia and noncardia GC. Design: prospective observational cohort study recruiting members from the American Association of Retired Persons (N = 311,115) from 8 US states. NSAID intake determine by mailed questionnaire. The subjects were followed-up for a mean of 6.7 y. Results: there were 182 cases of noncardia GC (N = 115 in aspirin users) and 178 cases of cardia GC (N = 130 in aspirin users). Aspirin was associated with a strong dose-dependent reduction of the development of noncardia GC with an HR of 0.64 (95% CI, 0.47–0.86) for any aspirin use (HR 0.74 for monthly use vs HR 0.57 for weekly or daily use; P = .0032). The HR for nonaspirin NSAIDs use with noncardia GC was 0.68 (95% CI, 0.51–0.92) with no clear dose-dependent trend. Conclusions: evidence that regular use of aspirin or nonaspirin NSAIDs may reduce the risk of noncardia gastric cancer. Limitations: observational study. Short duration of follow-up. Recall bias despite more detailed questionnaire. Aspirin and NSAID dosing unknown.
Epplein et al,[45] 2009	Aims: to determine the association between NSAID use (aspirin and nonaspirin) with the development of GC. Design: prospective observational cohort study recruiting members from the Multiethnic Cohort (N = 193,000) from 2 US states. NSAID intake determine by questionnaire. The subjects were followed-up for between 8 y and 11 y. Results: multivariate adjusted HR of 0.73 (95% CI, 0.61–0.89; P [trend] = .009) for risk of noncardia GC in regular vs nonaspirin users. Multivariate adjusted HR 1.00 (95% CI, 0.81–1.24; P [trend] = .99) for the development of noncardia GC in regular vs non-NSAID (not aspirin) users. Conclusions: regular aspirin use is associated with a reduced risk of noncardia intestinal-type GC. Regular nonaspirin NSAID use does not reduce noncardia GC. Limitations: observational study. Recall bias despite more detailed questionnaire. Aspirin and NSAID dosing unknown.

Table 4	
COX-2 inhibitor studies on the effect of precancerous gastric lesions	
Leung et al,[52] 2006	Aims: to determine the effect of COX-2 inhibition on gastric IM
	Design: prospective, randomized, double-blind, placebo-controlled study recruited 213 HP-negative patients with IM from a single center in Hong Kong. Patients randomized to rofecoxib (N = 106) or placebo for 2 y and patients followed for 5 y. IM was assessed by endoscopy annually.
	Results: the proportion of subjects with the regression of IM was not significantly different between rofecoxib and placebo groups (antrum, 24.5% vs 26.9%; P = .74; corpus, 4.3% vs 2.2%; P = .68). There was no significant difference in the severity of IM between the 2 treatment groups ($P \geq 0.3$) and in the proportion of patients who had no detectable IM in the stomach (19.1% vs 16.1%, P = .59, rofecoxib vs placebo, respectively)
	Conclusions: treatment with rofecoxib for 2 y did not result in the regression of gastric IM.
	Limitations: short duration of chemoprevention. Short follow up.
Wong et al,[51] 2012	Aims: to determine the association between COX-2 inhibition and/or HP eradication on regression of advanced gastric lesions
	Design: prospective, randomized, double-blind, placebo-controlled study recruited 1024 subjects from Linqu county, China, with HP infection and advanced gastric lesions. Subjects randomized to 2 interventions (celecoxib and/or HP eradication) or placebo in a 2 × 2 factorial design. COX-2 inhibition was given for 2 y. Patients followed up for up to 5 y.
	Results: 9 cases of GC were diagnosed during the follow-up period (5 in COX-2 inhibitor groups). Compared with placebo, the proportions of regression of gastric lesions significantly increased in the celecoxib treatment group (52.8% vs 41.2) (OR 1.72; 95% CI, 1.07–2.76) respectively. No statistically significant effect was found for HP eradication followed by celecoxib on the regression of advanced gastric lesions (OR 1.48; 95% CI, 0.91–2.40).
	Conclusions: celecoxib treatment had beneficial effects on the regression of advanced gastric lesions. No favorable effects were reported for HP eradication followed by celecoxib treatment.
	Limitations: short duration of chemoprevention. Short follow-up time. GC as a secondary outcome measure.

that reported death from cancer as an endpoint.[50] After 10 to 20 years of follow-up in the 3 trials that reported the primary site of cancer, aspirin use was found protective against gastric cancer (HR 0.42; 95% CI, 0.23–0.79).

Finally, although to date there has only been 1 RCT examining the risk of cancer in women randomized to aspirin, there have been no published RCTs designed to specifically examine aspirin, NSAIDs, or COX-2 inhibitor effects on the development of GC. The long lead times involved in gastric carcinogenesis have led researchers to consider the effects of these agents on advanced gastric lesions as a surrogate for GC development. Two RCTs have been performed examining the progression or regression of advanced gastric lesions in subjects randomized to COX-2 inhibitors.[51,52] Only the study by Wong and colleagues[51] reported GC outcomes, but no analysis was made due to the small numbers observed. The study by Leung and colleagues[52] found no effect of rofecoxib on IM after 5 years' follow-up. The investigators suggested that chemoprevention with COX-2 inhibitors may not be effective at the late stage of IM. By contrast, the study by Wong and colleagues, which included subjects with a range of advanced gastric lesions, found celecoxib treatment for 2 years was associated with regression of advanced gastric lesions after 5 years of follow-up.[51] In summary, the evidence from multiple case-control, cohort RCTs, a pooled analysis, and meta-analyses suggest there seems to be a preventive effect of aspirin and/or NSAIDs on the development of noncardia GC. Limited evidence from COX-2 inhibitors suggests there may be a role for these agents in promoting the regression of advanced gastric lesions. Before chemoprevention with these agents can be recommended, however, RCTs in populations at high risk of GC are warranted to confirm these associations and determine the dose of aspirin and/or NSAIDs and duration of chemoprevention, and, finally, ensure that no excess risk of gastrointestinal bleeding and hemorrhagic strokes are observed.

OTHER CHEMOPREVENTIVE AGENTS

In terms of environmental factors found in observational studies associated with GC, diets high in salt and nitrates, especially in the form of preserved fish and vegetables, seem to confer the highest risks. Conversely, a balanced diet rich in fresh fruits and vegetables is associated with a reduced risk of GC. Despite these observations, sustained measurable alterations in diet sufficient to affect GC prevalence are difficult to assess in a study population, particularly over the long lead times GC studies require. In an effort to replicate the presumed antioxidant effect of fresh fruits and vegetables, several groups have attempted to augment the diet with garlic supplements, multivitamins, and/or trace elements, including selenium. These studies have demonstrated conflicting results, which are compounded by the factorial designs that have been used to undertake these studies.[31,33,53–55]

Statins, although initially prescribed for their lipid-lowering agent via HMG-CoA reductase, have been observed to have several pleiotropic effects, including the potential to inhibit activation of Ras protein, which is involved in regulating cellular proliferation and differentiation, triggering the apoptosis of GC cells and inhibiting angiogenesis. Multiple studies and 2 meta-analyses have attempted to explore the association between statin therapy and GC development. Results have been conflicting, with 1 meta-analysis finding no benefit of statins on GC development and a second meta-analysis finding a 41% RR reduction of GC with statin therapy.[56–60]

SUMMARY

Chemoprevention may form the cornerstone in the management of GC of the future. HP eradication and aspirin and/or NSAID therapy have emerged as front-runner chemotherapeutic agents due to the putative pathogenic mechanisms that they address. Moreover, existing evidence supports their use. Before a population-based chemopreventive strategy can be recommended on a large scale, RCTs with follow-up of more than 10 years of these 2 agents in populations at high GC risk are urgently awaited.

REFERENCES

1. Parkin DM, Bray F, Ferlay J, et al. Global cancer statistics, 2002. CA Cancer J Clin 2005;55:74–108.
2. Fock KM, Katelaris P, Sugano K, et al. Second Asia-Pacific Consensus Guidelines for Helicobacter pylori infection. J Gastroenterol Hepatol 2009;24:1587–600.
3. Bang YJ, Van Cutsem E, Feyereislova A, et al. Trastuzumab in combination with chemotherapy versus chemotherapy alone for treatment of HER2-positive

advanced gastric or gastro-oesophageal junction cancer (ToGA): a phase 3, open-label, randomised controlled trial. Lancet 2010;376:687–97.

4. Ma BB, Hui EP, Mok TS. Population-based differences in treatment outcome following anticancer drug therapies. Lancet Oncol 2010;11:75–84.

5. Lello E, Furnes B, Edna TH. Short and long-term survival from gastric cancer. A population-based study from a county hospital during 25 years. Acta Oncol 2007; 46:308–15.

6. Cunningham SC, Kamangar F, Kim MP, et al. Survival after gastric adenocarcinoma resection: eighteen-year experience at a single institution. J Gastrointest Surg 2005;9:718–25.

7. Vakil N, Talley NJ, Veldhuyzen van Zanten S, et al. Cost of detecting malignant lesions by endoscopy in 2741 primary care dyspeptic patients without alarm symptoms. Clin Gastroenterol Hepatol 2009;7:756–61.

8. Roderick P, Davies R, Raftery J, et al. The cost-effectiveness of screening for *Helicobacter pylori* to reduce mortality and morbidity from gastric cancer and peptic ulcer disease: a discrete-event simulation model. Health Technol Assess 2003;7:1–86.

9. Correa P, Piazuelo MB, Camargo MC. The future of gastric cancer prevention. Gastric Cancer 2004;7:9–16.

10. Correa P. Human gastric carcinogenesis: a multistep and multifactorial process—First American Cancer Society Award Lecture on Cancer Epidemiology and Prevention. Cancer Res 1992;52:6735–40.

11. Correa P, Haenszel W, Cuello C, et al. A model for gastric cancer epidemiology. Lancet 1975;2:58–60.

12. Marshall BJ, Warren JR. Unidentified curved bacilli in the stomach of patients with gastritis and peptic ulceration. Lancet 1984;1:1311–5.

13. Forman D, Newell DG, Fullerton F, et al. Association between infection with *Helicobacter pylori* and risk of gastric cancer: evidence from a prospective investigation. BMJ 1991;302(6788):1302–5.

14. Parsonnet J, Friedman GD, Vandersteen DP, et al. *Helicobacter pylori* infection and the risk of gastric carcinoma. N Engl J Med 1991;325(16):1127–31.

15. International Agency for Research on Cancer. Schistosomes, Liver Flukes and *Helicobacter Pylori*. IARC Monogr Eval Carcinog Risks Hum 1994;61:177–241.

16. Webb PM, Yu MC, Forman D, et al. An apparent lack of association between *Helicobacter pylori* infection and risk of gastric cancer in China. Int J Cancer 1996;67(5):603–7.

17. Hansen S, Melby KK, Aase S, et al. *Helicobacter pylori* infection and risk of cardia cancer and non-cardia gastric cancer. A nested case-control study. Scand J Gastroenterol 1999;34(4):353–60.

18. Danesh J. *Helicobacter pylori* infection and gastric cancer: systematic review of the epidemiological studies. Aliment Pharmacol Ther 1999;13:851–6.

19. Helicobacter and Cancer Collaborative Group. Gastric cancer and *Helicobacter pylori*: a combined analysis of 12 casecontrol studies nested within prospective cohorts. Gut 2001;49(3):347–53.

20. Graham DY, Shiotani A. The time to eradicate gastric cancer is now. Gut 2005; 54(6):735–8.

21. Wu CY, Kuo KN, Wu MS, et al. Early *Helicobacter pylori* eradication decreases risk of gastric cancer in patients with peptic ulcer disease. Gastroenterology 2009;137(5):1641–8.

22. Uemura N, Okamoto S, Yamamoto S, et al. Schlemper RJ. *Helicobacter pylori* infection and the development of gastric cancer. N Engl J Med 2001;345(11):784–9.

23. Yanaoka K, Oka M, Ohata H, et al. Eradication of *Helicobacter pylori* prevents cancer development in subjects with mild gastric atrophy identified by serum pepsinogen levels. Int J Cancer 2009;125(11):2697–703.

24. Take S, Mizuno M, Ishiki K, et al. The long-term risk of gastric cancer after the successful eradication of *Helicobacter pylori*. J Gastroenterol 2011;46(3):318–24.

25. Fukase K, Kato M, Kikuchi S, et al, Japan Gast Study Group. Effect of eradication of *Helicobacter pylori* on incidence of metachronous gastric carcinoma after endoscopic resection of early gastric cancer: an open-label, randomised controlled trial. Lancet 2008;372:392–7.

26. Fuccio L, Zagari RM, Eusebi LH, et al. Meta-analysis: can *Helicobacter pylori* eradication treatment reduce the risk for gastric cancer? Ann Intern Med 2009; 151(2):121–8.

27. Ford AC. Chemoprevention for gastric cancer. Best Pract Res Clin Gastroenterol 2011;25(4–5):581–92.

28. Leung WK, Lin SR, Ching JY, et al. Factors predicting progression of gastric intestinal metaplasia: results of a randomised trial on *Helicobacter pylori* eradication. Gut 2004;53(9):1244–9.

29. Zhou L. Ten-year follow-up study on the incidence of gastric cancer and the pathological changes of gastric mucosa after *H. pylori* eradication in China [abstract]. Gastroenterology 2008;134:A233.

30. Saito D, Boku N, Fujioka T, et al. Impact of *H. pylori* eradication on gastric cancer prevention: endoscopic results of the Japanese Intervention Trial(JITHP-Study). A randomized multi-center trial [abstract]. Gastroenterology 2005;128:A4.

31. Ma JL, Zhang L, Brown LM, et al. Fifteen-year effects of *Helicobacter pylori*, garlic, and vitamin treatments on gastric cancer incidence and mortality. J Natl Cancer Inst 2012;104(6):488–92.

32. Mera R, Fontham ET, Bravo LE, et al. Long-term follow-up of patients treated for *Helicobacter pylori* infection. Gut 2005;54:1536–40.

33. You WC, Brown LM, Zhang L, et al. Randomized double-blind factorial trial of three treatments to reduce the prevalence of precancerous gastric lesions. J Natl Cancer Inst 2006;98(14):974–83.

34. Wong BC, Lam SK, Wong WM, et al. *Helicobacter pylori* eradication to prevent gastric cancer in a high-risk region of China: a randomized controlled trial. JAMA 2004;291(2):187–94.

35. Chen CN, Sung CT, Lin MT, et al. Clinicopathologic association of cyclooxygenase 1 and cyclooxygenase 2 expression in gastric adenocarcinoma. Ann Surg 2001;233:183–8.

36. Reddy BS, Rao CV, Rivenson A, et al. Inhibitory effects of aspirin on azoxymethane-induced colon carcinogenesis in F344 rats. Carcinogenesis 1993;14:1493–7.

37. Kune GA, Kune S, Watson LF. Colorectal cancer risk, chronic illnesses, operations and medications: case control results from the Melbourne Colorectal Cancer Study. Cancer Res 1988;48:4399–404.

38. Tan VP, Chan P, Hung IF, et al. Chemoprophylaxis in colorectal cancer: current concepts and a practical algorithm for use. Expert Opin Investig Drugs 2010; 19(Suppl 1):S57–66.

39. Cole BF, Logan RF, Halabi S, et al. Aspirin for the chemoprevention of colorectal adenomas: meta-analysis of the randomized trials. J Natl Cancer Inst 2009;101: 256–66.

40. Duan L, Wu AH, Sullivan-Halley J, et al. Nonsteroidal anti-inflammatory drugs and risk of esophageal and gastric adenocarcinomas in Los Angeles County. Cancer Epidemiol Biomarkers Prev 2008;17(1):126–34.

41. Lindblad M, Lagergren J, García Rodríguez LA. Nonsteroidal anti-inflammatory drugs and risk of esophageal and gastric cancer. Cancer Epidemiol Biomarkers Prev 2005;14(2):444–50.

42. Akre K, Ekström AM, Signorello LB, et al. Aspirin and risk for gastric cancer: a population-based case-control study in Sweden. Br J Cancer 2001;84(7):965–8.

43. Thun MJ, Namboodiri MM, Calle EE, et al. Aspirin use and risk of fatal cancer. Cancer Res 1993;53(6):1322–7.

44. Ratnasinghe LD, Graubard BI, Kahle L, et al. Aspirin use and mortality from cancer in a prospective cohort study. Anticancer Res 2004;24(5B):3177–84.

45. Epplein M, Nomura AM, Wilkens LR, et al. Nonsteroidal antiinflammatory drugs and risk of gastric adenocarcinoma: the multiethnic cohort study. Am J Epidemiol 2009;170(4):507–14.

46. Abnet CC, Freedman ND, Kamangar F, et al. Non-steroidal anti-inflammatory drugs and risk of gastric and oesophageal adenocarcinomas: results from a cohort study and a meta-analysis. Br J Cancer 2009;100(3):551–7.

47. Cook NR, Lee IM, Gaziano JM, et al. Low-dose aspirin in the primary prevention of cancer: the Women's Health Study: a randomized controlled trial. JAMA 2005;294(1):47–55.

48. Wang WH, Huang JQ, Zheng GF, et al. Non-steroidal anti-inflammatory drug use and the risk of gastric cancer: a systematic review and meta-analysis. J Natl Cancer Inst 2003;95:1784–91.

49. Yang P, Zhou Y, Chen B, et al. Aspirin use and the risk of gastric cancer: a meta-analysis. Dig Dis Sci 2010;55:1533–9.

50. Rothwell PM, Fowkes FG, Belch JF, et al. Effect of daily aspirin on long-term risk of death due to cancer: analysis of individual patient data from randomised trials. Lancet 2011;377(9759):31–41.

51. Wong BC, Zhang L, Ma JL, et al. Effects of selective COX-2 inhibitor and Helicobacter pylori eradication on precancerous gastric lesions. Gut 2012;61(6):812–8.

52. Leung WK, Ng EK, Chan FK, et al. Effects of long-term rofecoxib on gastric intestinal metaplasia: results of a randomized controlled trial. Clin Cancer Res 2006;12(15):4766–72.

53. Correa P, Fontham ET, Bravo JC, et al. Chemoprevention of gastric dysplasia: randomized trial of antioxidant supplements and anti-Helicobacter pylori therapy. J Natl Cancer Inst 2000;92:1881–8.

54. Blot WJ, Li JY, Taylor PR, et al. Nutrition intervention trials in Linxian, China: supplementation with specific vitamin/mineral combinations, cancer incidence, and disease-specific mortality in the general population. J Natl Cancer Inst 1993;85:1483–92.

55. Qiao YL, Dawsey SM, Kamangar F, et al. Total and cancer mortality after supplementation with vitamins and minerals:follow-up of the Linxian general population nutrition intervention trial. J Natl Cancer Inst 2009;101:507–18.

56. Browning DR, Martin RM. Statins and risk of cancer: a systematic reviewand meta-analysis. Int J Cancer 2006;120:833–43.

57. Kuoppala J, Lamminpaa A, Pukkala E. Statins and cancer: a systematic review and meta-analysis. Eur J Cancer 2008;44:2122–32.

58. Graaf MR, Beiderbeck AB, Egberts AC, et al. The risk of cancer in statin users. J Clin Oncol 2004;22:2388–94.

59. Kaye JA, Jick H. Statin use and cancer risk in the general Practice research database. Br J Cancer 2004;90:635–7.

60. Hippisley-Cox J, Coupland C. Unintended effects of statins in men and women in England and Wales: population based cohort study using the QResearch database. BMJ 2010;340:c2197.
61. Takenaka R, Okada H, Kato J, et al. *Helicobacter pylori* eradication reduced the incidence of gastric cancer, especially of the intestinal type. Aliment Pharmacol Ther 2007;25(7):805–12.
62. Ogura K, Hirata Y, Yanai A, et al. The effect of Helicobacter pylori eradication on reducing the incidence of gastric cancer. J Clin Gastroenterol 2008;42(3):279–83.

Screening and Treating Intermediate Lesions to Prevent Gastric Cancer

Noriya Uedo, MD[a],*, Kenshi Yao, MD[b], Ryu Ishihara, MD[a]

KEYWORDS

- Early gastric cancer • Screening • Endoscopy • Narrow-band imaging
- Endoscopic mucosal resection • Endoscopic submucosal dissection
- Mucosal high-grade neoplasia

KEY POINTS

- Early gastric cancer is defined as adenocarcinoma confined to the mucosa or submucosa irrespective of lymph node involvement. In Japan, mucosal high-grade neoplasia is diagnosed as intramucosal early gastric cancer.
- Some early gastric cancers progress to advanced gastric cancer after several years of follow-up.
- A proper endoscopic screening procedure would increase the detection of intramucosal early gastric cancer.
- Image-enhanced endoscopy (ie, chromoendoscopy), narrow-band imaging, and magnifying endoscopy increase the diagnostic yield for characterization of early gastric cancer.
- Endoscopic resection of intramucosal early gastric cancer with endoscopic mucosal resection or endoscopic submucosal dissection is currently performed in East Asian countries to prevent the development of advanced gastric cancer and to preserve patients' quality of life after treatment.

 A video of a case of superficial elevated early gastric cancer accompanies this article at http://www.gastro.theclinics.com/

Conflict of Interest: No conflict of interest or funding to be declared.

Author Contributions: Conception and design, Noriya Uedo; analysis and interpretation of the data, Noriya Uedo; drafting of the article, Noriya Uedo; critical revision of the article for important intellectual content, Ryu Ishihara and Kenshi Yao; final approval of the article, Noriya Uedo, Ryu Ishihara, and Kenshi Yao.

[a] Department of Gastrointestinal Oncology, Osaka Medical Center for Cancer and Cardiovascular Diseases, 3-3 Nakamichi 1-chome, Osaka 537-8511, Japan; [b] Department of Endoscopy, Fukuoka University Chikushi Hospital, Fukuoka, Japan

* Corresponding author. Department of Gastrointestinal Oncology, Osaka Medical Center for Cancer and Cardiovascular Diseases, 3-3 Nakamichi 1-chome, Higashinari-ku, Osaka 537-8511, Japan.

E-mail address: uedou-no@mc.pref.osaka.jp

BACKGROUND

Gastric cancer is currently the fourth most common malignancy and the second most common cause of cancer deaths worldwide. Half the global total of gastric cancer occurs in East Asia. Age-standardized mortality rate is estimated as the highest (28.1 per 100,000 in men and 13.0 per 100,000 in women) in East Asia, whereas that in the United States is low (2.8 per 100,000 in men and 1.5 per 100,000 in women).[1] Early detection and treatment are considered to be effective strategies in reducing mortality from gastric cancer as a secondary prevention. Thus, many attempts have been made in this direction, such as encouragement of mass screening[2,3] or the development of accurate diagnostic procedures in East Asian countries.

DEFINITION OF EARLY GASTRIC CANCER

Early gastric cancer (EGC) was first defined in 1962 by the Japanese Society of Gastroenterological Endoscopy as adenocarcinoma confined to the mucosa or submucosa irrespective of lymph node involvement.[4] The need for such a definition was based on the observation that this type of gastric cancer has a favorable prognosis; 5-year survival rates are greater than 95%.[5] The fact that lymph node or distant metastasis is uncommon explains the good prognosis for EGC. Lymph node invasion exists in 10% to 20% of cases; however, the metastatic lymph nodes of EGC are mostly restricted to a few regional nodes (N1).[6] Therefore, gastrectomy with lymph node dissection shows an excellent outcome in patients with EGC. Moreover, the presence of nodal metastases is closely related to the depth of local invasion. When EGC is confined to the mucosa, lymph node involvement is much less common ($\leq$3%).[7] With the increase in the detection rate of EGC throughout the country, the Japanese national records show that the percentage of EGC among resected cases was 40% in 1985.[8]

Many investigators attribute the high incidence of gastric carcinoma in East Asia to dietary[9,10] and genetic factors,[11,12] and to *Helicobacter pylori* infection.[13,14] The high detection rate of EGC in Japan and Korea is explained by the availability of population-based screening programs. In addition, there are differences between the Japanese and Western criteria for the diagnosis of EGC that are considered relevant.[15] In Western countries, gastric cancer is diagnosed when invasive growth of the neoplasm into the lamina propria of the mucosa or beyond is evident.[16] By contrast, Japanese pathologists often use the term EGC for intramucosal lesions that Western pathologists classify as precursor lesions termed dysplasia or adenoma.[17] In the authors' opinion, this discrepancy does not express a biological difference in the tumor itself, but represents a difference of conception and terminology. Western pathologists diagnose high-grade dysplasia as a lesion that does not yet have malignant potential, but probably could develop it over time. Japanese pathologists diagnose EGC as a lesion that has malignant potential but has not yet expressed it. In practice, a biopsy diagnosis of high-grade dysplasia in the West or carcinoma in Japan would lead to consideration of therapeutic resection in both scenarios. Recently, a new system of categories classifying gastrointestinal neoplasia (ie, the Vienna classification) has been proposed **(Table 1)** to bridge the East-West gap.[18] Intramucosal EGC in the Japanese classification corresponds to mucosal high-grade neoplasia (Category 4) in this revised Vienna classification. The classification is important in transferring interpretations of epidemiologic, clinical, and pathologic studies from one arena to the other. This article regards EGC, including intramucosal EGC, as "intermediate lesions" for developing gastric cancer.

Category	Diagnosis	Clinical Management
Table 1 The revised Vienna classification		
1	Negative for neoplasia	Optional follow-up
2	Indefinite for neoplasia	Follow-up
3	Mucosal low-grade neoplasia Low-grade adenoma Low-grade dysplasia	Endoscopic resection or follow-up[a]
4	Mucosal high-grade neoplasia 4.1 High-grade adenoma/dysplasia 4.2 Noninvasive carcinoma (carcinoma in situ) 4.3 Suspicious for invasive carcinoma 4.4 Intramucosal carcinoma	Endoscopic or surgical local resection[a]
5	Submucosal invasion by carcinoma	Surgical resection[a]

[a] Choice of treatment will depend on the overall size of the lesion; the depth of invasion as assessed endoscopically, radiologically, or ultrasonographically; and on general factors such as the patient's age and comorbid conditions. For gastric, esophageal, and nonpolypoid colorectal well-differentiated and moderately differentiated carcinomas showing only minimal submucosal invasion (sm1) without lymphatic involvement, local resection is sufficient. Likewise, for polypoid colorectal carcinomas with deeper submucosal invasion in the stalk/base but without lymphatic or blood vessel invasion, complete local resection is considered adequate treatment.

NATURAL HISTORY OF EARLY GASTRIC CANCER

Although EGC has a long natural history, some cases do progress to advanced cancer (**Fig. 1**). Rugge and colleagues[19] followed up 118 consecutive patients with noninvasive neoplasia for an average of 52 (range 12–206) months, and found that 20 (17%) evolved into invasive gastric cancer. Among patients who underwent surgery for invasive cancer, 13 were pathologically staged as EGC while 2 were staged as advanced gastric cancer. Tsukuma and colleagues[20] identified 56 patients with EGC (diagnosed as EGC with endoscopy and proved by biopsy) in whom neither endoscopic nor surgical resection was performed. Over a period of 6 to 137 months (mean 39 months), 20 remained in the early stage and 36 progressed to an advanced stage. The cumulative proportion of patients with advanced gastric cancer consistently increased with time, and the median time to develop advanced gastric cancer from EGC was 44 months.

SCREENING FOR THE DETECTION OF EARLY GASTRIC CANCER

At present, nationwide screening is undertaken in Japan and Korea, where gastric cancer is highly prevalent. Whether screening, especially that of the mass population, should be done remains controversial because the incidence of gastric cancer varies substantially among countries and within the same ethnic group. Even in a very high-risk area, there is only some evidence that mass screening reduces mortality from gastric cancer.[21] Therefore, identification of high-risk populations to undergo screening is fundamental for the early detection of gastric cancer in countries with medium to low incidence.

High-Risk Populations for Gastric Cancer

In general, the incidence of gastric cancer increases after 40 years of age and is higher in men than in women. Furthermore, the risk of gastric cancer is increased at least 1.5 times in siblings or offspring of patients with gastric cancer.[22,23] For the familial

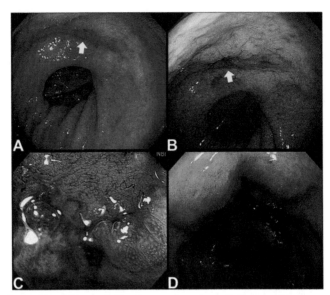

Fig. 1. A patient with a history of gastric resection. A small depressed lesion was noticed at the lesser curvature of the operated stomach (*yellow arrow, A* and *B*). Magnifying narrow-band imaging (NBI) revealed irregular microvessel and absent microstructure patterns in the well-demarcated area (*C*). One biopsy specimen was taken from the depressed lesion, but the result indicated "negative for neoplasia." The patient was asked for a follow-up examination after 3 months but did not come back. Three years later, the patient was found to have advanced gastric cancer at the same site (*D*).

aggregation of gastric cancer, the clustering of *H pylori* in family members may be an important contributory factor, in addition to genetic factors.[24,25] In multiethnic countries such as Malaysia and Singapore, gastric cancer is more common in Chinese people than in those of Malay and Indian origin.[26] In a study from Singapore, screening for gastric cancer was cost-effective in high-risk groups such as Chinese men aged 50 to 70 years.[27] Therefore, individuals with a high-risk ethnic background or those with a family history of gastric cancer may benefit most from screening and surveillance examination. Relatives with hereditary diffuse gastric cancer should be managed by specialists because genetic testing and prophylactic gastrectomy are sometimes advocated.

Despite the strong link between *H pylori* and gastric cancer, there are currently no data to suggest that a screen for gastric cancer should be limited to those infected with *H pylori*. Progression of intestinal metaplasia (IM) in the gastric mucosa can cause spontaneous eradication of *H pylori* or to an underestimation of *H pylori* infection[28,29]; therefore, patients with gastric cancer might no longer have detectable *H pylori* and, thus, the screening of only actively infected individuals is generally not effective.

Patients who have established precursor conditions such as mucosal atrophy or IM caused by chronic *H pylori* infection are at high risk for developing gastric cancer, especially the intestinal type.[30] A Dutch nationwide cohort study indicated that the annual incidence of gastric cancer was 0.1% for patients with atrophic gastritis, 0.25% for IM, 0.6% for mild to moderate dysplasia, and 6% for severe dysplasia within 5 years after diagnosis.[31] The potential benefits of endoscopic surveillance of gastric IM patients was suggested by a cancer incidence of 11% and improved survival in a retrospective study from the United Kingdom.[32] At present, the diagnosis of atrophy and IM is based on the histology of the biopsy specimens. As a result of uneven distribution and topography of atrophy and IM in the stomach, multiple biopsies are recommended from certain anatomic locations of the gastric mucosa, as indicated by the updated Sydney System[33] and the Operative Link on Gastritis Assessment (OLGA).[34]

Although atrophy or IM are histologic entities, their presence can be predicted by endoscopic findings. Kimura and Takemoto[35] suggested that the endoscopic findings of atrophic mucosa were the presence of a pale whitish mucosa and increased mucosal vessel visibility, indicating that it is related histologically to atrophy of the fundic gland (**Fig. 2**D). When the atrophic border remains on the lesser curvature of the corpus, the diagnosis is closed-type atrophic gastritis (antral predominant gastritis), whereas when the atrophic border no longer exists on the lesser curvature and extends along the anterior and posterior walls of the stomach, the diagnosis is open-type atrophic gastritis (pangastritis or corpus-predominant gastritis). These endoscopic diagnostic criteria are commonly accepted and are used in practice for the diagnosis of chronic atrophic gastritis in Japan and Korea. An association between the endoscopically diagnosed extent of atrophic gastritis and the risk for development of gastric cancer has been demonstrated in a large cohort study.[36,37] Recently, newer endoscopic imaging technologies such as autofluorescence imaging (AFI; see **Fig. 2**B, E),[38] magnifying narrow-band imaging (NBI; see **Fig. 2**C, F),[39] and confocal laser endomicroscopy[40] have been introduced, and these methods have been reported as useful for the diagnosis of atrophy or IM. In contrast to single-point evaluations of gastritis by biopsy, a possible advantage of these endoscopic imaging modalities is to enable evaluation of the prevalence, actual extent, and distribution of atrophy or IM in the gastric mucosa without taking multiple biopsies.[41,42]

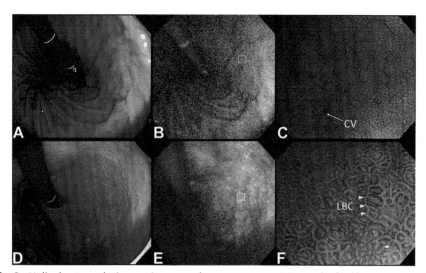

Fig. 2. *Helicobacter pylori*–negative normal corpus mucosa: Mucosa looked homogeneously reddish, and the gastric folds were observed circumferentially in the gastric corpus (*A*). On autofluorescence imaging (AFI), the color of the whole corpus mucosa appeared purple to dark green (*B*). Magnifying NBI image at the lesser curvature of the lower corpus (*white box* in *B*) showed regularly arranged collecting venule (CV) (*C*). (*D*) Atrophic gastritis mucosa. Whitish mucosa was seen in the lesser curvature of the corpus and gastric folds were absent in that area, which appeared bright green in the AFI image (*E*). Magnifying NBI image of the green mucosa in the corpus lesser curvature (*white box* in *E*) showed a ridged/villiform surface structure with light blue crest (LBC, *yellow arrowhead*) (*F*).

Screening Test Methods

Radiography using barium meal has been used in Japan for population-based screening for gastric cancer since 1960.[43] When suspicious lesions are identified on barium examination, endoscopy is used to analyze the detected lesions. Barium radiography is the only recommended population-based screening method in the Japanese guidelines for gastric cancer screening,[21] because several case-control studies have shown a 40% to 60% decrease in mortality from gastric cancer in those who have been screened with photofluorography.[21,44] However, data from prospective cohort studies that defined death from gastric cancer as an end point do not give consistent results.[45–47] The sensitivity of barium radiography for gastric cancer is reported to be 70% to 86%, but the sensitivity for advanced cancer is 92%, whereas for EGC it is only 32%.[48] Because of the low sensitivity in detecting early lesions, barium radiography is becoming less common in clinical practice.

Serum pepsinogen (PG) is a popular serologic screening test for gastric cancer, particularly in Japan. Serum PG consists of 2 types, PG I and PG II. PG I concentrations decrease with loss of fundic-gland mucosa, whereas PG II remains constant. Therefore, a low PG I level or a low PG I/II ratio, or both, are good serum indicators of the presence of atrophic gastritis.[49] In Japanese patients, a PG I/II ratio greater than 3.0 has a sensitivity of 93% and a specificity of 88% for the diagnosis of normal fundic glands.[50] Serum testing for H pylori alone could miss high-risk gastric cancer populations, because the bacteria can no longer colonize the gastric mucosa with extensive atrophy or IM. Thus, the PG test is used in combination with serum H pylori antibody to assess the risk of gastric cancer. In a large Japanese cohort study, more than 9000 people were stratified according to H pylori antibody status (positive vs negative) and serum pepsinogen test (normal vs atrophic), and followed up endoscopically for a mean duration of 4.7 years (**Table 2**).[51] In patients with nonatrophic fundic mucosa (as defined by serum PG testing), risk of gastric cancer did not increase

Table 2
Combining serum H pylori antibody and pepsinogen test, and risk of gastric cancer

Group	H pylori Antibody	Serum Pepsinogen	Interpretation	Estimated Gastric Cancer Risk	
				Annual Incidence of Gastric Cancer (%/y)	Adjusted Hazard Ratio[a]
A	Negative	Normal	H pylori–naive individual	0.04	1
B	Positive	Normal	Active H pylori infection but no corpus atrophy	0.06	1.1
C	Positive	Atrophic	Active H pylori infection with corpus atrophy	0.35	6.0
D	Negative	Atrophic	Undetectable or previous H pylori infection with extensive corpus atrophy	0.60	8.2

[a] Adjusted for age and sex.
    Data from Watabe H, Mitsushima T, Yamaji Y, et al. Predicting the development of gastric cancer from combining *Helicobacter pylori* antibodies and serum pepsinogen status: a prospective endoscopic cohort study. Gut 2005;54:764–8.

substantially, regardless of the presence of H pylori antibody. By contrast, in individuals with a low PG level that indicated atrophic gastritis, a significantly higher risk (6–8 times) of developing gastric cancer was found, compared with those with normal PG levels. Of note, among individuals with atrophic gastritis (as indicated with PG testing), those with negative H pylori serology had a higher risk than those with positive serology, presumably attributable to loss of H pylori in advanced gastric atrophy. Limitations of the serum PG test include suitability to detect mostly the intestinal type of gastric cancer, variation of cutoff values according to study or measurement kits, and normalization of test results after eradication of H pylori.[52] Despite these limitations, in Japan the PG test is currently the most realistic and reliable marker for identifying high-risk populations that warrant endoscopy or more intensive surveillance.

Endoscopy plays a pivotal role in screening for gastric cancer, because of its high lesion detection rate and the ability to remove biopsy specimens for histologic diagnosis. Endoscopy is particularly useful in identifying superficial lesions that may not be recognized by barium examination. A Japanese study comparing the diagnostic ability of endoscopy with barium meal examination in a mass screening population showed that the detection rate for gastric cancer was about 2.7 to 4.6 times higher with endoscopy than with barium studies or photofluorography.[53] Despite these favorable data, the capacity of endoscopy is restricted in Japan because of the availability of gastroscopes and the number of experienced endoscopists. Moreover, endoscopy carries some risks, including perforation, cardiopulmonary events, aspiration pneumonia, and bleeding, that are not negligible in the general population. Therefore, mass screening with endoscopy alone is probably not feasible. Consequently, selection of high-risk candidates for endoscopic examination is important in efficient screening for gastric cancer.

Recently, various advanced endoscopic techniques such as chromoendoscopy, magnifying endoscopy, AFI, NBI, and confocal laser endomicroscopy have been introduced. However, currently available data about the utility of these new imaging techniques for the diagnosis of EGC is mainly concerned with characterization of superficial lesions detected by conventional endoscopy. Accordingly, white-light endoscopy is still the primary method used to detect EGC in routine screening practice.

ENDOSCOPIC SCREENING PROCEDURE

The performance of endoscopy for detecting EGC depends heavily on the skill and knowledge of the endoscopist, so standardization and adequate training in endoscopic screening procedures are important.

Screening Procedure

To minimize the time and effort involved, methods have been developed to remove mucus and bubbles from the mucosal surface during the procedure to improve the detection of EGC. In Japan, a mixture of water with mucolytic and antifoaming agents (100 mL of water with 20,000 U pronase [Kaken Pharmaceutical, Tokyo, Japan], 1 g sodium bicarbonate, and 10 mL dimethylpolysiloxane [20 mg/mL; Horii Pharmaceutical, Osaka, Japan]) is administered before the procedure. An alternative mixture comprises 100 mL of water mixed with 2 mL of acetylcysteine (200 mg/mL Parvolex [Celltech, UK] or Mucomyst [Bristol-Myers Squibb, USA]), and 0.5 mL (40 mg/mL) activated dimethicone (Infacol; Forest Laboratories, Slough, Berkshire, UK) when pronase is not available. An anticholinergic agent, such as 10 to 20 mg scopolamine butylbromide (Buscopan, Nippon Boehringer Ingelheim Co, Ltd, Tokyo, Japan) or 1 mg glucagon (Glucagon G Novo; Eisai Co, Ltd, Tokyo, Japan), is given just before inserting the endoscope to inhibit peristalsis.

To avoid blind areas during gastroscopic observation, a standardized procedure to map the entire stomach is recommended. A basic technique for avoiding blind areas involves adequate air insufflation to extend the gastric wall to separate the folds, rinsing mucus and froth from the gastric mucosa through irrigation with defoaming agent solution, and mapping the entire stomach. The European Society of Gastrointestinal Endoscopy proposed a protocol for upper gastrointestinal endoscopy that includes taking 4 pictures in the stomach.[54] However, 4 images are not enough to cover and record the whole stomach. The Japanese Society of Gastroenterological Cancer Screening has also published a standard protocol,[55] however, with this protocol it is difficult to remember where to take pictures and how many pictures to take. Recently, Yao[56] has proposed a minimum required standard, the "systematic screening protocol for the stomach (SSS)," as shown in **Fig. 3**. With this method, images are arranged according to the order of the procedure, and pictures of 4 or 3 quadrant views are taken in either a clockwise or counterclockwise manner. Because the SSS is proposed as a minimum requirement, these images can be regarded as only checkpoints for the entire observation procedure.

Knowledge About Endoscopic Findings of Gastric Cancer

Even if endoscopic procedures are performed appropriately, EGC can still be missed if an endoscopist does not recognize the lesion. Superficial mucosal lesions mimicking gastritis (gastritis-like lesions) are difficult to detect even with optimum preparation and the best technique.[57] Accordingly, it is important to understand the characteristic findings of superficial mucosal neoplasias. The 2 distinct features for detecting superficial lesions are changes in surface (elevated or depressed) and color (reddish or whitish). These findings are usually subtle in superficial EGC, and may only be recognized as unevenness or as a faint discoloration of the mucosa. Spontaneous bleeding can be a clue to any abnormality. Image-enhanced endoscopy is useful for recognition and comprehension of lesion characteristics (**Fig. 4**). In the magnifying image, EGC is diagnosed with an irregular microvascular or irregular microsurface pattern with a demarcation line (the VS classification system).[58]

ENDOSCOPIC TREATMENT OF EARLY GASTRIC CANCER

Advances in the efficacy of EGC screening have increased the detection of intramucosal EGC. Although standard lymph node dissection is performed, lymph node metastases are rare in patients with intramucosal EGC. If lymphatic spread has been ruled out as far as possible, local therapy with endoscopic resection would be a reasonable approach in selected cases. The advantage of endoscopic resection over ablation techniques such as argon plasma coagulation, photodynamic therapy, or radiofrequency ablation is that the success of the endoscopic treatment can be assessed by histologic examination of the retrieved specimen.

Indications for Endoscopic Resection for Early Gastric Cancer

Patients with a small, differentiated intramucosal carcinoma without ulceration or scarring have a low risk of lymph node metastasis (**Table 3**). These tumors can be removed relatively easily in comparison with large lesions or lesions with a scar. Accordingly, the Japanese gastric cancer treatment guidelines[59] state that a differentiated adenocarcinoma without ulcerative findings, of which the depth of invasion is clinically diagnosed as intramucosal and the diameter is 2 cm or less, is a "guideline indication" for endoscopic resection (**Table 4**). In addition, data from 2 large Japanese cancer centers indicate that lymph node metastasis is absent in the following

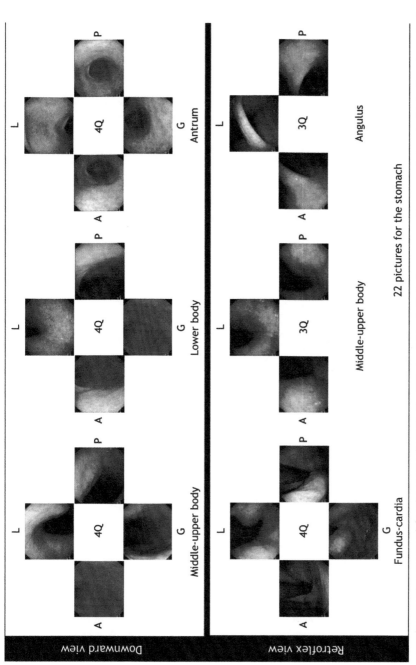

Fig. 3. Systematic screening protocol for the stomach (SSS). The SSS should be initiated as soon as the scope is inserted into the stomach. From the antegrade view, endoscopic photos of 4 quadrants of the middle-upper body, the lower body, and the antrum are taken. Then from the retroflex view, 3 quadrants of the gastric incisura and the middle-upper body, and photos of 4 quadrants of the gastric fundus and cardia are taken. Overall, the SSS series comprises 22 endoscopic photos. A, anterior wall; G, greater curvature; L, lesser curvature; P, posterior wall; Q, quadrant.

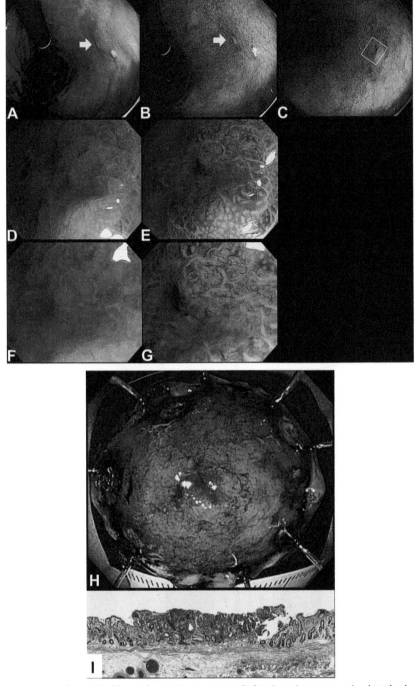

Fig. 4. A case of gastritis-like early gastric cancer. A slight elevation was noticed at the lesser curvature of the gastric body (*yellow arrow, A* and *B*). In the close view, a small depression was revealed (*C*). In the magnifying observation (*white box* in *C*), a demarcation line was observed between the depression and the surrounding mucosa (*D* and *E*). Irregular microvascular pattern and irregular microsurface pattern were evident in the maximum magnifying view (*F* and *G*). The lesion was removed with endoscopic submucosal dissection techniques (*H*). Histopathologic findings demonstrated the lesion to be an intramucosal early gastric cancer, that is, a mucosal high-grade neoplasia (*I*).

Table 3
Lymph node metastasis rate of early gastric cancer

Depth	Ulcer or Scar	Histologic Type			
		Differentiated		Undifferentiated	
Mucosa	(−)	≤2 cm[a] 0% (0%–0.8%) 0/437	>2 cm[a] 0% (0%–0.6%) 0/493	≤2 cm 0%[b] (0%–0.96%) 0/310	>2 cm 5.0%[b] (2.9%–7.0%) 21/423
	(+)	≤3 cm[a] 0% (0%–0.6%) 0/488	>3 cm[a] 3.0% (1.5%–6.1%) 7/230	5.9%[b] (4.6%–7.1%) 84/1430	
Submucosa		≤3 cm[a] 0% (0%–2.0%) 0/145	>3 cm[a] 2.6% (0.3%–9.0%) 2/78	10.6%[a] (5.0%–19.2%) 9/85	

[a] *Data from* Japanese Gastric Cancer Association. Japanese gastric cancer treatment guidelines 2010 (ver. 3). Gastric Cancer 2011;14:113–23; and Gotoda T, Yanagisawa A, Sasako M, et al. Incidence of lymph node metastasis from early gastric cancer: estimation with a large number of cases at two large centers. Gastric Cancer 2000;3:219–25.
[b] *Data from* Hirasawa T, Gotoda T, Miyata S, et al. Incidence of lymph node metastasis and the feasibility of endoscopic resection for undifferentiated-type early gastric cancer. Gastric Cancer 2009;12:148–52.

lesions[60,61]: (1) differentiated intramucosal carcinoma, 2 cm in size, without ulceration or scarring; (2) differentiated intramucosal carcinoma, 3 cm or less in size, with ulceration or scarring; and (3) undifferentiated intramucosal carcinoma, 2 cm or less in size, without ulceration or scarring (see **Table 3**). Hence, these lesions are regarded as "expanded indications" for endoscopic resection (see **Table 4**).

Pretreatment Diagnosis for Endoscopic Resection

In contrast to gastric surgical resection, the extent and depth of the tumor should be carefully assessed before an endoscopic resection, because only intramucosal lesions are indicated for endoscopic resection, and the risk of lymph node metastasis is closely associated with the size and depth of EGC. The types of tumor are classified according to the Japanese Classification of Gastric Carcinoma[62,63] as: type 0 I (protruded); type 0 IIa (slightly elevated); type 0 IIb (flat); type 0 IIc (slightly depressed); or type 0 III (excavated). The tumor extent is diagnosed using chromoendoscopy with 0.05% indigo carmine according to differences in color, height, and areae gastricae patterns between cancer and noncancer mucosa. Nagahama and colleagues[64] have indicated that around 80% of EGC was clearly delineated with chromoendoscopy, but the

Table 4
Indication for EMR/ESD according to endoscopic finding

	Depth of Invasion	Histology	Ulcer or Scar	Size
Guideline indication	Intramucosal	Differentiated type	(−)	≤2 cm
Expanded indication	=	=	=	>2 cm
	=	=	(+)	≤3 cm
	=	Undifferentiated type	=	=

=, same as guideline indication.

remainder of the tumors showed unclear margins. NBI using magnifying endoscopy successfully determined the tumor boundary in more than 70% of cases that showed unclear margins with chromoendoscopy. Magnifying NBI adds useful information for the diagnosis of tumor extent, but only a small area of mucosa is observable; therefore, chromoendoscopy is still essential for the diagnosis of tumor extent because it enables one to evaluate the tumor's gross appearance.[65]

The depth of the tumor is assessed mainly by morphologic features of conventional endoscopy and chromoendoscopy. In the case of inconclusive findings, endoscopic ultrasonography (EUS) with a standard echoendoscope (GIF-UMQ200; Olympus Medical Systems, Tokyo, Japan) or a miniprobe (UM-2R, UM-3R; Olympus Medical Systems) is used. A frequency of 20 MHz is recommended for assessment of the tumor depth, and 7.5 MHz is used to observe extramural lymph nodes. The diagnostic accuracy of conventional endoscopic findings for tumor depth by experienced endoscopists is comparable with that achieved with EUS.[66] EUS has a tendency to overestimate tumor depth, leading to unnecessary surgery in some cases.[67] Therefore, when all attempts are made at pretreatment diagnosis and there is a possibility of intramucosal carcinoma, with no definitive findings of massive submucosal invasion, endoscopic resection is usually carried out after explaining to the patient the possibility of additional surgery. Histologic analysis of the resected specimens provides the most accurate assessment of the tumor depth and lymphatic or venous involvement, which defines the requirement for subsequent surgery.

Method of Endoscopic Resection for Early Gastric Cancer

Endoscopic mucosal resection (EMR) was first developed in 1984 to obtain large specimens of gastric mucosa for the diagnosis of chronic gastritis.[68] Eventually EMR was used for endoscopic removal of intramucosal carcinoma. The strip biopsy EMR method, using a double-channel videoendoscopy, involves: (1) injection of normal saline into the submucosa to create a submucosal cushion, preventing perforation; (2) drawing the lesion into the snaring wire with a grasping forceps; and (3) electrocautery cutting. However, one of the main drawbacks of EMR is that the size of the removable specimen is restricted by the size of the snare. Moreover, it is sometimes difficult to remove the intended area precisely with EMR. Thus, when the lesions cannot be resected en bloc they are removed piecemeal, which makes it difficult to assess the completeness and curability of the resection by histopathology and increases the incidence of residual tumor.

In late 1990, Ohkuwa and colleagues[69] developed a new endoscopic electrosurgical knife that has a small insulated ceramic ball on its tip to prevent perforation (insulated-tip knife, IT knife, KD-610L; Olympus Medical Systems). Later, the endoscopic submucosal dissection (ESD) technique was developed using the IT knife.[70] The ESD technique consists of marking the margins of the area to be removed under image-enhanced endoscopy observation (**Fig. 5**A–D); mucosal incision outside the marking dots with an IT knife after injection of a solution (see **Fig. 5**E, F); and submucosal dissection with the IT knife (see **Fig. 5**G).[71] With the ESD method, the indicated mucosal lesion can be removed en bloc even if it is large or scarred. The rate of en bloc resection that was defined as 1-piece resection without tumor invasion to the resected margin was 50% to 70% for EMR, whereas it was almost 90% to 95% for ESD. The difference in the en bloc resection rate between EMR and ESD was more evident for expanded-indication lesions (EMR 20%–40% vs ESD 75%–85%) than for guideline-indication lesions (EMR 64% vs ESD 95%).[72] Refinements of equipment or accessories, such as development of various knives,[73,74] or use of a transparent hood or water-jet endoscope,[75] have continued to improve ESD in practice.

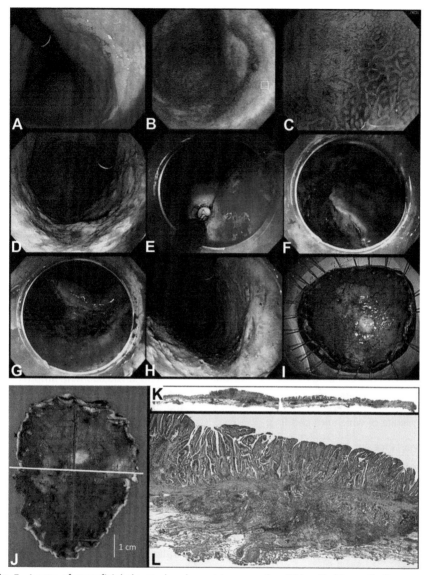

Fig. 5. A case of superficial elevated early gastric cancer (see Video 1). Biopsy findings were suspicious for neoplasia, but were regarded as an indication for endoscopic resection because the size exceeded 6 cm (*A*). AFI (*B*) and magnifying NBI of white box in (*C*) clearly showed the tumor boundary. Marking was performed under chromoscopic observation (*D*). Mucosal incision was performed with an insulated-tipped knife (*E* and *F*). Subsequently, the lesion was dissected (*G, H, I*). Histopathologic findings (section of yellow line in J) revealed submucosal invasion of carcinoma (*J, K, L*), so the patient underwent gastric resection with lymph node dissection.

Assessment of Curability by Histology

Retrieved specimens are pinned onto hard gum plates and immersed in 20% formalin. The fixed specimens are serially sectioned at 2-mm intervals for histologic examination (see **Fig. 5**J). According to the Japanese Classification of Gastric Carcinoma,[62] histologic type, depth of invasion, presence of ulcerative change, lymphatic and venous involvement, and tumor involvement to the horizontal (mucosal) and vertical (submucosal) margins are evaluated to estimate the curability of the resection. The lesion is considered to be curative when the completely resected specimen satisfies the following criteria.[59] No tumor invasion to horizontal and vertical margins, and no lymphatic or venous involvement, and: (1) differentiated intramucosal tumor without ulceration or scarring; (2) differentiated intramucosal adenocarcinoma with ulceration or scarring, tumor 3 cm or smaller; (3) differentiated adenocarcinoma with minimal submucosal invasion (SM1: $\leq$500 μm from the muscularis mucosae), 3 cm or smaller; and (4) undifferentiated intramucosal adenocarcinoma without ulceration or scarring, 2 cm or smaller (**Table 5**). When a differentiated carcinoma shows a positive horizontal (mucosal) margin but satisfies all the other curable criteria, repeated ESD could be proposed for residual tumor or when local recurrence is found during close observation, because it carries a very low risk of harboring lymph node metastasis.[76] In the case of possible lymph node metastasis, demonstrated by submucosal invasion or lymphatic or venous involvement, patients are subjected to gastric resection with lymph node dissection (see **Fig. 5**K, L).[77]

Long-Term Outcome

Excellent long-term outcomes after gastric EMR and ESD (5-year survival rate >90%) have been reported from several institutions.[78–80] However, all these single-center retrospective studies refer to a median follow-up of less than 5 years after endoscopic resection. EGC has a long natural history and incidence of disease-related death is low, therefore long-term survival should be investigated with a high follow-up rate. Moreover, intent-to-treat analysis in a prospective cohort study is desirable. The Japan Clinical Oncology Group is currently conducting a multicenter, prospective cohort study investigating 5-year survival rates of all ESD patients who had EGC that fulfilled the expanded indication criteria in the Japanese treatment guidelines, the results of which are pending.

Surveillance for Metachronous Multiple Cancers

In contrast to gastric surgical resection, endoscopic resection spares the stomach, which contains premalignant mucosal lesions such as atrophic gastritis, IM, and dysplasia. Therefore, metachronous cancers develop after endoscopic resection for EGC in 5.9% of cases within 3 years, and annual endoscopic surveillance is recommended.[81] Recently, the prophylactic effect of H pylori eradication on the incidence of metachronous gastric cancer after endoscopic resection of EGC has been demonstrated in a randomized controlled trial (odds ratio 0.35 in favor of eradication

Table 5
Criteria for curative resection in histologic findings

Predominant Histologic Type	Tumor Invasion to Resected Margin	Lymphatic or Venous Involvement	Depth of Invasion	Ulcerative Finding	Size
Differentiated	(−)	(−)	Intramucosal	(−)	Any
			Intramucosal	(+)	≤3 cm
			Minimal submucosal invasion	(−)	≤3 cm
Undifferentiated			Intramucosal	(−)	≤2 cm

therapy).[82] However, atrophic gastritis and IM usually continue after successful eradication of *H pylori* in patients undergoing EMR or ESD for EGC.[83] Therefore, surveillance endoscopy to detect metachronous multiple cancers is essential for the management of patients undergoing EMR and ESD, even if they have received *H pylori* eradication therapy, because such continuous atrophy and IM can be the background for further metachronous EGC in these patients.[84]

SUMMARY: PICK UP A LESION; OBSERVE IT, CUT IT OUT, OR PEEL IT OFF?

Proper endoscopic screening of high-risk populations can increase the detection of EGC. At present, accurate prediction of which EGCs will eventually become invasive within a certain period, if left untreated, is not possible. In the future, histologic or molecular markers may be established to predict the biological aggressiveness of EGC. Meanwhile, all EGC should be regarded as potentially progressive. If the risk of lymph node metastasis can be ruled out as far as possible, complete removal of EGC with EMR/ESD is a reasonable approach in selected cases. Careful histologic examination of the resected specimen and further endoscopic follow-up is mandatory after the endoscopic resection. The effectiveness of endoscopic detection and resection of EGC regarding improvement in gastric cancer mortality warrants definitive proof in a further study.

SUPPLEMENTARY DATA

Supplementary data related to this article can be found online at http://dx.doi.org/ 10.1016/j.gtc.2013.01.007.

REFERENCES

1. Ferlay J, Shin HR, Bray F, et al. Estimates of worldwide burden of cancer in 2008: GLOBOCAN 2008. Int J Cancer 2010;127:2893–917.
2. Hisamichi S. Screening for gastric cancer. World J Surg 1989;13:31–7.
3. Kim YS, Park HA, Kim BS, et al. Efficacy of screening for gastric cancer in a Korean adult population: a case-control study. J Korean Med Sci 2000;15: 510–5.
4. Murakami T. Pathomorphological diagnosis. Definition and gross classification of early gastric cancer. Gann Monogr Cancer Res 1971;11:53–5.
5. Yamazaki H, Oshima A, Murakami R, et al. A long-term follow-up study of patients with gastric cancer detected by mass screening. Cancer 1989;63:613–7.
6. Everett AM, Axon AT. Early gastric cancer in Europe. Gut 1997;41:142–50.
7. Sano T, Kobori O, Muto T. Lymph node metastasis from early gastric cancer: endoscopic resection of tumour. Br J Surg 1992;79:241–4.
8. Hirota T, Ming SC. Early gastric carcinoma. In: Ming SC, Goldman H, editors. Pathology of the gastrointestinal tract. Philadelphia: Saunders; 1992. p. 570–83.
9. Kobayashi M, Tsubono Y, Sasazuki S, JPHC Study Group. Vegetables, fruit and risk of gastric cancer in Japan: a 10-year follow-up of the JPHC Study Cohort I. Int J Cancer 2002;102:39–44.
10. Joossens JV, Hill MJ, Elliott P, et al. Dietary salt, nitrate and stomach cancer mortality in 24 countries. European Cancer Prevention (ECP) and the INTERSALT Cooperative Research Group. Int J Epidemiol 1996;25:494–504.
11. El-Omar EM, Rabkin CS, Gammon MD, et al. Increased risk of noncardia gastric cancer associated with proinflammatory cytokine gene polymorphisms. Gastroenterology 2003;124:1193–201.

12. Goto Y, Ando T, Yamamoto K, et al. Association between serum pepsinogens and polymorphism of PTPN11 encoding SHP-2 among *Helicobacter pylori* seropositive Japanese. Int J Cancer 2006;118:203–8.

13. The EUROGAST Study Group. An international association between *Helicobacter pylori* infection and gastric cancer. Lancet 1993;341:1359–62.

14. Schlemper RJ, van der Werf SDJ, Vandenbroucke JP, et al. Seroepidemiology of gastritis in Japanese and Dutch working populations: evidence for the development of atrophic gastritis that is not related to *Helicobacter pylori*. Gut 1995;37:199–204.

15. Schlemper RJ, Itabashi M, Kato Y, et al. Differences in diagnostic criteria for gastric carcinoma between Japanese and western pathologists. Lancet 1997; 349:1725–9.

16. Lansdown M, Quirke P, Dixon MF, et al. High grade dysplasia of the gastric mucosa: a marker for gastric carcinoma. Gut 1990;31:977–83.

17. Lewin KJ, Riddell RH, Weinstein WM. Gastrointestinal pathology and its clinical implications. New York: Igaku-Shoin; 1992.

18. Dixon MF. Gastrointestinal epithelial neoplasia: Vienna revisited. Gut 2002;51: 130–1.

19. Rugge M, Cassaro M, Di Mario F, et al, Interdisciplinary Group on Gastric Epithelial Dysplasia (IGGED). The long term outcome of gastric non-invasive neoplasia. Gut 2003;52:1111–6.

20. Tsukuma H, Oshima A, Narahara H, et al. Natural history of early gastric cancer: a non-concurrent, long term, follow up study. Gut 2000;47:618–21.

21. Hamashima C, Shibuya D, Yamazaki H, et al. The Japanese guidelines for gastric cancer screening. Jpn J Clin Oncol 2008;38:259–67.

22. Zanghieri G, Di Gregorio C, Sacchetti C, et al. Familial occurrence of gastric cancer in the 2-year experience of a population-based registry. Cancer 1990; 66:2047–51.

23. La Vecchia C, Negri E, Franceschi S, et al. Family history and the risk of stomach and colorectal cancer. Cancer 1992;70:50–5.

24. Brenner H, Bode G, Boeing H. *Helicobacter pylori* infection among off spring of patients with stomach cancer. Gastroenterology 2000;118:31–5.

25. Chang YW, Han YS, Lee DK, et al. Role of *Helicobacter pylori* infection among off spring or siblings of gastric cancer patients. Int J Cancer 2002;101:469–74.

26. Goh KL, Cheah PL, Md N, et al. Ethnicity and *H. pylori* as risk factors for gastric cancer in Malaysia: a prospective case control study. Am J Gastroenterol 2007; 102:40–5.

27. Dan YY, So JB, Yeoh KG. Endoscopic screening for gastric cancer. Clin Gastroenterol Hepatol 2006;4:709–16.

28. Testoni PA, Bonassi U, Bagnolo F, et al. In diffuse atrophic gastritis, routine histology underestimates *Helicobacter pylori* infection. J Clin Gastroenterol 2002;35:234–9.

29. Kang HY, Kim N, Park YS, et al. Progression of atrophic gastritis and intestinal metaplasia drives *Helicobacter pylori* out of the gastric mucosa. Dig Dis Sci 2006;51:2310–5.

30. Correa P. Chronic gastritis as a cancer precursor. Scand J Gastroenterol 1984; 104:131–6.

31. De Vries A, van Grieken N, Looman C, et al. Gastric cancer risk in patients with premalignant gastric lesions: a nationwide cohort study in the Netherlands. Gastroenterology 2008;134:945–52.

32. Whiting JL, Sigurdsson A, Rowlands DC, et al. The long term results of endoscopic surveillance of premalignant gastric lesions. Gut 2002;50:378–81.

33. Dixon MF, Genta RM, Yardley JH, et al. Classification and grading of gastritis. The updated Sydney System. International workshop on the histopathology of gastritis, Houston 1994. Am J Surg Pathol 1996;20:1161–81.

34. Rugge M, Meggio A, Pennelli G, et al. Gastritis staging in clinical practice: the OLGA staging system. Gut 2007;56:631–6.

35. Kimura K, Takemoto T. An endoscopic recognition of the atrophy border and its significance in chronic gastritis. Endoscopy 1969;3:87–97.

36. Tatsuta M, Iishi H, Nakaizumi A, et al. Fundal atrophic gastritis as a risk factor for gastric cancer. Int J Cancer 1993;53:70–4.

37. Uemura N, Okamoto S, Yamamoto S, et al. *Helicobacter pylori* infection and the development of gastric cancer. N Engl J Med 2001;345:784–9.

38. Inoue T, Uedo N, Ishihara R, et al. Autofluorescence imaging videoendoscopy in the diagnosis of chronic atrophic fundal gastritis. J Gastroenterol 2010;45:45–51.

39. Uedo N, Ishihara R, Iishi H, et al. A new method of diagnosing gastric intestinal metaplasia: narrow-band imaging with magnifying endoscopy. Endoscopy 2006; 38:819–24.

40. Wang P, Ji R, Yu T, et al. Classification of histological severity of *Helicobacter pylori*-associated gastritis by confocal laser endomicroscopy. World J Gastroenterol 2010;16:5203–10.

41. Uedo N. Do we need multiple biopsies for assessing gastric cancer risk? [editorial]. Dig Dis Sci 2011;56:926–8.

42. Kanzaki H, Uedo N, Ishihara R, et al. Comprehensive investigation of areae gastricae pattern in gastric corpus using magnifying narrow band imaging endoscopy in patients with chronic atrophic fundic gastritis. Helicobacter 2012;17: 224–31.

43. Tsubono Y, Hisamichi S. Screening for gastric cancer in Japan. Gastric Cancer 2000;3:9–18.

44. Leung WK, Wu MS, Kakugawa Y, et al. Screening for gastric cancer in Asia: current evidence and practice. Lancet Oncol 2008;9:279–87.

45. Ohata H, Oka M, Yanaoka K, et al. Gastric cancer screening of a high-risk population in Japan using serum pepsinogen and barium digital radiography. Cancer Sci 2005;96:713–20.

46. Mizoue T, Yoshimura T, Tokui N, et al. Prospective study of screening for stomach cancer in Japan. Int J Cancer 2003;106:103–7.

47. Lee KJ, Inoue M, Otani T, et al. Gastric cancer screening and subsequent risk of gastric cancer: a large-scale population-based cohort study, with a 13-year follow up in Japan. Int J Cancer 2006;118:2315–21.

48. Ichinose M, Mukaibayashi C, Enomoto S, et al. Current status of gastric cancer screening. Jpn J Clin Exp Med 2010;87:41–5.

49. Miki K, Morita M, Sasajima M, et al. Usefulness of gastric cancer screening using the serum pepsinogen test method. Am J Gastroenterol 2003;98:735–9.

50. Miki K. Gastric cancer screening using the serum pepsinogen test method. Gastric Cancer 2006;9:245–53.

51. Watabe H, Mitsushima T, Yamaji Y, et al. Predicting the development of gastric cancer from combining *Helicobacter pylori* antibodies and serum pepsinogen status: a prospective endoscopic cohort study. Gut 2005;54:764–8.

52. Kawai T, Kawakami K, Kataoka M, et al. Correlation of serum pepsinogen with histological atrophy following successful *Helicobacter pylori* eradication. Aliment Pharmacol Ther 2006;24(Suppl 4):23–30.

53. Tashiro A, Sano M, Kinameri K, et al. Comparing mass screening techniques for gastric cancer in Japan. World J Gastroenterol 2006;12:4874–5.

54. Rey JF, Lambert R, ESGE Quality Assurance Committee. ESGE recommendations for quality control in gastrointestinal endoscopy: guidelines for image documentation in upper and lower GI endoscopy. Endoscopy 2001;33:901–3.

55. The committee for standardizing screening gastroscopy. Gastric cancer screening techniques. In: JSGCS, editor. I to Cho Handbook. Tokyo: Igakushoin; 2010. p. 1–24 [in Japanese].

56. Yao K. The endoscopic diagnosis of early gastric cancer. Ann Gastroenterol 2013;26:11–22.

57. Gotoda T, Shimoda T, Fujishiro M, et al. Macroscopic feature of gastritis-like cancer with little malignant appearance in early gastric cancer [Japanese with English abstract]. Stomach and Intestine 1999;34:1495–503.

58. Yao K, Takaki Y, Matsui T, et al. Clinical application of magnification endoscopy and narrow-band imaging in the upper gastrointestinal tract: new imaging techniques for detecting and characterizing gastrointestinal neoplasia. Gastrointest Endosc Clin N Am 2008;18:415–33.

59. Japanese Gastric Cancer Association. Japanese gastric cancer treatment guidelines 2010 (ver. 3). Gastric Cancer 2011;14:113–23.

60. Gotoda T, Yanagisawa A, Sasako M, et al. Incidence of lymph node metastasis from early gastric cancer: estimation with a large number of cases at two large centers. Gastric Cancer 2000;3:219–25.

61. Hirasawa T, Gotoda T, Miyata S, et al. Incidence of lymph node metastasis and the feasibility of endoscopic resection for undifferentiated-type early gastric cancer. Gastric Cancer 2009;12:148–52.

62. Japanese Gastric Cancer Association. Japanese classification of gastric carcinoma: 3rd English edition. Gastric Cancer 2011;14:101–12.

63. Participants in the Paris Workshop The Paris endoscopic classification of superficial neoplastic lesions: esophagus, stomach, and colon: November 30 to December 1, 2002. Gastrointest Endosc 2003;58(Suppl 6):S3–43.

64. Nagahama T, Yao K, Maki S, et al. Usefulness of magnifying endoscopy with narrow-band imaging for determining the horizontal extent of early gastric cancer when there is an unclear margin by chromoendoscopy (with video). Gastrointest Endosc 2011;74:1259–67.

65. Uedo N, Fujishiro M, Goda K, et al. Role of narrow band imaging for diagnosis of early-stage esophagogastric cancer: current consensus of experienced endoscopists in Asia–Pacific region. Dig Endosc 2011;23(Suppl 1):58–71.

66. Choi J, Kim SG, Im JP, et al. Comparison of endoscopic ultrasonography and conventional endoscopy for prediction of depth of tumor invasion in early gastric cancer. Endoscopy 2010;42:705–13.

67. Yanai H, Noguchi T, Mizumachi S, et al. A blind comparison of the effectiveness of endoscopic ultrasonography and endoscopy in staging early gastric cancer. Gut 1999;44:361–5.

68. Tada M, Shimada M, Murakami F, et al. Development of strip-off biopsy (in Japanese with English abstract). Gastroenterol Endosc 1984;26:833–9.

69. Ohkuwa M, Hosokawa K, Boku N, et al. New endoscopic treatment for intramucosal gastric tumors using an insulated-tip diathermic knife. Endoscopy 2001; 33:221–6.

70. Ono H, Kondo H, Gotoda T, et al. Endoscopic mucosal resection for treatment of early gastric cancer. Gut 2001;48:225–9.

71. Takeuchi Y, Uedo N, Iishi H, et al. Endoscopic submucosal dissection with insulated-tip knife for large mucosal early gastric cancer: a feasibility study (with videos). Gastrointest Endosc 2007;66:186–93.

72. Uedo N, Takeuchi Y, Ishihara R. Endoscopic management of early gastric cancer: endoscopic mucosal resection or endoscopic submucosal dissection: data from a Japanese high-volume center and literature review. Ann Gastroenterol 2012;25: 1–10.

73. Ono H, Hasuike N, Inui T, et al. Usefulness of a novel electrosurgical knife, the insulation-tipped diathermic knife-2, for endoscopic submucosal dissection of early gastric cancer. Gastric Cancer 2008;11:47–52.

74. Toyonaga T, Man-I M, Fujita T, et al. The performance of a novel ball-tipped Flush knife for endoscopic submucosal dissection: a case-control study. Aliment Pharmacol Ther 2010;32:908–15.

75. Tatsumi K, Uedo N, Ishihara R, et al. A water-jet videoendoscope may reduce operation time of endoscopic submucosal dissection for early gastric cancer. Dig Dis Sci 2012;57:2122–9.

76. Yokoi C, Gotoda T, Hamanaka H, et al. Endoscopic submucosal dissection allows curative resection of locally recurrent early gastric cancer after prior endoscopic mucosal resection. Gastrointest Endosc 2006;64:212–8.

77. Oda I, Gotoda T, Sasako M, et al. Treatment strategy after non-curative endoscopic resection of early gastric cancer. Br J Surg 2008;95:1495–500.

78. Uedo N, Iishi H, Tatsuta M, et al. Longterm outcomes after endoscopic mucosal resection for early gastric cancer. Gastric Cancer 2006;9:88–92.

79. Chung IK, Lee JH, Lee SH, et al. Therapeutic outcomes in 1000 cases of endoscopic submucosal dissection for early gastric neoplasms: Korean ESD Study Group multicenter study. Gastrointest Endosc 2009;69:1228–35.

80. Gotoda T, Iwasaki M, Kusano C, et al. Endoscopic resection of early gastric cancer treated by guideline and expanded National Cancer Centre criteria. Br J Surg 2010;97:868–71.

81. Nakajima T, Oda I, Gotoda T, et al. Metachronous gastric cancers after endoscopic resection: how effective is annual endoscopic surveillance? Gastric Cancer 2006;9:93–8.

82. Fukase K, Kato M, Kikuchi S, et al, Japan Gast Study Group. Effect of eradication of *Helicobacter pylori* on incidence of metachronous gastric carcinoma after endoscopic resection of early gastric cancer: an open-label, randomised controlled trial. Lancet 2008;372:392–7.

83. Shiotani A, Uedo N, Iishi H, et al. *H. pylori* eradication did not improve dysregulation of specific oncogenic miRNAs in intestinal metaplastic glands. J Gastroenterol 2012;47(9):988–98.

84. Hanaoka N, Uedo N, Shiotani A, et al. Autofluorescence imaging for predicting development of metachronous gastric cancer after *Helicobacter pylori* eradication. J Gastroenterol Hepatol 2010;25:1844–9.

Surgical Considerations in the Treatment of Gastric Cancer

Andrew M. Blakely, MD[a], Thomas J. Miner, MD[b],*

KEYWORDS

- Gastric cancer • Staging • Resection • Margins • Palliation
- Neoadjuvant chemotherapy

KEY POINTS

- Surgical resection remains the only potentially curative treatment of gastric cancer.
- Newer staging modalities aid in minimizing unnecessary laparotomy in noncurative disease.
- Adequate lymphadenectomy may improve outcomes, similar to selective resection of adjacent organs based on tumor invasion.
- Lymph node involvement and positive surgical margins are associated with poorer overall survival.
- Neoadjuvant chemotherapy may downstage responsive tumors and may improve survival even with extensive lymphatic disease.
- Palliative surgery for advanced gastric cancer remains important in providing symptom relief in appropriately selected patients.

INTRODUCTION

Despite steady declines in the incidence and mortality, gastric cancer is the 5th most common malignancy diagnosed in developed countries in both men and women, with more than 270,000 new diagnoses in 2011. More than 180,000 deaths from gastric cancer were reported for the same year, reflecting a high cancer-related mortality rate.[1] Fatality rates are high in most countries (overall mortality approximately 70%–90%) except in Japan (40%), and stomach cancer ranks 2nd as a cause of cancer-related death. Surgical resection remains the treatment of choice for gastric cancer. Improvements in multimodal chemotherapy and radiotherapy, however, have influenced clinical decision making and treatment algorithms. The largest reported

Disclosures: None to declare.
[a] Department of Surgery, Warren Alpert Medical School of Brown University, 593 Eddy Street, APC 4, Providence, RI 02903, USA; [b] Department of Surgery, Warren Alpert Medical School of Brown University, 593 Eddy Street, APC 443, Providence, RI 02903, USA
* Corresponding author.
E-mail address: tminer@usasurg.org

Gastroenterol Clin N Am 42 (2013) 337–357
http://dx.doi.org/10.1016/j.gtc.2013.01.010
0889-8553/13/$ – see front matter © 2013 Elsevier Inc. All rights reserved.

experience in the surgical treatment of gastric cancer originates from the East Asia, especially Japan and Korea. New data from Western centers have reproduced many of these findings. This review aims to evaluate the role of surgery in the staging, resection, and palliation of gastric cancer.

GASTRIC CANCER STAGING
Histologic Staging

Staging of gastric cancer is according to depth of invasion (T stage), number of lymph node metastases (N stage), and presence of distant disease (M stage). Starting January 1, 2010, newly diagnosed gastric cancers were to be staged using the 7th edition of the TNM staging system (**Table 1**).[2,3] The differences between the 6th and 7th editions specifically regarding gastric cancer pertain mostly to depth of tumor invasion, including

- T1 subdivided to delineate mucosal versus submucosal lesions
- T2a and T2b changed to T2 and T3 to represent muscularis propria and subserosa invasion, respectively
- T3 and T4 changed to T4a and T4b to represent serosal perforation and invasion of adjacent structures, respectively

Historically, the Siewert criteria published in 1998 have been used to classify adenocarcinomas arising at or near the gastroesophageal junction (GEJ)[4]:

- Type I: lesion of the distal esophagus, 1–5 cm proximal to the GEJ
- Type II: lesion arising within the GEJ, within 1 cm proximal and 2 cm distal to the GEJ
- Type III: Lesion arising 2 cm to 5 cm distal to the GEJ with invasion into the esophagus

As part of the 7th edition of the TNM staging system, GEJ adenocarcinomas were also reclassified as follows:

- A lesion with its center within 5 cm of the GEJ and with extension into the esophagus is staged using esophageal carcinoma criteria.
- A lesion with its center within 5 cm of the GEJ but without extension into the esophagus, and a lesion with its center greater than 5 cm away from the GEJ are staged using gastric carcinoma criteria.

Table 1
TNM staging classification, 7th edition; stages 0 to IIIC are M0

T Stage	N Stage	Stage
Tis: carcinoma in situ	N1: 1–2 nodes	Stage 0: TisN0
T1a: lamina propria T1b: submucosa	N2: 3–6 nodes	Stage IA: T1N0 Stage IB: T2N0, T1N1
T2: muscularis propria	N3a: 7–15 nodes N3b: >15 nodes	Stage IIA: T3N0, T2N1, T1N2 Stage IIB: T4aN0, T3N1, T2N2, T1N3
T3: subserosa		Stage IIIA: T4aN1, T3N2, T2N3 Stage IIIB: T4bN0, T4bN1, T4aN2, T3N3 Stage IIIC: T4bN2, T4bN3, T4aN3
T4a: perforates serosa T4b: invades adjacent structures		Stage IV: any T, any N, M1 Positive cytology is M1 disease

To evaluate the clinical effects of the new TNM staging system, Suh and colleagues[5] retrospectively reviewed adenocarcinoma of the GEJ in 497 patients operated on with curative intent based on Siewert classification, from 2003 to 2009. On analysis of staging, 11 of 230 (4.6%) lesions that before would have been classified as TNM stage I under gastric guidelines were upstaged to TNM stage II esophageal lesions. The 5-year survival rates of gastric TNM stage I and esophageal TNM stage II in this study were 92.1% and 90.6%, respectively. Meanwhile, 20 of 125 (16.0%) gastric TNM stage II cancers were upstaged to esophageal TNM stage III cancers. The 5-year survival rates of gastric TNM stage II and esophageal TNM stage III in this study were 84.6% and 51.4%, respectively. The investigators argued that the new guidelines did not adequately distinguish GEJ tumors, because upstaging did not correlate with clinical outcomes.

Surgical Staging

Two-thirds of patients with gastric cancer in the United States present with advanced disease, and the majority show no significant findings on physical examination. The development of specific physical signs usually indicates metastatic disease.

For years, laparotomy was the standard surgical procedure for staging. On gross inspection, the decision between a resection with curative intent versus a nontherapeutic or noncurative procedure was made based on nodal disease, extension into adjacent organs, or distant metastasis. Preoperative CT scans and MRI have not been able to detect noncurative disease in all patients. As technology has progressed, new staging modalities have emerged, including staging laparoscopy, endoscopic and intraoperative ultrasound, and peritoneal washings for cytology. With advances made in neoadjuvant chemotherapy, minimally invasive staging methods have become more important for optimal management.

Staging laparoscopy was compared with preoperative staging CT scan by Burke and colleagues.[6] Between 1990 and 1995, 103 patients with newly diagnosed gastric adenocarcinoma and no evidence of intra-abdominal metastatic disease on CT scan underwent staging laparoscopy. Sixty contemporary patients who underwent staging laparotomy were selected from the same prospective database as a control. Frozen sections were taken of suspicious lesions to evaluate for metastasis: 32 (31.1%) had biopsy-proved metastatic disease and 71 had no laparoscopic evidence of metastasis, of whom 6 (8.5%) had metastases on laparotomy (n = 3) or in distant lymph nodes after resection (n = 3). In this study, staging laparoscopy had a sensitivity of 94% and a specificity of 100%. Patients with metastatic disease confirmed during laparoscopy avoided the unnecessary morbidity of laparotomy. Karanicolas and colleagues[7] reviewed the Surveillance, Epidemiology and End Results cancer database to analyze frequency of staging laparoscopy in the general population. Patients over 65 years of age diagnosed with gastric adenocarcinoma between 1998 and 2005 who underwent a surgical procedure related to gastric cancer were identified. Of 6388 patients, 506 (8%) underwent staging laparoscopy, of whom 306 (60%) underwent therapeutic intervention, 49 (10%) proceeded to laparotomy but no therapeutic procedure, and 151 (30%) underwent only laparoscopy. Use of staging laparoscopy increased over time (5.5% in 1998 to 11.1% in 2005, $P<.01$), and patients tended to be young and white, living in the Northeast, and with proximal cancers, and they had fewer comorbidities than those who did not undergo staging laparoscopy. Although increasing in use, staging laparoscopy seems to remain underutilized in its potential benefit of avoiding unnecessary laparotomy.

To evaluate endoscopic ultrasound (EUS) compared with staging laparoscopy, Power and colleagues[8] prospectively reviewed patients being evaluated for neoadjuvant chemotherapy. Between 2003 and 2005, 94 patients without evidence of metastatic disease on staging CT scan or MRI were analyzed. Those with T1–2 and N0 lesions on EUS were considered low risk for M1 disease (n = 26), and those with T3–4 or N+ were considered high risk (n = 68). Those deemed high risk by EUS most often had tumors at the GE junction or gastric cardia. Staging laparoscopy detected M1 disease in 18 (19%) patients, of whom 17 had been high risk by EUS; the other patient was low risk by EUS but had linitis plastica, which some investigators consider high risk in and of itself. In this study, EUS was 89% sensitive (95% CI, 67%–99%) and 100% specific (95% CI, 95%–100%) in predicting M1 disease when followed by staging laparoscopy. This compared favorably with staging laparoscopy alone, with sensitivity 95% (74%–100%) and specificity 100% (95%–100%). The investigators suggest that in centers with sufficient experience, high-risk lesions on EUS may be a deciding factor in who requires a staging laparoscopy to limit unnecessary or low-yield procedures. Often-present esophageal strictures, however, may limit the application of EUS.

EUS cannot assess the presence of liver or retroperitoneal metastasis. Smith and colleagues[9] prospectively evaluated the benefit of laparoscopic ultrasound (LUS) when added to staging laparoscopy for esophageal and gastric cancers. After standard noninvasive staging work-up, patients with potentially resectable disease underwent complete staging laparoscopy followed by LUS. Of 93 patients, 18 (19.4%) were considered unresectable on staging laparoscopy. Of the remaining 75 patients, 9 (12.0%) were determined unresectable on LUS—4 with esophageal cancer had celiac and para-aortic lymph node disease and 5 with gastric cancer had liver metastases, liver or pancreatic invasion, or celiac and para-aortic lymph node disease. Staging laparoscopy and LUS had a combined 29.0% reduction in unnecessary laparotomy. The investigators concluded that LUS provides a small added benefit to staging laparoscopy in preventing low-yield laparotomy. Hulscher and colleagues[10] narrowed their evaluation of LUS to adenocarcinoma of the gastric cardia with distal esophageal involvement. Between 1995 and 1999, 48 patients with potentially resectable disease on preoperative imaging underwent staging laparoscopy with LUS. Laparoscopy detected distant metastases in 7 (14.6%) and LUS detected distant metastases in an additional 4 (8.3%) patients, resulting in a combined 23% reduction in unnecessary laparotomy.

Bentrem and colleagues[11] evaluated peritoneal cytology as a predictor of poor outcomes before attempted gastric cancer resection. Between 1993 and 2002, 371 patients underwent staging laparoscopy with peritoneal lavage cytology performed before undergoing R0 resection; 24 (6.5%) had positive cytology, which was associated with T stage (10% of T3–4 vs 2% of T1–2; $P = .02$) and overall stage (11% of stage III, 7% of stage II, 2% of stage I; $P = .002$). On multivariate analysis, poorer overall survival was associated with positive cytology (relative risk 2.7, $P<.001$), distal tumor location, and preoperative T stage and N stage. The investigators suggest that peritoneal lavage cytology should be considered in assessing a patient's prognosis after attempted curative resection. Mezhir and colleagues[12] re-evaluated outcomes of gastric cancer patients with positive cytology, because the TNM 7th edition considers positive peritoneal lavage equivalent to M1 disease. Patients who had undergone staging laparoscopy with positive peritoneal lavage between 1993 and 2009 were included whereas those with ascites or who had undergone chemotherapy were excluded. Of the 291 patients included, 198 (68%) had gross peritoneal disease or visceral metastases seen on staging laparoscopy. In the remaining 93 patients, only positive peritoneal cytology indicated M1 disease. Median overall survival was 1 year, with 80% mortality at that time. Patients with gross metastatic disease had poor disease-specific survival, and those with positive cytology fared only slightly better. Peritoneal cytology, particularly for patients without evidence of gross metastasis, should be factored into the decision of whether to proceed with resection.

EXTENT OF GASTRIC RESECTION
Distal Disease

For years, there was debate over subtotal gastrectomy (SG) versus total gastrectomy (TG) as the optimal procedure for gastric antrum malignancies. Gouzi and colleagues[13] published the first randomized study comparing SG and TG for distal lesions in 1989. From 1980 to 1985, 169 patients of any age with a potentially curable distal gastric malignancy underwent either SG or TG, without routine splenectomy. SG and TG were similar in terms of perioperative morbidity (34% vs 33%) and mortality (3.2% vs 1.6%). Overall 5-year survival was 48%, similar to contemporary Western retrospective studies. Nodal involvement and serosal invasion were associated with survival, whereas extent of resection was not. Although the trial suffered from a small study population, the investigators concluded that SG was a viable treatment option for distal gastric cancer.

Bozzetti and colleagues[14] conducted a larger randomized controlled trial to compare SG and TG. Patients with distal cancers underwent staging laparotomy to confirm that the location of the primary lesion was at least 6 cm away from the gastric cardia and that there was no N3 disease or unresectable disease. From 1982 to 1993, 624 patients were included, 320 in the SG group and 306 in the TG group. All underwent D2 dissection, splenectomy was optional, and 6-cm margins were obtained when possible. Although perioperative mortality was similar between SG and TG (1.3% vs 2.3%, $P = .27$), morbidity was greater in the TG group (15.5% vs 10.3%, $P = .05$), which was attributed to complications associated with splenectomy. Mean length of stay was improved in the SG group (13.8 days vs 15.4 days, $P<.001$). Bozzetti and colleagues[15] subsequently published 5-year survival data as well as descriptive data. Results of permanent sections revealed R1 resection in 15 (4.7%) patients in the SG group versus 6 (2%) patients in the TG group. Only 10 patients overall received adjuvant chemotherapy. Patients with larger tumors, higher tumor grade, and nodal involvement fared worse. Five-year survival rates between SG and TG were similar (65.3% vs 62.4%; hazard ratio [HR] 95% CI not significant).

Because the aforementioned studies did not include data on number of lymph nodes dissected and because the range of tumor grade was variable, de Manzoni and colleagues[16] conducted a prospective multicenter trial comparing SG with TG in patients with a T3 lesion of the gastric antrum. During 1996, 117 patients who underwent potentially curative surgery with D2 dissection were analyzed; 77 (65.8%) underwent SG whereas 40 underwent TG without splenectomy. Overall perioperative morbidity (14.5%) and mortality (2.6%) were not associated with extent of resection. The median number of lymph nodes dissected was 30. Median survival was improved in the SG group (38 months vs 23 months, $P = .011$) as was 5-year survival (36% vs 22%). On multivariate analysis, only nodal disease was independently associated with survival. The study was limited in that it was not randomized, and surgeon preference had an effect in that elderly patients were more likely to undergo SG instead of TG. It seemed, however, that even in distal lesions involving the serosa, performing SG instead of TG had no adverse effect on survival.

One of the primary arguments in favor of SG over TG when possible was the effect on quality of life. Davies and colleagues[17] evaluated 47 consecutive patients who had presented with gastric cancer and underwent potential R0 resection. TG was performed for lesions of the proximal and middle thirds of the stomach (n = 26), and SG was performed for those of the distal third (n = 21). D2 dissection was performed, and the spleen and pancreas were preserved when possible. No patient received adjuvant chemotherapy. Quality of life was assessed preoperatively and at 1, 3, 6, and 12 months postoperatively using 5 validated questionnaires. The interviewer was blinded to the procedure the patient had received. Of the 5 assessment tools used, only the Rotterdam symptom checklist and the Troidl index achieved a statistically significant difference between the SG and TG groups through 12 months postoperatively. Each one indicated improved quality of life in the SG group over the TG group.

Based on approximately equivalent long-term survival rates, generally higher operative morbidity and mortality of patients undergoing TG, and improved quality of life for patients undergoing SG, for distal gastric cancer the procedure of choice is SG, provided that adequate proximal margins of 5 cm to 6 cm are able to be obtained.

Proximal Disease

The adequacy of proximal gastrectomy (PG) versus TG for tumors of the proximal one-third of the stomach has been the subject of various studies. Harrison and colleagues[18] published one of the first studies to evaluate the long-term outcomes of each procedure. Between 1985 and 1995, 98 patients underwent surgery other than esophagogastrectomy for proximal tumors; 65 (66%) patients underwent PG and 33 underwent TG, all via an abdominal approach. Tumor differentiation and stage were similar between the groups, but tumor size was larger in the TG group (7 cm vs 4 cm, $P = .02$) and more lymph nodes were harvested. Proximal margins were similar between the groups, but distal margins were improved in the TG group (6.5 ± 1.2 cm vs 3.9 ± 0.5 cm, $P<.05$). Overall 5-year survival was similar (41% in TG vs 43% in PG). Kim and colleagues[19] retrospectively reviewed patients who underwent either PG or TG for proximal gastric cancer. PG was performed only when the cancer was limited to the proximal one-third. Between 1992 and 2000, 43 patients underwent PG and 104 underwent TG. Thoracotomy was performed in 3 PG (7.0%) and 7 TG (6.7%), splenectomy and distal pancreatectomy in 18 PG (41.8%) and 15 TG (14.4%), and splenectomy alone in 8 PG (18.6%) and 13 TG (12.5%). The groups were fairly well matched for tumor characteristics, including size and differentiation, although all T4 lesions were resected via TG. The majority of the PG group underwent D1 dissection, whereas the majority of the TG group underwent at least D2 dissection. The PG group experienced higher perioperative morbidity (48.8% vs 14.4%, $P<.001$), most commonly anastomotic strictures, and higher rate of recurrence (39.5% vs 4.8%, $P<.001$). Overall 5-year survival was similar (48.6% in TG vs 46.0% in PG, $P = .972$). This remained true for stage I or stage II disease; however, for stage III disease, 5-year survival after TG was significantly improved (38.4% vs 17.1%, $P = .035$). Therefore, given higher rates of concomitant organ resection and perioperative morbidity as well as more challenging D2 dissection, PG could only be recommended for early gastric cancer with adequate margins and limited nodal involvement.

Regarding management specifically of proximal early gastric cancer, An and colleagues[20] compared PG with TG. From 2000 to 2005, 423 patients underwent PG (n = 89 [21.0%]) or TG (n = 334 [79.0%]) for stage I or stage II proximal gastric adenocarcinoma. The TG group had larger tumors (4.0 cm vs 2.5 cm, $P<.001$) and more mean lymph nodes harvested (39.1 vs 22.4, $P<.001$). PG was associated with higher morbidity (61.8% vs 12.6%, $P<.001$), most often anastomotic stenosis and esophageal reflux, and these were successfully treated with balloon dilatation. Five-year survival was similar between the 2 groups (99.2% in PG vs 98.5% in TG, $P = .57$), as were long-term body weight and nutritional markers. The investigators could not recommend PG over TG for proximal early gastric cancer based on the frequency of postoperative complications.

Resection of Adjacent Organs

Although direct tumor involvement of the spleen or distal pancreas warrants resection to achieve potential R0 resection and remove pathologic lymph nodes, routine splenectomy and distal pancreatectomy as part of a D2 dissection adds early morbidity without a proven long-term survival benefit. The most common complications cited are postoperative infection and pancreatic fistula. Yu and colleagues[21] made one of the clearest arguments against routine splenectomy. Between 1995 and 1999, patients undergoing TG for proximal gastric adenocarcinoma were randomized to undergo splenic resection versus preservation. Those with pancreas or spleen invasion, gastrosplenic ligament involvement, or hilar or splenic artery lymph node disease were excluded. Of 207 patients who met criteria, 104 (50.2%) underwent splenectomy. The resection and preservation groups had similar perioperative morbidity (15.4% vs 8.7%, $P = .142$) and mortality (1.9% vs 1.0%), median length of stay (11 days in each group), median number of harvested lymph nodes (40 in each group), and overall 5-year survival (54.8% vs 48.8%, $P = .503$). With no survival benefit or improved lymph node yield, routine splenectomy could not be recommended.

To evaluate extension of gastric cancer resection to adjacent organs, Shchepotin and colleagues[22] retrospectively reviewed 353 patients who underwent multiorgan resection of T4 gastric cancers between 1974 and 1994. Resection of adjacent organs was based on gross appearance; permanent section revealed that 39 (11%) had desmoplastic reactions instead of direct tumor invasion. Patients with tumors localized to the distal one-third or the cardia underwent SG (n = 237, 67.1%) and the remainder underwent TG (n = 116, 32.9%). N1 or N2 lymph node involvement was present in 137 (38.8%) patients. Transverse colectomy was performed in 159 (45.0%) patients, combined splenectomy and distal pancreatectomy in 150 (42.5%), left hepatic lobectomy in 101 (28.5%), and proximal pancreatectomy in 37 (10.5%). Overall, 254 (71.9%) had 1 extra organ removed, 73 (20.7%) had 2 removed, and 26 (7.4%) had 3 or more resected. Perioperative morbidity was 31.2% (most commonly intra-abdominal abscess) and mortality was 13.6%. Overall 5-year survival was 25%, 37% among node-negative patients versus 15% among node-positive patients. Number or type of organ resected did not affect survival.

Martin and colleagues[23] retrospectively reviewed adjacent organ resection among R0 resections from 1985 to 2000. Of 1133 patients who underwent PG, SG, or TG, 865 underwent gastrectomy alone whereas 268 underwent gastrectomy with additional organ resection. Additional organ resection was more common with proximal cancers, and more often TG was performed. The most common additional organs resected were spleen (45.9%), spleen and pancreas (14.2%), spleen and colon (6.7%), colon (6.0%), pancreas (4.5%), and other (22.8%). Additional organ resection was associated with more-invasive cancers and increased nodal involvement. Postoperative mortality was similar even with additional organ resections (3.7% vs 3.6%). Five-year survival for the additional organ resection group was 32%, similar to contemporary studies; on multivariate analysis, T stage and N stage were independently associated with survival, whereas number or type of additional organs resected was not. Risk of recurrence was, however, higher in the additional resection group (52% vs 42%, $P = .003$). With appropriate identification of T3 or T4 tumors, the investigators recommended additional organ resection due to its potential benefit and low additional morbidity and mortality.

Several subsequent series have supported the role of extended organ resection for patients who have potentially curable disease (**Table 2**). Kobayashi and colleagues[24] retrospectively reviewed patients presenting between 1993 and 2000, 82 of whom had invasion into adjacent organs. Extended resections included distal pancreatectomy and splenectomy (n = 36), transverse colectomy (n = 35), and other (n = 34). Some patients underwent noncurative resections due to peritoneal dissemination or liver or distant lymph node involvement. The most common postoperative complication was pancreatic fistula. Kunisaki and colleagues[25] retrospectively reviewed 117 patients with T4 gastric adenocarcinoma undergoing surgery from 1994 to 1999. Thirty-eight (32.5%) were attempted curative resections, whereas the remainder were noncurative in intent due to peritoneal dissemination, liver or para-aortic involvement, positive margins, distant metastasis, or unresectable bulky lymph node disease. The most commonly involved organs were pancreas (52.1%), transverse colon (37.6%), and liver (8.5%). Fifteen (12.8%) patients underwent multiple additional organ resections. The most common postoperative complication was pancreatic fistula. Carboni and colleagues[26] performed a similar retrospective review, identifying 65 patients with advanced gastric adenocarcinoma undergoing surgery between 1979 and 2004. Extended resections included spleen (n = 31), pancreas (n = 28), colon (n = 16), and other (n = 24). Desmoplastic reaction instead of tumor invasion was confirmed in 13 (20%) patients. Medical complications produced half of the operative morbidity and an additional 7 perioperative deaths. Other small series have been published but do not report 5-year mortality, limiting comparison.

Resection of Gastroesophageal Junction Tumors

Although it is generally accepted that Siewert type I tumors are best treated by esophagectomy, the optimal surgical management of proximal gastric tumors, grades II and III, has been debated. Ito and colleagues[27] retrospectively reviewed the charts of all patients with Siewert type II or III lesions presenting between 1991 and 2001; 82 patients were included for analysis, 59 (72.0%) had Siewert type II lesions and 23 (28.0%) had type III lesions. Operative management consisted of 27 (33%) total esophagectomy (mostly transthoracic), 24 (29%) extended gastrectomy with thoracotomy, and 31 (38%) extended gastrectomy without thoracotomy. More patients with type II cancer had received neoadjuvant chemotherapy than those with type III cancer. Overall perioperative mortality was 2.4% and morbidity was 20%. Morbidity among the esophagectomy group was higher (33% vs 11%, $P = .014$), and thoracotomy had no

Author	Patients	Tumor Grade	30-Day Mortality	30-Day Morbidity	R0 Resection	5-Year Survival	R0 5-Year Survival	Recurrence Rate
Table 2 Multiple organ resections in treatment of invasive gastric cancer								
Kobayashi et al,[24] 2004	82	T3, T4	1.2%	28%	50 (61.0%)	31.1%	36.9% ($P = .004$)	NR
Kunisaki et al,[25] 2006	117	T4	4.3%	22.2%	38 (32.5%)	16.0%	32.2% ($P<.0001$)	50%
Carboni et al,[26] 2005	65	T3, T4	1.5%	27.7%	40 (61.5%)	21.8%	30.6% ($P = .001$)	NR

Abbreviation: NR, not reported.

significant effect on morbidity in the extended gastrectomy group (13% with vs 10% without, $P = .74$). There was no significant difference in tumor grade, T stage, or N stage between esophagectomy and gastrectomy groups. Overall mean number of lymph nodes resected was suboptimal (median 6), but 65% were determined to have an R0 resection. Those who underwent extended gastrectomy had positive margins more frequently (38% vs 7%, $P = .04$), and this was associated with T3 and T4 lesions. Margin information was used to determine that the optimal proximal gross margin length was 6 cm and the distal margin length 4 cm. Five-year mortality was similar among the 3 groups (esophagectomy 30%, extended gastrectomy with thoracotomy 23%, extended gastrectomy without thoracotomy 34%; $P = .16$). On multivariate analysis, positive margins, increased patient age, and nodal disease were independently associated with poorer survival. The investigators recommended whichever surgical approach would best achieve adequate gross margins and improved lymph node harvesting.

Laparoscopic Gastric Resection

In recent years, surgeons have been performing laparoscopic-assisted or robotic-assisted gastric cancer resections, but laparoscopic extended lymph node dissection is technically challenging and requires experience. To assess the adequacy of totally laparoscopic SG, Huscher and colleagues[28] conducted a randomized prospective trial comparing laparoscopic and open approaches. Between 1992 and 1996, 59 patients with distal gastric cancer underwent either open or laparoscopic SG with D1 or D2 dissection and Roux-en-Y or Billroth II reconstructions. No patient from the laparoscopic group was reported to have port site metastasis on follow-up. The laparoscopic group had less operative blood loss (229 mL vs 391 mL, $P<.001$), shorter length of stay (10.3 days vs 14.5 days, $P<.001$), and quicker return to diet (5.1 days vs 7.4 days, $P<.001$). Differences in perioperative morbidity (26.7% vs 27.6%) and mortality (3.3% vs 6.7%) and overall 5-year survival (58.9% vs 55.7%) were not statistically significant. Lee and colleagues[29] demonstrated similar benefits by prospectively analyzing 34 patients with distal lesions less than 5 cm and without significant serosal involvement who had undergone potentially curative laparoscopic gastrectomy between 1998 and 2005, matching them to 34 patients who had undergone open surgery for similar pathology. No patients were converted from laparoscopic to open. Mean operative time (283 minutes vs 195 minutes, $P<.001$) was longer in the laparoscopic group, whereas estimated blood loss (74 mL vs 190 mL, $P<.001$), return of bowel function (2.9 days vs 4.9 days, $P<.01$), and length of stay (8.5 days vs 12.1 days, $P<.001$) were all improved in the laparoscopic approach compared with open surgery. Perioperative morbidity and survival during follow-up were similar.

To compare laparoscopic with open SG and TG, Moisan and colleagues[30] prospectively analyzed 31 patients who had undergone laparoscopic SG or TG for adenocarcinoma between 2005 and 2010. The 31 patients were case-matched by randomly selecting patients from the open surgery group with similar T stage, extent of gastrectomy, age, and gender. All included patients who lived longer than 30 days postoperatively, achieved R0 resection, had at least D1 dissection, did not undergo splenectomy or pancreatectomy, and did not have neoadjuvant chemotherapy. Patients were fairly evenly distributed by stage (I–III) and tumor location (upper vs middle vs lower third); 22 patients in each group underwent TG and 9 underwent SG. As before, the laparoscopic group experienced longer mean operative time (250 minutes vs 210 minutes, $P = .007$), less mean estimated blood loss (100 mL vs 300 mL, $P<.001$), faster return to diet (4 days vs 7 days, $P<.001$), and shorter length of stay (7 days vs 10.5 days, $P = .001$). Perioperative morbidity was identical (12.9%) and the difference in median number of retrieved nodes was nonsignificant (35 vs 39). Overall 3-year survival was not significantly different (82.3% vs 86.9%, $P = .557$).

The laparoscopic approach specifically for proximal gastric tumors was retrospectively reviewed by Ahn and colleagues.[31] Between 2003 and 2009, 131 patients underwent either laparoscopic PG (LAPG) or laparoscopic TG (LATG). Fifty patients underwent LAPG and 81 underwent LATG; a common reason to perform LATG instead was a tumor size too large to provide a remnant of sufficient capacity to allow return of postoperative gastric function. Patient demographics between the groups were similar. LAPG patients experienced shorter operative time and less blood loss as well as lower rate of splenectomy (0 vs 6). All LAPG and most LATG patients (86.4%) underwent D1 dissection. The LAPG group had similar staging compared with the LATG group but smaller tumors (2.8 ± 1.3 cm vs 4.0 ± 2.7 cm, $P = .002$), shorter proximal margins (3.5 ± 2.3 cm vs 4.4 ± 2.3 cm, $P = .038$) and distal margins (4.0 ± 1.6 cm vs 14.3 ± 4.2 cm, $P<.001$), and fewer mean harvested lymph nodes (33.1 vs 47.4, $P<.001$). Return to diet, return of bowel function, hospital length of stay, and early morbidity were similar. Late morbidity among the LAPG group, however, was higher (44.0% vs 22.2%, $P = .005$), most commonly reflux symptoms or anastomotic stenosis. This joins a growing body of data that demonstrates similar long-term outcomes between open and laparoscopic approaches for the resection of gastric tumors.

Role of Endoscopic Resection

Two endoscopic treatment modalities are in wide use today in Eastern centers and selectively used in Western centers: endoscopic mucosal resection (EMR) and endoscopic submucosal dissection (ESD). Originally, Japanese guidelines indicated EMR for less than 2 cm, well-differentiated, nonulcerated gastric cancer lesions confined to the mucosa before they invaded the submucosa and subsequently the lymphatic system.[32] Later, guidelines were expanded to include differentiated, nonulcerated mucosal cancer greater than 2 cm; differentiated, ulcerated mucosal cancer up to 3 cm; and undifferentiated, nonulcerated, mucosal cancer up to 2 cm. After excision of the lesion using these techniques, histologic staging is used to determine adequacy of the excision and need for subsequent surgery.

These endoscopic techniques must be carefully applied, however. Ishikawa and colleagues[33] retrospectively reviewed the histology specimens of resections with D2 dissections for early gastric adenocarcinoma from 1980 to 2004. Of 278 specimens, 156 were mucosal and 122 were submucosal lesions. Ulceration was present in 41 (26.3%) of mucosal cancers, of which 6 (14.6%) also had lymph node metastasis, all only to the N1 tier. Ulceration was present in 21 (18.3%) of submucosal cancers, of which 10 (47.6%) had lymph node involvement. Of the 101 nonulcerated submucosal cancers, however, 18 (17.8%) had nodal disease. Overall, 3 cases that would have met extended criteria for EMR or ESD were found to have lymph node metastasis, which has been shown the major prognostic factor in early gastric cancer. The investigators suggest that the safest use of EMR/ESD is for nonulcerated mucosal lesions of any size and ulcerated mucosal lesions less than 2 cm in diameter.

LYMPH NODE DISSECTION

One of the best-known and earliest randomized trials to evaluate extent of lymph node dissection is by the Dutch Gastric Cancer Group. Bonenkamp and colleagues[34] published initial results of the Dutch D1D2 trial, a prospective, randomized controlled trial conducted from 1989 to 1993. Inclusion required histologic confirmation of gastric adenocarcinoma without evidence of distant metastasis. Eleven supervising surgeons were involved, determining if curative resection was possible based on gross appearance and frozen section of para-aortic lymph node biopsy. Patients underwent either SG, if 5-cm margins could be achieved, or TG. D1 dissection was defined as including the N1 tier (perigastric) lymph nodes whereas D2 dissection included dissection of lymph nodes in the N2 tier. Of 1078 patients originally randomized, 711 were operated on with curative intent, 380 in the D1 group and 331 in the D2 group; 41 (11%) of the D1 group underwent splenectomy compared with 124 (38%) of the D2 group, and distal pancreatectomy was performed in 10 (3%) of the D1 group versus 98 (30%) of the D2 group. Perioperative mortality was significantly higher in D2 patients (10% vs 4%, $P = .004$), as was morbidity (43% vs 25%, $P<.001$), rate of reoperation (18% vs 8%, $P<.001$), and average length of stay (25 days vs 18 days, $P<.001$). Bonenkamp and colleagues[35] later published 5-year survival data. Of 589 patients who achieved R0 resection and survived the operative hospital stay, 324 underwent D1 and 265 underwent D2 dissection. The risk of relapse at 5 years in the D1 group was higher (43% vs 37%), but the 95% CI failed to achieve statistical significance ($P = .22$). Overall survival rates between the 2 groups were similar (45% in D1 vs 47% in D2), and the HR 95% CI failed to achieve significance. At this point, resection with D2 dissection showed no clear benefit over D1 dissection for curative resection of gastric cancer in Western countries. Hartgrink and colleagues[36] published 10-year survival data and Songun and colleagues[37] reported 15-year survival data. Overall survival rates were similar between D1 and D2 dissection at 10 years (30% vs 35%, $P = .53$) and 15 years (21% vs 29%, $P = .34$). The long-term follow-up data confirmed the previous conclusion of no clear survival benefit of D2 dissection over D1 dissection.

Cuschieri and colleagues[38] reported initial results of the Medical Research Council (MRC) prospective, randomized controlled trial evaluating D1 versus D2 dissection, a parallel United Kingdom study. Inclusion criteria were histologically confirmed gastric adenocarcinoma with potential for curative resection. All patients underwent staging laparotomy, including examination of para-aortic lymph nodes. Those with potentially curable disease were randomized intraoperatively to resection with either D1 or D2 dissection. D1 dissection involved those nodes within 3 cm of the primary tumor along with omentum, whereas D2 dissection added celiac axis, hepatoduodenal, retroduodenal, splenic, and peripancreatic lymph nodes. SG was performed for antral tumors if a 2.5-cm proximal margin was possible; all others underwent TG. Over a 7-year period, 400 patients were deemed eligible at laparotomy and were randomized. As with the Dutch trial, the D2 group experienced higher perioperative morbidity (46% vs 28%, $P<.001$) and mortality (10.5% vs 4.5%, $P<.04$) and longer length of stay (23 days vs 18 days, $P = .01$). Cuschieri and colleagues[39] later reported survival data, showing similar overall 5-year survival between D1 and D2 (35% vs 33%, $P = .43$). This correlated with conclusions from the Dutch trial.

The aforementioned trials were performed when D2 dissection frequently involved splenectomy and/or distal pancreatectomy, the portions of the procedure to which the higher morbidity and mortality of D2 versus D1 dissection had been attributed. Subsequent studies have analyzed a limited or modified D2 dissection compared with either D1 or standard D2 dissection. Edwards and colleagues[40] prospectively evaluated D1 versus spleen-preserving D2 dissection. The study consecutively enrolled patients with histologically confirmed gastric adenocarcinoma with potential for curative resection based on staging laparoscopy. Of 118 potentially curable patients, 36 presented to one surgeon and were treated with resection plus D1 dissection, whereas

82 presented to the other surgeon and were treated with resection and modified D2 dissection. Extent of dissection for each group was similar to previous studies, except that nodes were dissected off the splenic artery, and splenectomy was only performed for hilar involvement. In this limited study, perioperative mortality was similar between the D1 and modified D2 groups (8.3% vs 7.3%, P = 0.848), but 5-year survival was improved in the modified D2 group (59% vs 32%, P = .039). On univariate analysis, splenectomy and pancreatectomy were not associated with survival. On multivariate analysis, however, extent of lymphadenectomy was associated with survival, suggesting a survival benefit of the modified D2 dissection over the standard D1 dissection.

Degiuli and colleagues[41] published initial results of the Italian Gastric Cancer Study Group's experience in pancreas-preserving D2 dissections. The study was conducted from 1994 to 1996, in an effort to decrease the Western operative morbidity and mortality of standard D2 dissections with distal pancreatectomy. After staging laparotomy demonstrated no gross metastatic disease or pathologic N3 or N4 lymph nodes, 191 patients underwent SG or TG with D2 lymph node dissection. The distal pancreas was spared in TG when there was no direct tumor invasion. Perioperative morbidity (20.9%) and mortality (3.1%) compared favorably with contemporary Eastern center results. Degiuli and colleagues[42] later published 5-year survival data. Overall survival was 55% and disease-free survival was 65%, which were improved compared with the Dutch and MRC results. Specific data on how many distal pancreatectomies were performed, however, were not included and the effect of European surgeons' increased experience in performing D2 dissection was unable to be assessed.

Building on previous experience, Degiuli and colleagues[43] designed a multicenter randomized controlled trial to evaluate D1 versus modified D2 dissection in specialized Western centers. From 1998 to 2005, 267 patients with potentially curable disease based on staging laparotomy, using peritoneal lavage and lymph node biopsy at the left renal vein, were randomized to SG or TG with either D1 or modified D2 dissection. The study faced some difficulty with enrollment due to the perception that D2 dissection was the superior treatment, causing many eligible patients to decline randomization. Only surgeons involved with the previous Italian Gastric Cancer Study Group trial were included. Of patients who underwent TG with D2 dissection, 12 of 31 underwent splenectomy and 2 of 31 underwent distal pancreatectomy. The study found no significant differences between D1 and D2 dissection in perioperative morbidity (12.0% vs 17.9%, P = .178) or mortality (3.0% vs 2.2%, P = .722) or length of stay (12.8 days vs 13.1 days, P = .732). These results were improved over the earlier Dutch and UK trials.

The standard of care in Eastern centers, such as in Japan and Korea, consists of SG or TG with at least a D2 lymph node dissection, because a D1 dissection is considered an inadequate oncologic procedure. Because of their referral system, where patients with gastric cancer are evaluated by and operated on by foregut specialists, the reported perioperative morbidity and mortality of the standard D2 dissection is less than what was reported in the Dutch and MRC trials. More recent data generated from specialized Western centers compare more favorably with Eastern data, so it may be concluded that the learning curve for performing a D2 gastrectomy may have been responsible for such disparate results from the 1990s.

As to whether more extensive lymph node dissection provides a survival benefit, Sasako and colleagues[44] evaluated the addition of para-aortic lymph node dissection (PAND) to D2 dissection. Between 1995 and 2001, patients with potentially curable T2b, T3, or T4 gastric adenocarcinoma were included, because para-aortic nodal involvement may only occur once the subserosa is invaded. Of 523 patients, 263 underwent standard D2 dissection whereas 259 underwent D2 dissection with PAND. Each treatment arm was well matched for extent of gastric resection and frequency of splenectomy and distal pancreatectomy. Patients who underwent PAND experienced longer operative times (300 minutes vs 237 minutes, $P<.001$), greater median blood loss (660 mL vs 430 mL, $P<.001$), and more transfusions (30.0% vs 14.1%, $P<.001$). Twenty-two of 259 patients (8.5%) who underwent PAND had positive lymph nodes. Morbidity was higher in the PAND group but did not achieve statistical significance (28.1% vs 20.9%, $P = .07$). Overall survival rates were similar between the standard D2 dissection and D2 dissection plus PAND (69.2% vs 70.3%), as were recurrence-free survival rates (62.6% vs 61.7%). Thus, the investigators could not recommend routine para-aortic node dissection as part of resection of potentially curable gastric malignancies.

POSITIVE MARGINS

Positive resection margins for potentially curative gastric cancer are associated with poorer outcomes. Shen and colleagues[45] retrospectively reviewed patients with primary tumors in the gastric cardia, Siewert type II or III, who had undergone TG with curative intent between 1995 and 2000. Frozen sections were not done, D2 dissection was performed, and adjuvant fluorouracil-based chemotherapy was administered except for tumor grade T2N0M0. Of 191 patients, 16 (8.4%) had positive margins at permanent section, 15 of whom were stage III or IV. Characteristics that were associated with positive margins included tumor size greater than 5 cm ($P = .001$), depth of tumor invasion ($P<.001$), node involvement ($P<.001$), and stage ($P<.001$). On multivariate analysis, only tumor stage was independently associated with survival ($P<.001$); positive margins were not associated ($P = .23$). Median survival in those with positive margins, however, was poorer (33.9 months vs 62.4 months, $P<.001$).

Cho and colleagues[46] also retrospectively reviewed the clinical impact of positive margin status. Between 1987 and 2001, 2740 consecutive patients presented for potentially curable advanced gastric cancer, defined as at least T2. All patients underwent intraoperative frozen section and D2 or D3 lymph node dissection. Positive margins were those that were positive on permanent section despite negative frozen section. Forty-nine patients (1.8%) had positive margins, of whom 1 underwent relaparotomy, 43 underwent chemotherapy, and 5 received no further treatment. Factors associated with positive resection margins included greater stomach involvement by the tumor ($P = .001$), signet ring morphology and poor differentiation ($P = .019$), TNM stage of IIIB or IV ($P = .001$), and tumor depth of T3 or T4 ($P = .001$). Five-year overall survival was poorer with positive margins (28% vs 51%, $P = .0028$). In the presence of positive lymph nodes, survival was similar between negative and positive margins (37 months vs 33 months, $P = .259$). In node-negative disease, however, positive margins were associated with poorer 5-year survival (29% vs 80%, $P = .0001$). Sun and colleagues[47] performed a similar retrospective review from 1980 to 2006. Frozen section was performed if margins were considered insufficient, and reresection of margins was performed after positive frozen section. Of 2269 patients who underwent an intended R0 resection, 110 (4.8%) had a positive margin on permanent section. Positive margins were associated with worse outcomes for less invasive tumors (T1 or T2) ($P<.001$), limited nodal involvement (N0 or N1) ($P<.001$), and lower-stage malignancies (stage I or II) ($P = .006$). Although 5-year overall survival was worse with positive margins (25.8% vs 52.6%, $P<.001$), this association did not hold up on multivariate analysis. This indicates that negative margins are more important when resecting lower-stage tumors, because advanced tumors have likely progressed beyond the primary site.

PALLIATIVE SURGERY

Palliative surgery is defined as procedures that are performed with noncurative intent to improve quality of life or to relieve symptoms secondary to an advanced malignancy.[48] Worse outcomes after palliative surgery have been associated with poor functional status, recent weight loss, and low serum albumin. Appropriate selection of patients with advanced cancer of any type for palliative surgery can yield several months of symptom relief at the end of life while minimizing operative morbidity and mortality. Involvement of the patient, patient's family members, and operating surgeon in the palliative decision-making process, known as the palliative triangle, has been associated with more successful relief of symptoms and fewer postoperative complications.[49] The importance of explicitly defining procedures performed on patients with advanced gastric cancer as palliative has been emphasized by Miner and colleagues.[50] Among 307 patients who underwent R1 or R2 resection for noncurable disease, 147 (47.9%) underwent procedures that were performed with palliative intent whereas the remainder were nonpalliative. Patients undergoing palliative procedures more frequently had distal cancers, nodal involvement, and metastatic disease on staging. Perioperative morbidity (49% vs 61%, $P = .25$) and mortality (7% vs 4%, $P = .46$) were similar, but palliative patients had a lower rate of high-grade complications (22% vs 29%, $P = .049$), likely due to less extensive surgical procedures performed. Median overall survival was 10.6 months but was significantly decreased among palliative patients (8.3 months vs 13.5 months, $P<.001$).

The natural history of metastatic gastric cancer has been analyzed in terms of need for palliative intervention by Sarela and colleagues.[51] Between 1993 and 2002, 147 patients with metastatic disease diagnosed on staging laparoscopy and 18 patients with metastatic disease discovered on laparotomy after negative laparoscopy were included. Disease most commonly involved the peritoneum, with some patients with liver and/or distant lymph node involvement. All patients started single-agent or multi-agent chemotherapy after diagnosis of metastatic disease. Of 97 patients who were treated only at the investigators' institution, 48 (49.5%) underwent palliative procedures; 29 had a procedure involving the GEJ or stomach, 7 had a procedure on a distant anatomic site, and 12 patients had a combination of the 2 types of surgery. Median overall survival was 10 months; however, median survival after any palliative procedure was 3 months. On multivariate analysis, survival was improved in patients with better baseline performance status and limited peritoneal metastasis. The investigators argued that palliative procedures often did not improve survival and that preemptive palliative procedures before symptomatic presentation were not necessary.

The benefit of palliative resection for incurable gastric cancer has been debated (**Table 3**). These arguments are often limited by emphasis on survival data or morbidity and mortality rates rather than the more appropriate palliative endpoints of symptom resolution or potential quality-of-life benefits. Hartgrink and colleagues[52] compared exploratory laparotomy with or without surgical bypass to palliative gastric resection in unresectable patients identified in the prospective Dutch D1D2 trial. Of 285 patients with unresectable tumors (T^+), hepatic (H^+) or peritoneal (P^+) metastasis, or distal lymph node involvement (N^+), 156 (54.7%) underwent palliative resection. Median survival in resected patients was improved over those who had exploratory laparotomy with or without gastroenterostomy (8.1 months vs 5.4 months, $P<.001$);

Table 3
Survival benefit of palliative resection compared with laparotomy with or without bypass

Author	Number of Patients	Resected Patients	30-Day Mortality	30-Day Morbidity	Unresected Median Survival	Resected Median Survival
Hartgrink et al,[52] 2002	285	156 (54.7%)	12%	38%	5.4 mo	8.1 mo (P<.001)
Samarasam et al,[53] 2006	151	107 (70.9%)	NR	NR	12 mo	24 mo (P = .0003)
Saidi et al,[54] 2006	105	24 (22.9%)	8.3%	33.3%	5.5 mo (mean)	13.2 mo (mean) (P = .006)
Huang et al,[55] 2010	516	365 (70.7%)	3.3%	18%	4.5 mo	10.2 mo (P<.001)
Zhang et al,[56] 2011	377	197 (52.3%)	3.0%	24.3%	5.8 mo bypass 4.7 mo no bypass	16.4 mo (P<.05)

Abbreviation: NR, not reported.

however, they had higher morbidity (38% vs 12%, $P<.001$) and length of stay (15 days vs 10 days, $P<.001$). Perioperative mortality was similar (12% vs 10%). The investigators concluded that patients under 70 years of age with only 1 of the 4 criteria for unresectability obtained a survival benefit from resection, whereas older patients or those with more than one manifestation of unresectable disease had no survival benefit. Samarasam and colleagues[53] retrospectively reviewed consecutive patients from 1999 to 2003 who underwent palliative surgery for gastric adenocarcinoma. Of 151 patients, 107 (70.9%) underwent either SG or TG if macroscopic free margins could be obtained; the remaining 44 underwent laparotomy with or without gastrojejunostomy. All patients received adjuvant chemotherapy. Resectability decreased with increasing number of criteria for unresectability (T^+, H^+, P^+, and N^+). Median survival was improved in resected patients (24 months vs 12 months, $P = .0003$); however, the survival benefit disappeared with more than one criterion for unresectability. Median survival was similar between SG and TG (24 months and 20 months, respectively). Saidi and colleagues[54] compared no resection with palliative resection for patients with stage IV gastric cancer between 1990 and 2000. Of 105 patients, 24 (22.9%) underwent palliative resection, whereas the remainder underwent laparotomy with or without bypass. Some patients received adjuvant chemotherapy. Mean survival was improved in the resected group (13.2 months vs 5.5 months, $P = .006$), mostly in the group who also received adjuvant chemotherapy. Huang and colleagues[55] compared outcomes of palliative gastrectomy to exploratory laparotomy with or without bypass in unresectable gastric cancer. From 1988 to 2008, 365 patients underwent palliative SG (71.5%) or TG (28.5%) and 151 patients underwent exploratory laparotomy with or without gastrojejunostomy. Median overall survival was improved in the resected group (10.2 months vs 4.5 months, $P<.001$), and it was similar between SG and TG (10.3 months vs 8.7 months, $P = .135$). Palliative resection was tolerated better in younger patients. Survival was improved in resected patients even with more than 1 criterion for unresectability having been met. Zhang and colleagues[56] compared outcomes of palliative TG with exploratory laparotomy with or without gastrojejunostomy or no surgery for advanced proximal malignancy. Of 377 patients undergoing surgery, 197 (52.3%) underwent TG, whereas 180 underwent laparotomy with (n = 78) or without (n = 102) bypass. Median survival was improved in the resected group (16.4 months vs 5.8 months gastrojejunostomy, 4.7 months laparotomy only, 5.5 months no surgery; $P<.05$). Based on these data, palliative gastric resection improves median survival, and modern surgical techniques have been able to reduce perioperative morbidity and mortality to acceptable levels. This benefit is presumably due to reduction in overall tumor burden.

The apparent survival benefit from noncurative gastrectomy from these series is attributable to them being performed on patients without widely disseminated disease. Often, survival is worse in patients operated on with palliative intent compared with those who had noncurative nonpalliative resection. This highlights the importance of patient selection for palliative surgery, because increased survival is not a goal of treatment but rather durable symptom improvement. In an effort to more fully evaluate potential benefits from palliative surgery in gastric cancer, Miner and Karpeh[57] performed a partitioned survival analysis, which assesses state of health in relation to treatment, toxicity, and relapse over time. Patient health state was defined in terms of time without symptoms or toxicity (TWiST). Of 307 noncurative resections included in the analysis, 147 (48%) were performed with palliative intent. In the palliative subgroup, patients experienced an average of 8.5 months in the TWiST state. This time was significantly reduced due to high-grade complications, such as unplanned reintervention, ICU admission, or permanent disability (2.1 months, $P = .04$). In addition, patients with multiple sites of metastasis trended toward less time in the TWiST state (4.9 months, $P = .08$). These data demonstrates the importance of appropriate patient selection, indicating that perhaps the most symptomatic patients have the greatest potential benefit. Preoperative counseling is critical in defining treatment goals and minimizing unnecessary treatment toxicity.

Recently, endoscopic stent placement for malignant gastric outlet obstruction (GOO) has gained attention. Maetani and colleagues[58] retrospectively reviewed palliative stent placement versus gastrojejunostomy for GOO; 22 patients with gastric adenocarcinoma and GOO who underwent endoscopic stenting between 1994 and 2004 were compared with 22 contemporary patients who had undergone gastrojejunostomy. Exclusion criteria were prophylactic intervention and the indication for procedure being recurrent cancer. Morbidity was higher among the gastrojejunostomy group (18.2% vs 4.5%, $P = .20$) whereas median survival was similar (90 days vs 65 days, $P = .79$). The stent group, however, had faster return to diet (2 days vs 8 days, $P<.0001$) and shorter median length of stay (19 days vs 28 days, $P = .056$). In this underpowered study, the procedures seemed approximately equivalent in outcomes. Jeurnink and colleagues[59] conducted a multicenter, randomized trial to compare palliative stent placement to gastrojejunostomy for GOO. Between 2006 and 2008, 21 patients underwent stent placement and 18 patients underwent gastrojejunostomy for GOO secondary to various gastrointestinal malignancies, most commonly pancreatic. Despite early advantages in the stent group, such as return to diet (5 days vs 8 days, $P<.01$) and shorter length of stay (7 days vs 15 days, $P = .04$), stents more often had recurrent obstructive symptoms (23.8% vs 5.6%, $P = .02$) and need for reintervention (33.3% vs 11.1%, $P<.01$). In addition, quality of life was initially approximately equal but slightly improved at 5 months in the gastrojejunostomy group. Therefore, stenting is likely more beneficial for patients with a short life expectancy, whereas gastrojejunostomy more often provides durable symptom improvement. Kim and colleagues[60] compared covered and noncovered stents in a prospective, randomized study; 80 patients with gastric adenocarcinoma but no prior gastric surgery were enrolled between 2003 and 2007, 40 in each group. Patency at 8 weeks was similar between covered and noncovered stents (61.3% vs 61.1%). Stent migration, detected by endoscopy, was increased in the covered stent group (25.8% vs 2.8%, $P = .009$), but restenosis from tumor ingrowth was decreased

(0% vs 25.0%, $P = .003$). The investigators could not recommend one type of stent over the other due to their respective trade-offs.

NEOADJUVANT CHEMOTHERAPY

In recent years, much attention has been given to neoadjuvant chemotherapy as an adjunct to potentially curative gastric cancer surgery in an effort to improve outcomes. Hartgrink and colleagues[61] first presented results of a randomized trial to evaluate neoadjuvant administration of 5-fluorouracil, doxorubicin, and methotrexate (FAMTX) in potentially curable gastric cancer. Between 1993 and 1996, 56 eligible patients were enrolled in the study, 27 of whom received preoperative FAMTX. Due to poor enrollment, the study was terminated early. Subsequent analysis showed a lower overall 5-year survival rate in the FAMTX group (21% vs 34%, $P = .17$); this was more pronounced for those who underwent R0 resection (32% vs 53%, $P = .07$). The study was limited by the small sample size, which was an effect of unwillingness to proceed both on providers' and patients' parts. At the time of the study, FAMTX was the chemotherapy regimen of choice, but cisplatin-based regimens soon supplanted it. Cunningham and colleagues[62] were the first to report results of such a regimen in a randomized trial, known as the MAGIC (Medical Research Council Adjuvant Gastric Infusional Chemotherapy) trial, conducted between 1994 and 2002. Patients with potentially curable, at least stage II gastric and distal esophageal adenocarcinoma were randomized to surgery alone (n = 253) or neoadjuvant and adjuvant epirubicin, cisplatin, and 5-fluorouracil (n = 250). Of 209 patients who completed 3 cycles of preoperative chemotherapy and underwent surgery, only 137 (65.6%) began postoperative chemotherapy and only 104 (49.8%) completed all 3 cycles of postoperative chemotherapy. Five-year overall survival was improved in the chemotherapy group (36.3% vs 23.0%, $P = .009$) as was progression-free survival. The neoadjuvant portion was likely responsible for a good deal of the survival benefit seen in this study, because fewer than half of patients assigned to chemotherapy completed all 3 postoperative cycles, and other studies at the time failed to show significant benefit from adjuvant chemotherapy. Schuhmacher and colleagues[63] conducted a randomized trial of cisplatin, folinic acid, and 5-fluorouracil as neoadjuvant treatment. Patients with stages III or stage IV gastric or distal esophageal adenocarcinoma without distant metastasis were randomized to surgery alone (n = 72) or preoperative cisplatin, folinic acid, and 5-fluorouracil (n = 72) between 1999 and 2004. The study was terminated early due to poor enrollment. Of the 72 patients in the chemotherapy group, 70 underwent surgery, but only 45 completed both preoperative cycles of chemotherapy. Intraoperative R0 resection rates were considered equal, but pathology demonstrated an improvement in the chemotherapy group (81.9% vs 66.7%, $P = .036$). However, 5-year overall survival was similar (HR 0.84; 95% CI, 0.52–1.35; $P = .466$). The investigators attributed a lack of demonstrated survival benefit to poor study power, more extensive lymphadenectomy, overall higher tumor stage, and lower rates of completion of neoadjuvant therapy. A similar trial evaluating neoadjuvant 5-fluorouracil and cisplatin was performed by Ychou and colleagues.[64] Between 1995 and 2003, 219 patients who were randomized to surgery alone (n = 110) or surgery with perioperative 5-fluorouracil and cisplatin (n = 109) were eligible for analysis. Some patients in each group underwent postoperative chemotherapy or radiotherapy. The chemotherapy group had improved 5-year overall survival (HR 0.69; 95% CI, 0.50–0.95; $P = .02$) and disease-free survival (HR 0.65; 95% CI, 0.48–0.89; $P = .003$); the overall survival rates were 38% versus 24%, respectively. Yoshikawa and colleagues[65] prospectively evaluated the effectiveness of neoadjuvant chemotherapy in gastric cancer with significant nodal involvement. Patients with gastric adenocarcinoma and bulky N2 disease and/or para-aortic nodal involvement but without more distant disease received preoperative irinotecan and cisplatin between 2000 and 2003. Fifty-patients were enrolled, of whom 41 received the full neoadjuvant course and then underwent radical gastrectomy. The trial was closed prematurely due to high treatment-related mortality (5%). The 3-year overall survival rate was 27%, however, which was better than expected for patients with significant nodal involvement. A prospective randomized phase II trial (COMPASS-D) comparing neoadjuvant S-1 and cisplatin versus S-1, cisplatin, and docetaxel has recently been proposed by Yoshikawa and colleagues.[66]

SUMMARY

Surgical resection remains the only potentially curative treatment of gastric cancer. Newer staging modalities aid in minimizing unnecessary laparotomy in noncurative disease. Adequate lymphadenectomy may improve outcomes, similar to selective resection of adjacent organs based on tumor invasion. Lymph node involvement and positive surgical margins are associated with poorer overall survival. Neoadjuvant chemotherapy may downstage responsive tumors and may improve survival even with extensive lymphatic disease. Palliative surgery for advanced gastric cancer remains important in providing symptom relief in appropriately selected patients.

REFERENCES

1. Jemal A, Bray F, Center MM, et al. Global cancer statistics. CA Cancer J Clin 2011;61(2):69–90.
2. Sobin LH, Compton CC. TNM seventh edition: what's new, what's changed: communication from the International Union Against Cancer and the American Joint Committee on Cancer. Cancer 2010;116(22):5336–9.
3. Washington K. 7th Edition of the AJCC Cancer Staging Manual: Stomach. Ann Surg Oncol 2010;17(12):3077–9.
4. Siewert JR, Stein HJ. Classification of adenocarcinoma of the oesophagogastric junction. Br J Surg 1998;85(11):1457–9.
5. Suh YS, Han DS, Kong SH, et al. Should adenocarcinoma of the esophagogastric junction be classified as esophageal cancer? A comparative analysis according to the seventh AJCC TNM classification. Ann Surg 2012;255(5):908–15.
6. Burke EC, Karpeh MS, Conlon KC, et al. Laparoscopy in the management of gastric adenocarcinoma. Ann Surg 1997;225(3):262–7.
7. Karanicolas PJ, Elkin EB, Jacks LM, et al. Staging laparoscopy in the management of gastric cancer: a population-based analysis. J Am Coll Surg 2011; 213(5):644–51, 651.e1.
8. Power DG, Schattner MA, Gerdes H, et al. Endoscopic ultrasound can improve the selection for laparoscopy in patients with localized gastric cancer. J Am Coll Surg 2009;208(2):173–8.
9. Smith A, Finch MD, John TG, et al. Role of laparoscopic ultrasonography in the management of patients with oesophagogastric cancer. Br J Surg 1999;86(8):1083–7.
10. Hulscher JB, Nieveen van Dijkum EJ, de Wit LT, et al. Laparoscopy and laparoscopic ultrasonography in staging carcinoma of the gastric cardia. Eur J Surg 2000;166(11):862–5.
11. Bentrem D, Wilton A, Mazumdar M, et al. The value of peritoneal cytology as a preoperative predictor in patients with gastric carcinoma undergoing a curative resection. Ann Surg Oncol 2005;12(5):347–53.

12. Mezhir JJ, Shah MA, Jacks LM, et al. Positive peritoneal cytology in patients with gastric cancer: natural history and outcome of 291 patients. Ann Surg Oncol 2010;17(12):3173–80.

13. Gouzi JL, Huguier M, Fagniez PL, et al. Total versus subtotal gastrectomy for adenocarcinoma of the gastric antrum. A French prospective controlled study. Ann Surg 1989;209(2):162–6.

14. Bozzetti F, Marubini E, Bonfanti G, et al. Total versus subtotal gastrectomy: surgical morbidity and mortality rates in a multicenter Italian randomized trial. The Italian Gastrointestinal Tumor Study Group. Ann Surg 1997;226(5):613–20.

15. Bozzetti F, Marubini E, Bonfanti G, et al. Subtotal versus total gastrectomy for gastric cancer: five-year survival rates in a multicenter randomized Italian trial. Italian Gastrointestinal Tumor Study Group. Ann Surg 1999;230(2):170–8.

16. de Manzoni G, Verlato G, Roviello F, et al. Subtotal versus total gastrectomy for T3 adenocarcinoma of the antrum. Gastric Cancer 2003;6(4):237–42.

17. Davies J, Johnston D, Sue-Ling H, et al. Total or subtotal gastrectomy for gastric carcinoma? A study of quality of life. World J Surg 1998;22(10):1048–55.

18. Harrison LE, Karpeh MS, Brennan MF. Total gastrectomy is not necessary for proximal gastric cancer. Surgery 1998;123(2):127–30.

19. Kim JH, Park SS, Kim J, et al. Surgical outcomes for gastric cancer in the upper third of the stomach. World J Surg 2006;30(10):1870–6 [discussion: 1877–8].

20. An JY, Youn HG, Choi MG, et al. The difficult choice between total and proximal gastrectomy in proximal early gastric cancer. Am J Surg 2008;196(4):587–91.

21. Yu W, Choi GS, Chung HY. Randomized clinical trial of splenectomy versus splenic preservation in patients with proximal gastric cancer. Br J Surg 2006; 93(5):559–63.

22. Shchepotin IB, Chorny VA, Nauta RJ, et al. Extended surgical resection in T4 gastric cancer. Am J Surg 1998;175(2):123–6.

23. Martin RC 2nd, Jaques DP, Brennan MF, et al. Extended local resection for advanced gastric cancer: increased survival versus increased morbidity. Ann Surg 2002;236(2):159–65.

24. Kobayashi A, Nakagohri T, Konishi M, et al. Aggressive surgical treatment for T4 gastric cancer. J Gastrointest Surg 2004;8(4):464–70.

25. Kunisaki C, Akiyama H, Nomura M, et al. Surgical outcomes in patients with T4 gastric carcinoma. J Am Coll Surg 2006;202(2):223–30.

26. Carboni F, Lepiane P, Santoro R, et al. Extended multiorgan resection for T4 gastric carcinoma: 25-year experience. J Surg Oncol 2005;90(2):95–100.

27. Ito H, Clancy TE, Osteen RT, et al. Adenocarcinoma of the gastric cardia: what is the optimal surgical approach? J Am Coll Surg 2004;199(6):880–6.

28. Huscher CG, Mingoli A, Sgarzini G, et al. Laparoscopic versus open subtotal gastrectomy for distal gastric cancer: five-year results of a randomized prospective trial. Ann Surg 2005;241(2):232–7.

29. Lee WJ, Wang W, Chen TC, et al. Totally laparoscopic radical BII gastrectomy for the treatment of gastric cancer: a comparison with open surgery. Surg Laparosc Endosc Percutan Tech 2008;18(4):369–74.

30. Moisan F, Norero E, Slako M, et al. Completely laparoscopic versus open gastrectomy for early and advanced gastric cancer: a matched cohort study. Surg Endosc 2012;26(3):661–72.

31. Ahn SH, Lee JH, Park DJ, et al. Comparative study of clinical outcomes between laparoscopy-assisted proximal gastrectomy (LAPG) and laparoscopy-assisted total gastrectomy (LATG) for proximal gastric cancer. Gastric Cancer 2012. [Epub ahead of print].

32. Nakajima T. Gastric cancer treatment guidelines in Japan. Gastric Cancer 2002; 5(1):1–5.

33. Ishikawa S, Togashi A, Inoue M, et al. Indications for EMR/ESD in cases of early gastric cancer: relationship between histological type, depth of wall invasion, and lymph node metastasis. Gastric Cancer 2007;10(1):35–8.

34. Bonenkamp JJ, Songun I, Hermans J, et al. Randomised comparison of morbidity after D1 and D2 dissection for gastric cancer in 996 Dutch patients. Lancet 1995; 345(8952):745–8.

35. Bonenkamp JJ, Hermans J, Sasako M, et al. Extended lymph-node dissection for gastric cancer. N Engl J Med 1999;340(12):908–14.

36. Hartgrink HH, van de Velde CJ, Putter H, et al. Extended lymph node dissection for gastric cancer: who may benefit? Final results of the randomized Dutch gastric cancer group trial. J Clin Oncol 2004;22(11):2069–77.

37. Songun I, Putter H, Kranenbarg EM, et al. Surgical treatment of gastric cancer: 15-year follow-up results of the randomised nationwide Dutch D1D2 trial. Lancet Oncol 2010;11(5):439–49.

38. Cuschieri A, Fayers P, Fielding J, et al. Postoperative morbidity and mortality after D1 and D2 resections for gastric cancer: preliminary results of the MRC randomised controlled surgical trial. The Surgical Cooperative Group. Lancet 1996; 347(9007):995–9.

39. Cuschieri A, Weeden S, Fielding J, et al. Patient survival after D1 and D2 resections for gastric cancer: long-term results of the MRC randomized surgical trial. Surgical Co-operative Group. Br J Cancer 1999;79(9–10):1522–30.

40. Edwards P, Blackshaw GRJC, Lewis WG, et al. Prospective comparison of D1 vs modified D2 gastrectomy for carcinoma. Br J Cancer 2004;90(10):1888–92.

41. Degiuli M, Sasako M, Ponti A, et al. Morbidity and mortality after D2 gastrectomy for gastric cancer: results of the Italian Gastric Cancer Study Group prospective multicenter surgical study. J Clin Oncol 1998;16(4):1490–3.

42. Degiuli M, Sasako M, Ponti A, et al. Survival results of a multicentre phase II study to evaluate D2 gastrectomy for gastric cancer. Br J Cancer 2004;90(9): 1727–32.

43. Degiuli M, Sasako M, Ponti A. Morbidity and mortality in the Italian Gastric Cancer Study Group randomized clinical trial of D1 versus D2 resection for gastric cancer. Br J Surg 2010;97(5):643–9.

44. Sasako M, Sano T, Yamamoto S, et al. D2 lymphadenectomy alone or with para-aortic nodal dissection for gastric cancer. N Engl J Med 2008;359(5):453–62.

45. Shen JG, Cheong JH, Hyung WJ, et al. Influence of a microscopic positive proximal margin in the treatment of gastric adenocarcinoma of the cardia. World J Gastroenterol 2006;12(24):3883–6.

46. Cho BC, Jeung HC, Choi HJ, et al. Prognostic impact of resection margin involvement after extended (D2/D3) gastrectomy for advanced gastric cancer: a 15-year experience at a single institute. J Surg Oncol 2007;95(6):461–8.

47. Sun Z, Li DM, Wang ZN, et al. Prognostic significance of microscopic positive margins for gastric cancer patients with potentially curative resection. Ann Surg Oncol 2009;16(11):3028–37.

48. Miner TJ, Brennan MF, Jaques DP. A prospective, symptom related, outcomes analysis of 1022 palliative procedures for advanced cancer. Ann Surg 2004; 240(4):719–26 [discussion: 726–7].

49. Miner TJ, Cohen J, Charpentier K, et al. The palliative triangle: improved patient selection and outcomes associated with palliative operations. Arch Surg 2011; 146(5):517–22.

50. Miner TJ, Jaques DP, Karpeh MS, et al. Defining palliative surgery in patients receiving noncurative resections for gastric cancer. J Am Coll Surg 2004;198(6): 1013–21.

51. Sarela AI, Miner TJ, Karpeh MS, et al. Clinical outcomes with laparoscopic stage M1, unresected gastric adenocarcinoma. Ann Surg 2006;243(2):189–95.

52. Hartgrink HH, Putter H, Kranenbarg EK, et al. Value of palliative resection in gastric cancer. Br J Surg 2002;89(11):1438–43.

53. Samarasam I, Chandran S, Sitaram V, et al. Palliative gastrectomy in advanced gastric cancer: is it worthwhile? ANZ J Surg 2006;76(1–2):60–3.

54. Saidi RF, ReMine SG, Dudrick PS, et al. Is there a role for palliative gastrectomy in patients with stage IV gastric cancer? World J Surg 2006;30(1):21–7.

55. Huang KH, Wu CW, Fang WL, et al. Palliative resection in noncurative gastric cancer patients. World J Surg 2010;34(5):1015–21.

56. Zhang JZ, Lu HS, Huang CM, et al. Outcome of palliative total gastrectomy for stage IV proximal gastric cancer. Am J Surg 2011;202(1):91–6.

57. Miner TJ, Karpeh MS. Gastrectomy for gastric cancer: defining critical elements of patient selection and outcome assessment. Surg Oncol Clin N Am 2004;13(3): 455–66, viii.

58. Maetani I, Akatsuka S, Ikeda M, et al. Self-expandable metallic stent placement for palliation in gastric outlet obstructions caused by gastric cancer: a comparison with surgical gastrojejunostomy. J Gastroenterol 2005;40(10):932–7.

59. Jeurnink SM, Steyerberg EW, van Hooft JE, et al. Surgical gastrojejunostomy or endoscopic stent placement for the palliation of malignant gastric outlet obstruction (SUSTENT study): a multicenter randomized trial. Gastrointest Endosc 2010; 71(3):490–9.

60. Kim CG, Choi IJ, Lee JY, et al. Covered versus uncovered self-expandable metallic stents for palliation of malignant pyloric obstruction in gastric cancer patients: a randomized, prospective study. Gastrointest Endosc 2010;72(1):25–32.

61. Hartgrink HH, van de Velde CJH, Putter H, et al. Neo-adjuvant chemotherapy for operable gastric cancer: long term results of the Dutch randomised FAMTX trial. Eur J Surg Oncol 2004;30(6):643–9.

62. Cunningham D, Allum WH, Stenning SP, et al. Perioperative chemotherapy versus surgery alone for resectable gastroesophageal cancer. N Engl J Med 2006; 355(1):11–20.

63. Schuhmacher C, Gretschel S, Lordick F, et al. Neoadjuvant chemotherapy compared with surgery alone for locally advanced cancer of the stomach and cardia: European Organisation for Research and Treatment of Cancer randomized trial 40954. J Clin Oncol 2010;28(35):5210–8.

64. Ychou M, Boige V, Pignon JP, et al. Perioperative chemotherapy compared with surgery alone for resectable gastroesophageal adenocarcinoma: an FNCLCC and FFCD multicenter phase III trial. J Clin Oncol 2011;29(13):1715–21.

65. Yoshikawa T, Sasako M, Yamamoto S, et al. Phase II study of neoadjuvant chemotherapy and extended surgery for locally advanced gastric cancer. Br J Surg 2009;96(9):1015–22.

66. Yoshikawa T, Taguri M, Sakuramoto S, et al. A comparison of multimodality treatment: two and four courses of neoadjuvant chemotherapy using S-1/CDDP or S-1/CDDP/docetaxel followed by surgery and S-1 adjuvant chemotherapy for macroscopically resectable serosa-positive gastric cancer: a randomized phase II trial (COMPASS-D trial). Jpn J Clin Oncol 2012;42(1):74–7.

Modern Oncological Approaches to Gastric Adenocarcinoma

Roopma Wadhwa, MD, MHA, Takashi Taketa, MD,
Kazuki Sudo, MD, Mariela A. Blum, MD, Jaffer A. Ajani, MD*

KEYWORDS

- Gastric cancer • Gastric adenocarcinoma • Multidisciplinary approach
- Perioperative • Chemoradiation • Adjuvant therapy

KEY POINTS

- Gastric cancer (GC) is the fourth most common cancer in men and the fifth most common cancer in women worldwide.
- Surgery is the key for curing patients with localized GC. However, surgery alone is insufficient to achieve the highest possible cure rate, which can be obtained by the addition of adjunctive therapies.
- Advanced GC is an incurable condition; however, it is now possible to prolong survival with oncologic therapies.
- Patients with advanced GC with Her2-neu protein overexpression can benefit from the addition of trastuzumab to combination chemotherapy.
- Improved therapy will likely result from a better understanding of the molecular pathways in GC.

INTRODUCTION

GC is frequently diagnosed in the advanced stage and is associated with a poor prognosis. The incidence of GC still remains high, and there are many endemic areas in the world. Annually, the estimated number of new GC cases worldwide is 640,600 for men and 349,000 for women.[1] In 2012, approximately 21,320 new cases were likely to be diagnosed and 10,540 patients were expected to die in the United

---

This work was supported in part by The Park Family, Caporella Family, Bikoff Family, Cantu Family, Fairman Family, Dallas Family, Oaks Family, Sultan Family, Dio Family, Frazier Family, the Kevin Fund, the Schecter Private Foundation, and the Rivercreek Foundation.
Department of Gastrointestinal Medical Oncology, The University of Texas MD Anderson Cancer Center, 1515 Holcombe Boulevard, Houston, TX 77030, USA
* Corresponding author. Department of Gastrointestinal Medical Oncology, Unit 426, The University of Texas MD Anderson Cancer Center, 1515 Holcombe Boulevard, Houston, TX 77030.
E-mail address: jajani@mdanderson.org

Gastroenterol Clin N Am 42 (2013) 359–369
http://dx.doi.org/10.1016/j.gtc.2013.01.011
0889-8553/13/$ – see front matter © 2013 Elsevier Inc. All rights reserved.

gastro.theclinics.com

States.[2] Localized GC (LGC) is a potentially curable condition, and surgery plays a major role in the achievement of cure. The cure rates from surgery vary considerably with regions but are predominantly based on the surgical stage of LGC; however, surgical technique and surgical volume (of a center and surgeon) highly contribute to the cure rates (as well as the rates of complications and mortality). Advanced GC (AGC) is a treatable but not curable condition. AGC and LGC are highly heterogeneous (driven by patient and tumor genetic differences). In this regard, discovery of tumor subsets defined by their molecular subtypes (eg, Her2-neu overexpressing tumors vs those that do not overexpress Her2-neu) is likely to drive the direction of future research and to set the stage for improved and individualized therapies. This review highlights the current therapeutic strategies for LGC and AGC.

LOCALIZED GASTRIC CANCER (LGC)

Baseline clinical stage should be established meticulously.[3] Although baseline clinical stage is not as highly associated with long-term outcome as the surgical pathology stage,[4] the baseline clinical stage does help to define the short-term therapeutic strategy. It is important to emphasize that physician(s) from one discipline (eg, a gastroenterologist or a surgeon) should not decide the initial therapeutic strategy of LGC but that a consensus decision, derived from a multidisciplinary discussion of the baseline staging of patients with LGC, should be reached because this is likely to provide the highest benefit to a patient.[3,5]

Once it is established that the patient has LGC, the therapeutic plan should include adjunctive strategy for most patients (an example of an exception would be an LGC <3 cm in diameter and ≤T1bN0). The preferred adjunctive strategy differs by region worldwide, reflecting differences in practice patterns. The extent of lymphadenopathy also varies, and it is usually suboptimal in most areas of the world where GC is not highly prevalent. Surgery remains the best contributor to the cure rate, and when surgery is not done or not possible, one can anticipate a dismal outcome.[6] In the following section we discuss adjunctive strategies.

ADJUNCTIVE STRATEGIES
Postoperative Adjuvant Chemoradiation

The most important study that established this strategy firmly in the West is the Intergroup 0116 trial, headed by the Southwest Oncology Group.[7] This trial was based on prior nonrandomized observations in patients with LGC who received chemoradiation therapy. This trial was a phase 3 study that compared observation after surgery (control) with chemoradiation adjuvant after following surgery (experimental arm).[7]

Three other relevant studies are worth mentioning. The CALGB-driven intergroup adjuvant trial did not take advantage of improving chemoradiation efforts and instead compared fluorouracil to the combination of epirubicin/cisplatin/fluorouracil and demonstrated no advantage with the latter.[9] The second study was a retrospective comparison of 2 patient populations (one group had surgery and the other had surgery plus chemoradiation), and this comparison demonstrated benefit for the chemoradiation group.[10] However, the use of a retrospective design greatly limits this conclusion. The third study was a prospective comparison in patients with LGC who had an excellent D2 dissection (median number of nodes evaluated was >30). In this ARTIST trial (Adjuvant Chemoradiation Therapy in Stomach Cancer), both group of patients were treated after surgery (chemotherapy vs chemoradiation).[11] The primary analysis of

---

Key points about the INT0116 trial

- Recruitment duration: 1991–1998

- Total number of patients enrolled: 603

- Number of eligible patients: 559

- Criteria for eligibility: R0 resection for LGC (clinical stage ranged from IA to IV [but M0])

- High-risk LGC; 85% patients had lymph node metastases and more than 65% had a T3 primary

- Of the 559 patients, 282 were randomized to the experimental arm and 227 were randomized to the control arm

- The cure rate was significantly higher in the experimental arm (median 36 vs 27 months, $P = .005$) and included improved local control (30 vs 19 months, $P = .001$)

- Inadequate surgery (54% having a D0 nodal dissection) reflected the standard of surgery at the community level in the United States at that time

- Results have prevailed after more than 10 years of follow-up[8]

---

this study demonstrated no benefit for the group that received chemoradiation; however, an unplanned subgroup analysis (an ad hoc strategy that is generally questionable and often considered unreliable) demonstrated benefit for node-positive patients.[11] The ARTIST trial therefore casts doubt on the benefit from chemoradiation when high-quality surgery is performed.

Postoperative Chemotherapy

In the West, where surgery is often suboptimal, trials have not shown a significant benefit for adjuvant chemotherapy.[12] In addition to having inadequate surgery, most studies in the West have been underpowered and suboptimally conceived and/or executed.

In Southeast Asia, where the GC surgical standards are usually excellent, 2 prospective randomized well-conceived and well-executed trials have demonstrated benefit from adjuvant chemotherapy. The ACTS-GC trial (Adjuvant Chemotherapy Trial of TS-1 for Gastric Cancer) was conducted in 1059 Japanese patients with LGC, and patients were randomized to 1 year of an oral fluoropyrimidine, S-1, or observation only. The primary analysis demonstrated a 33% improvement in overall survival for the S-1 group.[13] In addition, these results held up with longer follow-up.[14] The CLASSIC trial (Capecitabine and Oxaliplatin Adjuvant Study in Stomach Cancer) randomized 1035 patients with LGC to capecitabine plus cisplatin as adjuvant for 6 months follow-up after surgery and demonstrated 44% improvement in disease-free survival (its primary end point) for the chemotherapy group versus the group that underwent surgery only.[15] Overall survival data are still pending.

Although meta-analyses have demonstrated some benefit for systemic adjuvant chemotherapy, they do not establish a standard of care and are limited by multiple design weaknesses.[16]

Perioperative or Preoperative Chemotherapy

The MAGIC (Medical Research Council Adjuvant Gastric Infusional Chemotherapy) trial established the evidence for the use of perioperative (or preoperative) chemotherapy over surgery alone in the West.[17]

Key points about the MAGIC trial

- Total number of patients randomized: 504
- Eligibility: R0 resection of LGC or gastroesophageal junction adenocarcinoma (15%) patients
- Experimental arm: epirubicin, cisplatin, and fluorouracil before and after surgery
- Control arm: follow-up after surgery
- Results: a 25% reduction in risk of death and 13% improvement in 5-year survival rates (hazard ratio = 1.31, 95% confidence interval = 1.08–1.61)

This trial had several limitations including inadequate staging, poor surgical technique, and poor outcome of the control group. Also, it confirmed previous findings that this group of patients cannot tolerate postoperative combination chemotherapy.

A second trial of preoperative chemotherapy was terminated prematurely because of poor accrual. This French trial (ACCORD07-FFCD 9703) had relatively few (25%) patients with LGC, and it randomized patients to cisplatin/fluorouracil versus observation after surgery.[18] Even with a small sample size, patients who had chemotherapy benefited.

Whether a preoperative treatment strategy is applicable to patients with LGC who have excellent surgery is the subject of the PRODIGY (Docetaxel+Oxaliplatin+S-1 [DOS] Regimen as Neoadjuvant Chemotherapy in Advanced Gastric Cancer) trial (preoperative docetaxel, oxaliplatin, and S-1 followed by postoperative S-1 vs postoperative S-1 for patients with D2 resection; NCT01515748; also see **Table 1**).

A hybrid trial is now enrolling patients combining the preoperative chemotherapy and postoperative chemoradiation strategies. The CRITICS (ChemoRadiotherapy after Induction chemo Therapy in Cancer of the Stomach) trial[19] is randomly assigning patients to perioperative (preoperative) chemotherapy with or without adjuvant chemoradiation.

Even with adjunctive approaches, the outcome of patients with LGC remains unsatisfactory and more research remains to be done.

ADVANCED GC (AGC)

There are only a few agents that are associated with level 1 evidence for an overall survival advantage in AGC. These are docetaxel,[20] cisplatin,[21] and trastuzumab.[22]

It is also clear that giving 2 cytotoxic agents together is better than giving one alone.[21] Whether there is an additional advantage from combining 3 cytotoxic agents is often debated, but it is likely minor. From a drug development perspective, most regulatory agencies currently accept a 2-cytotoxic-agent combination of a platinum compound and a fluoropyrimidine.

The subject of future research should be to establish patient subsets, based on the molecular subtypes of GC. The following section provides a rationale for this approach in focusing on the genes and pathways that seem important in GC.

IMPORTANT GENES AND PATHWAYS IN GC

Alterations in the following pathways seem important in the pathobiology of GC: ERBB2 (Her-2), angiogenesis, phosphatidyl inositol-3-kinase (PI3K)-AKT-mammalian target of rapamycin (mTOR), c-MET, and fibroblast growth factor receptor 2 (FGFR2). However, further research is expected to uncover more targets.

Anti-EGFR Therapy/Anti-Her2 Therapy

The epidermal growth factor receptor (EGFR) belongs to the erbB receptor family. EGFR is a prognosticator in GC, but targeting EGFR has proven to be fruitless in AGC. On the contrary, the Her-2 neu protein is overexpressed in 9% to 38% of AGCs[23–25] and has turned out to be not only prognostic[26] but also a good target for gaining therapeutic advantage.[22] The ToGA trial (Trastuzumab for Gastric Cancer)[22] enriched patients with AGC by Her-2 overexpression and randomized patients to chemotherapy versus chemotherapy plus trastuzumab. Of 810 Her-2 positive patients, 584 were randomized. Overall survival was prolonged from 10 to 13 months (hazard ratio 0.77) with the addition of trastuzumab. The tolerance was excellent. However, an updated survival analysis of the ToGA data performed by the US Food and Drug Administration shows a much reduced overall survival benefit for patients who received trastuzumab. (http://www.fda.gov/AboutFDA/CentersOffices/OfficeofMedicalProductsandTobacco/CDER/ucm230418.htm; viewed January 1, 2013).

Lapatinib, an orally active tyrosine kinase inhibitor of EGFR types 1 and 2, is currently under investigation (ClinicalTrials.gov identifier:NCT00486954).

c-MET Pathway

Met is a membrane receptor that is required for wound healing and embryogenesis. Hepatocyte growth factor (scatter factor) has tyrosine kinase activity and is the ligand for c-MET. c-MET, being an oncogene facilitates invasion, migration, and angiogenesis. c-MET gene amplification (3%–10%), mutation (2%–5%), and total c-MET overexpression (40%) have all been described in GC.[27] Patients with AGC with c-MET amplification have shorter disease-free interval after resection.[28]

Graziano and colleagues[29] in a retrospective study of 230 cases showed that about 10% of these patients had c-MET amplification and that a higher copy number was associated with poor outcome. Drugs such as PHA-665752 and foretinib, a tyrosine kinase inhibitor, among others are under development.[30,31]

Rilotumumab, a monoclonal antibody, has shown activity against GCs that have total c-MET overexpression.[32] This agent has entered a phase 3 trial.

FGFR Pathway

FGFR, another oncogene, regulates cell proliferation, differentiation, and survival and thus plays a role in angiogenesis and wound repair.[33] GC cells with FGFR overexpression are sensitive to FGFR inhibitors.[34] Dovitinib, a vascular endothelial growth factor receptor/FGFR2 inhibitor has also shown efficacy in FGFR-amplified GCs.[35] Other genes in this pathway, including *GATA4, GATA6, and KLF5*, are frequently amplified in GC.[35]

Vascular Endothelial Growth Factor-Targeted Therapy/Angiogenesis Inhibitors

The AVAGAST (Avastin in Gastric Cancer) trial, conducted on 774 patients, that randomized patients to chemotherapy with or without bevacizumab did not demonstrate a benefit from the addition of bevacizumab.[36] In contrast with the ToGA trial, AVAGAST did not enrich patients by any specific biomarker. Validated angiogenesis biomarkers do not currently exist and need to be developed.

In addition to these pathways, the PI3K/AKT/mTOR axis seems very important in GC. This axis is not described in detail in this review because of its complexity. This axis is being targeted in patients with AGC, although a phase 3 trial of everolimus has given negative results in patients with AGC.[37]

Table 1
Ongoing Phase 3 Clinical Trials for Gastric Cancer

Trial	Intervention	Primary Outcome, Enrollment	Estimated Start Date–End Date	Location (Countries)
CRITICS study NCT00407186	Chemoradiotherapy(45 Gy in 5 wk with daily CDDP and XELODA) after preoperative chemotherapy (3x ECC) and adequate (D1+) surgery vs postoperative chemotherapy (3x ECC)	OS 788	December 2006–June 2013	Netherlands
NCT01512745	Oral apatinib vs placebo	PFS, OS 270	January 2011–June 2012	China
NCT01671449	SC vs SOX	PFS 338	December 2012–December 2015	Republic of Korea
NCT01099085	XELODA/CDDP + simvastatin vs XELODA/CDDP + placebo	PFS 244	February 2009–May 2013	Republic of Korea
NCT01534546	Perioperative SOX vs SOX or XELOX as postoperative chemotherapy	3-yr DFS 1059	March 2012–September 2014	China
Japan Clinical Oncology Group Study (JCOG 0501) NCT00252161	Surgery vs neoadjuvant chemotherapy (TS-1 + CDDP) + surgery	OS 316	November 2005–April 2015	Japan
NCT01711242	XELOX vs XELOX + radiotherapy	3-yr DFS 300	January 2012–December 2015	China
NCT01470742	XELOX vs XELODA	OS 200	September 2010–???	Republic of Korea
PRODIGY trial NCT01515748	DOS + surgery + S-1 vs surgery + adjuvant S-1	3-yr PFS 640	January 2012–December 2017	Republic of Korea
NCT01248403	Paclitaxel + placebo vs paclitaxel + RAD001	OS 500	October 2011–January 2016	Germany

NCT number	Intervention	Outcome / N	Dates	Location
NCT01283217	DS vs SP	3-yr DFS 166	March 2010–March 2016	Republic of Korea
NCT01468389	Taxanes or platinum in combination with XELODA vs chemotherapy followed by XELODA alone	PFS 300	Nov 2011–January 2013	China
NCT01285557	S-1/CDDP vs fluorouracil/CDDP	OS 500	February 2011–June 2014	Multinational; United States and others
NCT01662869	Drug: onartuzumab Drug: placebo Drug: FOLFOX6	OS 800	November 2012–February 2016	Multinational
NCT01697072	Drug: rilotumumab Other: placebo	OS 450	October 2012–December 2015	United States, Australia, Canada
NCT01641939	Trastuzumab emtansine vs taxane	OS 412	September 2012–September 2015	Multinational
NCT00450203	ECX + bevacizumab vs ECX	Safety, efficacy, OS 1100	October 2007–December 2014	United Kingdom
NCT01516944	Perop S-1 + oxaliplatin vs XELOX	DFS 729	February 2012–December 2015	China
NCT01523015	Preoperative chemotherapy- and chemoradiotherapy followed by surgery vs surgery	Pathologic response to treatment 100	January 2012–December 2015	Poland
NCT01450696	Drug: trastuzumab [Herceptin] Drug: XELODA Drug: CDDP	OS 400	December 2011–June 2020	multinational
NCT01748851	XELOX vs FOLFOX	PFS 438	December 2012–December 2015	Republic of Korea

Abbreviations: CDDP, cisplatin; DFS, disease-free survival; DOS, docetaxel + oxaliplatin + S-1; DS, docetaxel and S1; ECC, epirubicin, cisplatin, and capecitabine; ECX, epirubicin hydrochloride, cisplatin, and capecitabine; FOLFOX6, 5-fluorouracil, folinic acid, and oxaliplatin; OS, overall survival; PFS, progression-free survival; RAD001, everolimus; S-1, tegafur, gimeracil, and oteracil potassium; SC, S-1 and cisplatin; SOX, S-1 and oxaliplatin; SP, S1 and cisplatin; XELODA, capecitabine; XELOX, oxaliplatin with capecitabine; 3x, 3 cycles.

SUMMARY

When evaluating newly diagnosed patients with GC, one must first establish whether a patient has AGC or LGC. Patients with LGC must undergo multidisciplinary evaluation and discussion before starting therapy. Surgery alone is inadequate in most patients with LGC, and adjunctive therapies should be considered. Surgery should be performed by an experienced high-volume surgeon, and at least 15 nodes must be evaluated.

For patients with AGC, much more research focusing on the molecular biology of GC and the patient's underlying genetics is needed. At present, palliative therapy consists of combination cytotoxic therapy (2 cytotoxic drugs are preferred over 3 cytotoxic drugs in most patients), and trastuzumab should be added if the GC overexpresses the Her2 protein. **Table 1** highlights the currently ongoing phase 3 trials for patients with LGC or AGC.

REFERENCES

1. Siegel R, Ward E, Brawley O, et al. Cancer statistics, 2011: the impact of eliminating socioeconomic and racial disparities on premature cancer deaths. CA Cancer J Clin 2011;61(4):212–36. http://dx.doi.org/10.3322/caac.20121. Available at: http://www.ncbi.nlm.nih.gov/pubmed/21685461. Accessed November 19, 2012.
2. Siegel R, Naishadham D, Jemal A. Cancer statistics, 2012. CA Cancer J Clin 2012;62(1):10–29. http://dx.doi.org/10.3322/caac.20138. Available at: http://www.ncbi.nlm.nih.gov/pubmed/22237781. Accessed November 19, 2012.
3. Ajani JA, Barthel JS, Bekaii-Saab T, et al. Gastric cancer. J Natl Compr Canc Netw 2010;8(4):378–409. Available at: http://www.jnccn.org/content/8/4/378.long. Accessed October 24, 2012.
4. Rohatgi PR, Mansfield PF, Crane CH, et al. Surgical pathology stage by American Joint Commission on Cancer criteria predicts patient survival after preoperative chemoradiation for localized gastric carcinoma. Cancer 2006;107(7):1475–82. Available at: http://www.ncbi.nlm.nih.gov/pubmed/16944539. Accessed October 23, 2012.
5. Stephens MR, Lewis WG, Brewster AE, et al. Multidisciplinary team management is associated with improved outcomes after surgery for esophageal cancer. Dis Esophagus 2006;19(3):164–71. http://dx.doi.org/10.1111/j.1442-2050.2006.00559.x. Available at: http://www.ncbi.nlm.nih.gov/pubmed/16722993. Accessed November 12, 2012.
6. Suzuki A, Xiao L, Taketa T, et al. Localized gastric cancer treated with chemoradiation without surgery: UTMD Anderson Cancer Center experience. Oncology 2012;82(6):347–51. http://dx.doi.org/10.1159/000338318 000338318. Available at: http://www.ncbi.nlm.nih.gov/pubmed/22677933.
7. Macdonald JS, Smalley SR, Benedetti J, et al. Chemoradiotherapy after surgery compared with surgery alone for adenocarcinoma of the stomach or gastroesophageal junction. N Engl J Med 2001;345(10):725–30. Available at: http://www.ncbi.nlm.nih.gov/pubmed/11547741. Accessed October 10, 2012.
8. Smalley SR, Benedetti JK, Haller DG, et al. Updated analysis of SWOG-directed intergroup study 0116: a phase III trial of adjuvant radiochemotherapy versus observation after curative gastric cancer resection. J Clin Oncol 2012;30(19):2327–33. http://dx.doi.org/10.1200/jco.2011.36.7136. Available at: http://jco.ascopubs.org/content/30/19/2327.full.pdf; http://www.ncbi.nlm.nih.gov/pubmed/22585691. Accessed November 12, 2012.

9. Fuchs CS, Tepper JE, Niedzwiecki D, et al. Postoperative adjuvant chemoradiation for gastric or gastroesophageal junction adenocarcinoma using epirubicin, cisplatin, infusional fluourouracil before and after infusional fluorouracil and radiotherapy compared with bolus fluorouracil/leucovorin before and after chemoradiation. Intergroup trial CALGC 80101 [abstract no. 4003]. J Clin Oncol 2011;29.

10. Kim S, Lim DH, Lee J, et al. An observational study suggesting clinical benefit for adjuvant postoperative chemoradiation in a population of over 500 cases after gastric resection with D2 nodal dissection for adenocarcinoma of the stomach. Int J Radiat Oncol Biol Phys 2005;63(5):1279–85. http://dx.doi.org/10.1016/j.ijrobp.2005.05.005. Available at: http://www.ncbi.nlm.nih.gov/pubmed/16099596. Accessed November 15, 2012.

11. Lee J, Lim do H, Kim S, et al. Phase III trial comparing capecitabine plus cisplatin versus capecitabine plus cisplatin with concurrent capecitabine radiotherapy in completely resected gastric cancer with D2 lymph node dissection: the ARTIST rial. J Clin Oncol 2012;30(3):268–73. http://dx.doi.org/10.1200/JCO.2011.39.1953. Available at: http://www.ncbi.nlm.nih.gov/pubmed/22184384. Accessed November 1, 2012.

12. Yao JC, Ajani JA. Gastric cancer. Curr Opin Gastroenterol 2000;16(6):516–21. Available at: http://www.ncbi.nlm.nih.gov/pubmed/17031130. Accessed October 23, 2012.

13. Sakuramoto S, Sasako M, Yamaguchi T, et al. Adjuvant chemotherapy for gastric cancer with S-1, an oral fluoropyrimidine. N Engl J Med 2007;357(18):1810–20. Available at: http://www.ncbi.nlm.nih.gov/pubmed/17978289. Accessed November 12, 2012.

14. Sasako M, Sakuramoto S, Katai H, et al. Five-year outcomes of a randomized phase III trial comparing adjuvant chemotherapy with S-1 versus surgery alone in stage II or III gastric cancer. J Clin Oncol 2011;29(33):4387–93. http://dx.doi.org/10.1200/JCO.2011.36.5908. Available at: http://www.ncbi.nlm.nih.gov/pubmed/22010012. Accessed December 1, 2012.

15. Bang YJ, Kim YW, Yang HK, et al. Adjuvant capecitabine and oxaliplatin for gastric cancer after D2 gastrectomy (CLASSIC): a phase 3 open-label, randomised controlled trial. Lancet 2012. http://dx.doi.org/10.1016/S0140-6736(11)61873-4. Available at: http://www.ncbi.nlm.nih.gov/pubmed/22226517. Accessed October 2, 2012.

16. Paoletti X, Oba K, Burzykowski T, et al. Benefit of adjuvant chemotherapy for resectable gastric cancer: a meta-analysis. JAMA 2010;303(17):1729–37. http://dx.doi.org/10.1001/jama.2010.534. Available at: http://www.ncbi.nlm.nih.gov/pubmed/20442389. Accessed November 12, 2012.

17. Cunningham D, Allum WH, Stenning SP, et al. Perioperative chemotherapy versus surgery alone for resectable gastroesophageal cancer. N Engl J Med 2006;355(1):11–20.

18. Ychou M, Boige V, Pignon JP, et al. Perioperative chemotherapy compared with surgery alone for resectable gastroesophageal adenocarcinoma: an FNCLCC and FFCD multicenter phase III trial. J Clin Oncol 2011;29(13):1715–21. http://dx.doi.org/10.1200/JCO.2010.33.0597. Available at: http://www.ncbi.nlm.nih.gov/pubmed/21444866; http://jco.ascopubs.org/content/29/13/1715.full.pdf. Accessed November 12, 2012.

19. Dikken JL, van Sandick JW, Maurits Swellengrebel HA, et al. Neo-adjuvant chemotherapy followed by surgery and chemotherapy or by surgery and chemoradiotherapy for patients with resectable gastric cancer (CRITICS). BMC Cancer 2011;11:329. http://dx.doi.org/10.1186/1471-2407-11-329. Available

at: http://www.ncbi.nlm.nih.gov/pubmed/21810227; http://www.biomedcentral. com/1471-2407/11/329. Accessed October 2, 2012.

20. Van Cutsem E, Moiseyenko VM, Tjulandin S, et al. Phase III study of docetaxel and cisplatin plus fluorouracil compared with cisplatin and fluorouracil as first-line therapy for advanced gastric cancer: a report of the V325 Study Group. J Clin Oncol 2006;24(31):4991–7. Available at: http://www.ncbi.nlm.nih.gov/pubmed/ 17075117. Accessed November 19, 2012.

21. Koizumi W, Narahara H, Hara T, et al. S-1 plus cisplatin versus S-1 alone for first-line treatment of advanced gastric cancer (SPIRITS trial): a phase III trial. Lancet Oncol 2008;9(3):215–21. Available at: http://www.ncbi.nlm.nih.gov/pubmed/ 18282805. Accessed November 20, 2012.

22. Bang YJ, Van Cutsem E, Feyereislova A, et al. Trastuzumab in combination with chemotherapy versus chemotherapy alone for treatment of HER2-positive advanced gastric or gastro-oesophageal junction cancer (ToGA): a phase 3, open-label, randomised controlled trial. Lancet 2010;376(9742):687–97. http: //dx.doi.org/10.1016/S0140-6736(10)61121-X. Available at: http://www.ncbi.nlm. nih.gov/pubmed/20728210. Accessed October 2, 2012.

23. Grabsch H, Sivakumar S, Gray S, et al. HER2 expression in gastric cancer: rare, heterogeneous and of no prognostic value - conclusions from 924 cases of two independent series. Cell Oncol 2010;32(1–2):57–65. http://dx.doi.org/ 10.3233/clo-2009-0497.

24. Gravalos C, Jimeno A. HER2 in gastric cancer: a new prognostic factor and a novel therapeutic target. Ann Oncol 2008;19(9):1523–9. http://dx.doi.org/ 10.1093/annonc/mdn169.

25. Warneke VS, Behrens HM, Boger C, et al. Her2/neu testing in gastric cancer: evaluating the risk of sampling errors. Ann Oncol 2012. http://dx.doi.org/ 10.1093/annonc/mds528. Available at: http://www.ncbi.nlm.nih.gov/pubmed/ 23139264. Accessed November 28, 2012.

26. Wu Y, Grabsch H, Ivanova T, et al. Comprehensive genomic meta-analysis iden-tifies intra-tumoural stroma as a predictor of survival in patients with gastric cancer. Gut 2012. http://dx.doi.org/10.1136/gutjnl-2011-301373. Available at: http://www.ncbi.nlm.nih.gov/pubmed/22735568. Accessed October 23, 2012.

27. Lennerz JK, Kwak EL, Ackerman A, et al. MET amplification identifies a small and aggressive subgroup of esophagogastric adenocarcinoma with evidence of responsiveness to crizotinib. J Clin Oncol 2011;29(36):4803–10. http: //dx.doi.org/10.1200/jco.2011.35.4928.

28. Lee J, Seo JW, Jun HJ, et al. Impact of MET amplification on gastric cancer: possible roles as a novel prognostic marker and a potential therapeutic target. Oncol Rep 2011;25(6):1517–24. http://dx.doi.org/10.3892/or.2011.1219.

29. Graziano F, Galluccio N, Lorenzini P, et al. Genetic activation of the MET pathway and prognosis of patients with high-risk, radically resected gastric cancer. J Clin Oncol 2011;29(36):4789–95. http://dx.doi.org/10.1200/jco.2011.36.7706.

30. Smolen GA, Sordella R, Muir B, et al. Amplification of MET may identify a subset of cancers with extreme sensitivity to the selective tyrosine kinase inhibitor PHA-665752. Proc Natl Acad Sci U S A 2006;103(7):2316–21. http: //dx.doi.org/10.1073/pnas.0508776103.

31. Kataoka Y, Mukohara T, Tomioka H, et al. Foretinib (GSK1363089), a multi-kinase inhibitor of MET and VEGFRs, inhibits growth of gastric cancer cell lines by blocking inter-receptor tyrosine kinase networks. Invest New Drugs 2012;30(4): 1352–60. http://dx.doi.org/10.1007/s10637-011-9699-0. Available at: http://www. ncbi.nlm.nih.gov/pubmed/21655918. Accessed November 26, 2012.

32. Oliner kS, Tang R, Anderson A, et al. Evaluation of MET pathway biomarkers in a phase II study of rilotumumab or placebo in combination with epirubicin, cisplatin, and capecitabine in patients with locally advanced or metastatic gastric or esophagogastric junction cancer [abstract 4005]. J Clin Oncol 2012;30.

33. Turner N, Grose R. Fibroblast growth factor signalling: from development to cancer. Nat Rev Cancer 2010;10(2):116–29. http://dx.doi.org/10.1038/nrc2780.

34. Matsumoto K, Arao T, Hamaguchi T, et al. FGFR2 gene amplification and clinico-pathological features in gastric cancer. Br J Cancer 2012;106(4):727–32. http://dx.doi.org/10.1038/bjc.2011.603.

35. Deng N, Goh LK, Wang H, et al. A comprehensive survey of genomic alterations in gastric cancer reveals systematic patterns of molecular exclusivity and co-occurrence among distinct therapeutic targets. Gut 2012;61(5):673–84. http://dx.doi.org/10.1136/gutjnl-2011-301839.

36. Ohtsu A, Shah MA, Van Cutsem E, et al. Bevacizumab in combination with chemotherapy as first-line therapy in advanced gastric cancer: a randomized, double-blind, placebo-controlled phase III study. J Clin Oncol 2011;29(30):3968–76. http://dx.doi.org/10.1200/JCO.2011.36.2236. Available at: http://www.ncbi.nlm.nih.gov/pubmed/21844504; http://jco.ascopubs.org/content/29/30/3968.full.pdf. Accessed October 2, 2012.

37. Van Cutsem E, Yeh KH, Bang YJ, et al. Phase II trial of everolimus in previously treated patients with advanced gastric cancer: GRANITE-I [abstract LBA3]. J Clin Oncol 2012;30.

Gastric Mucosal-Associated Lymphoid Tissue Lymphoma

Wolfgang Fischbach, MD, PhD

KEYWORDS

- Gastric mucosal-associated lymphoid tissue lymphoma • Pathogenesis • Diagnosis
- Treatment

KEY POINTS

- Gastric marginal zone B-cell lymphoma of mucosal-associated lymphoid tissue (MALT) is the predominant entity within the primary gastrointestinal lymphomas.
- *Helicobacter pylori* represents the decisive pathogenetic factor for gastric MALT lymphoma.
- The goal of treating gastric MALT lymphoma should be complete cure.
- The first choice of treatment is *H pylori* eradication.
- Patients with histologically persistent residual lymphoma after successful *H pylori* eradication and normalization of endoscopic findings should be managed by a watch-and-wait strategy.
- Patients who do not respond to *H pylori* eradication should be referred for radiation or chemotherapy.

INTRODUCTION

Malignant lymphomas are divided into Hodgkin disease and the heterogeneous group of non-Hodgkin lymphomas (NHLs) (**Fig. 1**). Sixty percent of the latter arise in lymph nodes (nodal lymphoma), while 40% are of an extranodal origin. The gastrointestinal tract is by far the most frequent site of manifestation for extranodal NHL (primary gastrointestinal lymphoma). A secondary involvement of the gastrointestinal tract (secondary gastrointestinal lymphoma) by disseminated nodal NHL can be found in up to 20% of cases when investigated systematically.[1]

CLASSIFICATION OF GASTROINTESTINAL LYMPHOMA

Box 1 represents the World Health Organization (WHO) classification as established in 2002 and updated in 2008.[2] More than 70% of primary gastrointestinal lymphomas

Department of Internal Medicine and Palliative Care Unit, Klinikum Aschaffenburg–Academic Teaching Hospital of the University of Würzburg, Am Hasenkopf, Aschaffenburg D-63739, Germany
E-mail address: med2-aschaffenburg@t-online.de

Gastroenterol Clin N Am 42 (2013) 371–380
http://dx.doi.org/10.1016/j.gtc.2013.01.008
0889-8553/13/$ – see front matter © 2013 Elsevier Inc. All rights reserved.

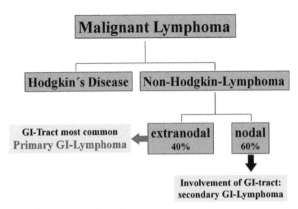

Fig. 1. Classification of malignant lymphoma.

present as gastric lymphoma. In terms of numbers, marginal zone B-cell lymphomas of mucosa-associated-lymphoid tissue (MALT) are predominant. The second most common types of gastric lymphoma are the diffuse large B-cell lymphomas with or without MALT components. T-cell lymphomas are extremely rare in the stomach but comprise a considerable part of intestinal lymphoma (EATCL: enteropathy-associated T-cell lymphoma). The various lymphoma entities are characterized by differences in pathogenesis, biologic behavior, and treatment options. This article exclusively focuses on extranodal gastric marginal zone B-cell lymphoma of MALT, subsequently named MALT lymphoma.

PATHOGENESIS OF GASTRIC MALT LYMPHOMA

Intensive basic research and clinical research during the last 2 decades has substantially enriched the understanding of the development and progression of gastric MALT lymphoma. MALT is acquired in a secondary process against a background of chronic antigen stimulation. As early as in the late 1980s, attention had been drawn to

---

Box 1
WHO classification of gastrointestinal lymphoma

B-Cell Lymphoma

Extranodal gastric marginal zone B-cell-lymphoma (MZBCL) of MALT

Follicular lymphoma (grades 1–3)

Mantle cell lymphoma (lymphomatous polyposis)

Diffuse large B-cell lymphoma with/without MALT components

Burkitt lymphoma

Immunodeficiency-associated lymphoma

T-Cell Lymphoma

Enteropathy-associated

T-cell lymphoma (EATCL)

Peripheral T-cell- lymphoma (previously: non-EATCL)

Helicobacter pylori, which was then still referred to as *Campylobacter pylori*.[3,4] The bacterium causes chronic gastritis and leads to the formation of intramucosal lymph follicles showing the morphologic characteristics of MALT. These changes proved to be reversible after bacterial eradication treatment.[5] There are convincing data from histomorphological, molecular biologic, epidemiological, and experimental studies that *H pylori* is the decisive pathogenetic factor for the development of gastric MALT lymphoma. Up to 98% of patients with gastric MALT lymphoma are *H pylori* positive when tested by serology.[6] However, only a small minority of all *H pylori*-infected individuals develops gastric MALT lymphoma. Virulence factors of the bacterium do not obviously determine this risk. There is, however, growing evidence that genetic host factors may play an important role in this context.

If any further evidence were needed for the pathogenic significance of *H pylori* for the development of gastric MALT lymphoma, it has been provided by experience with eradication treatment. In the first series of 6 patients with stage I gastric MALT lymphoma, successful eradication of *H pylori* led to a complete and lasting regression of the lymphoma.[7] The authors concluded that *H pylori* eradication should be the first choice of treatment. This was a quite audacious statement at that time considering the small number of patients treated in this way. However, it turned out to be right.

CLINICAL FEATURES OF GASTRIC MALT LYMPHOMA

The clinical features of gastric MALT lymphoma are nonspecific, including abdominal symptoms, pain, vomiting, diarrhea, weight loss, and overt or occult gastrointestinal bleeding.[8] However, gastric MALT lymphomas are also often found incidentally at endoscopy. Complications such as obstruction, perforation, or bleeding are rarely observed.

PROGNOSTIC FACTORS IN GASTRIC MALT LYMPHOMA

In the early 1990s, Cogliatti and colleagues[9] and Radaszkiewicz and colleagues[10] for the first time analyzed 2 large retrospective series of MALT lymphomas. Their main findings were that the grade of malignancy (MALT lymphoma vs diffuse large B-cell-lymphoma [DLBCL] with or without MALT components) and stage of the disease are the 2 major prognostic factors and therapeutic determinants. This conclusion has since been confirmed by several prospective studies.[11–16] Accurate staging requires a thorough endoscopic biopsy protocol (gastric mapping) and other staging procedures as outlined in this article and demonstrated in **Fig. 2** and **Box 2**.

Translocation t(11;18) is the most common genetic aberration in gastric MALT lymphoma. It is found in 25% of cases, more frequently in cases at stage II or above

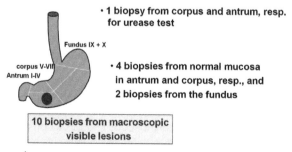

Fig. 2. Gastric mapping.

Box 2
Staging of gastric MALT lymphoma according to the EGILs Consensus Report

Absolute Requirements

Physical examination

    Laboratory tests: Blood count, lactate dehydrogenase (LDH), beta2-microglobulin, electrophoresis, hepatitis B virus (HBV), hepatitis C virus (HCV), human immunodeficiency virus (HIV)

Thoracic/abdominal computed tomography (CT) scan

Upper endoscopy with gastric mapping

Strongly Recommended

Endoscopic ultrasound

Bone marrow puncture

Should be Considered

Ileocolonoscopy

Abbreviation: EGILs; European Gastrointestinal Lymphoma Study Group.

---

than in stage I. T(11;18) has also been proven to be of prognostic value as it strongly predicts the response of gastric MALT lymphoma to *H pylori* eradication.[17,18] Nevertheless, routine testing for t(11;18) within the staging process is not mandatory, as *H pylori* eradication is recommended as the initial treatment irrespective of the bacterial status.[19,20]

DIAGNOSIS AND STAGING

In view of the nonspecific appearance of gastric MALT lymphoma[8] and potential sources of error in endoscopic and biopsy diagnosis, it is necessary to obtain a sufficient number of biopsies from macroscopic lesions and normal-appearing mucosa. This procedure, named gastric mapping (see **Fig. 2**), is strongly recommended in the German S3 guideline[19] as well as in the European EGILs Consensus Report of 2011.[20] In general, such a biopsy protocol is not performed during a routine diagnostic endoscopy. Therefore, a second esophagogastroduodenoscopy will be necessary in most cases.

Lymphoepithelial lesions represent the histomorphological characteristic of gastric MALT lymphoma. Additional criteria include a diffuse infiltrate of small to medium-sized B-lymphocytes that are similar to centrocytes ('centrocytoid').[21] Immunophenotypically, these cells express pan-B-cell markers (CD20), while they show no immunoreactivity for CD5, CD10, and CD11c. Staining for Ki67 may help in identifying large cell components. There is a widely accepted consensus that the diagnosis of gastric MALT lymphoma is based on histomorphological criteria according to the WHO classification.[19,20]

Once the diagnosis of gastric MALT lymphoma is established and confirmed by a reference pathologist, a staging procedure follows. **Box 2** summarizes the various examinations that must be done.[20] Endoscopic ultrasound and bone marrow puncture are strongly recommended, while ileocolonoscopy should be considered. For staging, the Ann Arbor classification is still used, with Musshoff's modification[22] and taking the Radaszkiewicz differentiation of stage I into I1 and I2 into account (**Table 1**).[10] The

Table 1
Staging systems for gastrointestinal lymphoma

Ann Arbor System[10,20]	TNM Classification[21]	Spread of Lymphoma
E I 1	T1 N0 M0	Mucosa, submucosa
E I 2	T2 N0 M0	Muscularis propria, subserosa
E I 2	T3 N0 M0	Serosal penetration
E I 2	T4 N0 M0	Infiltration of neighboring organs
E II 1	T1-4 N1 M0	Regional lymph nodes (compartments I + II)
E II 2	T1-4 N2 M0	Distant intra-abdominal lymph nodes
E III	T1-4 N3 M0	Lymph nodes on both sides of diaphragm
E IV	T1-4 N0-3 M1 B1	Distant or extragastrointestinal organs Bone marrow

Abbreviation: E, extranodal.

Paris staging system is an alternative based on the well-known TNM classification system.[23] However, this system has not yet been validated by prospective studies.

THERAPEUTIC OPTIONS IN GASTRIC MALT LYMPHOMA

Fig. 3 summarizes the treatment recommendations of the German S3 guideline[19] and the European EGILs consensus report of 2011.[20] It has to be emphasized that the goal of gastric MALT lymphoma should always be a complete cure. In a recent large prospective study from Japan, an excellent outcome was demonstrated with an

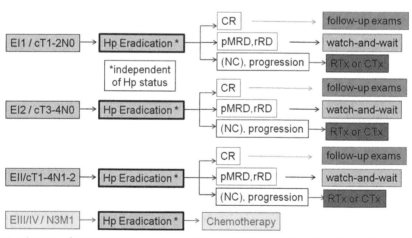

Fig. 3. Therapy of gastric MALT lymphoma. CR, complete remission; CTx, chemotherapy; Hp, *H pylori*; NC, no change; pMRD, probable minimal residual disease; rRD, responding residual disease; RTx, radiotherapy. (*Data from* Fischbach W, Malfertheiner P, Hoffmann JC, et al. S3-guideline "*Helicobacter pylori* and gastroduodenal ulcer disease" of the German Society for Digestive and Metabolic Diseases (DGVS) in cooperation with the German Society for Hygiene and Microbiology, Society for Pediatric Gastroenterology and Nutrition e.V., German society for rheumatology, AWMF-registration-no. 021/001. Z Gastreoenterol 2009;47(12):1230–63; and Ruskoné-Fourmestraux A, Fischbach W, Aleman BM, et al. EGILS consensus report. Gastric extranodal marginal zone B cell lymphoma of MALT. Gut 2011;60:747–58.)

overall 10-year survival rate of 95% and a disease-free survival rate of 86%.[24] The treatment strategies used in this study were very similar to those outlined in **Fig. 3**, and were based upon the data reviewed in this article.

H PYLORI ERADICATION

For stage I and stage II disease, H pylori eradication is the initial treatment of choice, with curative intent. According to a recent meta-analysis, 77.5% of patients with gastric MALT lymphoma achieve complete regression after successful eradication of H pylori.[25] Complete regression of lymphoma was more often observed in stage I than in stage II tumors (78% vs 56%) and was more common in Asian than in European populations (84% vs 55%). A relapse occurred in 7.2% of patients (2.2% per year). High-grade transformation into aggressive lymphoma was an extremely rare event (0.05%). A necessary precondition for lymphoma regression is the success of eradication therapy for H pylori. In a pooled data analysis, Zullo and colleagues reported a success rate of first-line eradication therapy in 91% of patients.[26] Including second- to fifth-line treatment protocols, a definite eradication rate of 98.3% was achieved. Interestingly, these data emphasize the effect of compliance on the eradication success. Although there is no evidence from the literature that H pylori eradication may also cure gastric MALT lymphoma of stages III and IV, eradication therapy is now recommended in all stages to eliminate a possible immunoproliferative stimulus.[20]

Even patients with a negative H pylori status should undergo eradication therapy.[20] Although this recommendation may seem initially illogical, small series have demonstrated that complete lymphoma regression can also be observed with eradication therapy in individual cases even if H pylori-negative,[27,28] perhaps because of microorganisms other than H pylori driving lymphoma cell proliferation.

LONG-TERM OUTCOME AFTER SUCCESSFUL ERADICATION

For many years, the positive effect of H pylori eradication on the long-term outcome of patients with gastric MALT lymphoma was regarded with some skepticism. It seems clear, however, that this therapeutic attempt cures most patients.[29,30] Recently, the 10-year follow-up data of a large prospective trial were published. Of 120 patients with gastric MALT lymphoma of stage I1, 96 (80%) achieved complete remission after successful H pylori eradication,[31] 80% of whom (77 of 96 patients) remained disease-free.

HISTOLOGICALLY RESIDUAL OF MALT LYMPHOMA AFTER SUCCESSFUL ERADICATION OF H PYLORI

Patients with histologically residual MALT lymphoma after successful eradication therapy used to be regarded as treatment failures and referred for radiation or chemotherapy until recently. In 2002, the author and colleagues reported for the first time on 7 patients who had histologically residual MALT lymphoma after successful H pylori eradication with normalization of their endoscopic findings.[32] These patients refused to undergo surgery, radiation or chemotherapy, but agreed to regular endoscopic surveillance. Up until now (follow-up >10 years), a clinical relapse of lymphoma, dissemination, or high-grade transformation has not been observed in any of these patients. Observing their favorable course of disease, the author and colleagues began to speculate that a watch-and-wait strategy might be a safe alternative to oncological treatment in such a situation. Within the EGILs study group, the author and colleagues subsequently reported the same experience in a large series of 108 patients.[33] All the cases had been diagnosed with a stage I gastric lymphoma and underwent *H pylori* eradication therapy. Twelve months later, *H pylori* was absent, but residual lymphoma was still present histologically. Despite the patients not receiving any further therapy, 35 of them (32%) developed late (>1 year) complete remission of their lymphoma, while 67 patients (62%) revealed histologic residuals during the median follow-up of almost 3 years. Only 5 patients (6%) needed oncological therapy, because of local progression of the lymphoma in 4 cases, and high-grade transformation in 1 case.

Patients with successful eradication of *H pylori* and normalization of the endoscopic findings but persisting histologic infiltrates can, therefore no more be regarded as treatment failures and regular candidates for radiation or chemotherapy. In the author's opinion, most can be successfully managed by a watch-and-wait strategy with regular endoscopic biopsies.[19,20] Only those patients revealing no change or progression of lymphoma despite successful *H pylori* eradication should be referred for radiation or chemotherapy (see **Fig. 3**).[34]

NONRESPONDERS TO *H PYLORI* ERADICATION

Patients not responding to *H pylori* eradication (those classified as no change or progression according to the GELA grading system for posteradication evaluation) (see **Fig. 3**)[34] should be treated by radiation or chemotherapy.

Radiation

Radiation offers a curative option to patients in stages I and II not responding to *H pylori* eradication.[12,15,16] Involved field radiation with 40 Gy is recommended in stage I, while a reduced extended field and extended field radiation with doses of 30–40 Gy are preferred in stages II1 and II2, respectively. In some European countries, chemotherapy is considered an alternative to radiation in MALT lymphoma of stages I/II.[20] In other countries, chemotherapy is restricted to MALT lymphoma in disseminated stages III and IV. It has to be emphasized that there is currently no generally accepted standard chemotherapy in gastric MALT lymphoma. The anti-CD20 antibody rituximab with Cyclophosphamid, Vincristin, Prednison (COP), Cyclophosphamid, Doxorubicin, Vincristin, Prednison (CHOP), bendamustine or fludarabin plus cyclophosphamide are possible choices.

Surgery

Surgery cannot be found any more in the list of treatment recommendations (see **Fig. 3**). Indeed, surgery is nowadays restricted to the treatment of rare complications such as perforation or bleeding that cannot be controlled endoscopically.[19,20] This may astonish some readers who have in mind that surgical resection was the standard therapeutic approach in gastric MALT lymphoma for many decades. It, indeed, offered an excellent long-term survival.[13] However, conservative organ-preserving therapeutic strategies have been shown to be equally effective.[14–16] A recent meta-analysis comparing surgical and medical treatment in 5 studies and 700 patients demonstrated the superiority of medical therapy.[35] There are mainly 2 arguments for such a recommendation: equal treatment outcomes after surgical or conservative strategies and a better quality of life by avoiding gastrectomy. The latter has been clearly demonstrated by a prospective randomized trial with 10-year follow-up.[36]

FOLLOW-UP EXAMINATIONS

Those patients having achieved complete remission after *H pylori* eradication or oncological treatment should continue to be followed, although the exact time interval and the duration of surveillance are not yet known.[20] The rationale for follow-up endoscopies is to detect local relapse of MALT lymphoma relatively early; this occurs in about 7% of cases.[25] Furthermore a sixfold elevated risk for gastric carcinoma has been reported for patients with MALT lymphoma in an epidemiologic survey from the Netherlands.[37] In a prospective multicenter trial published recently, there was a significantly higher incidence of gastric cancer (standardized morbidity ratio 8.567; 95% confidence interval, 3.566–20.582) or NHL (standardized morbidity ratio 18.621; 95% confidence interval, 8.365–41.448) compared with the general German population.[31]

REFERENCES

1. Fischbach W, Kestel W, Kirchner T, et al. Malignant lymphoma of the upper gastrointestinal tract. Results of a prospective study in 103 patients. Cancer 1992;70:1075–80.
2. Swerdlow SH, Campo E, Harris NL, et al. WHO classification of tumours of haematopoetic and lymphoid tissues. Lyon (France): IARC Press; 2008. p. 158–66, 214–7.
3. Stolte M, Eidt S. Lymphoid follicles in antral mucosa: Immune response to Campylobacter pylori? J Clin Pathol 1989;42:1269–71.
4. Wyatt JI, Rathbone BJ. Immune response of the gastric mucosa to Campylobacter pylori. Scand J Gastroenterol 1988;23(Suppl):135–40.
5. Stolte M. Helicobacter pylori gastritis and gastric MALT-lymphoma. Lancet 1992; 339:745.
6. Eck M, Schmaußer W, Haas R, et al. MALT-type lymphoma of the stomach is associated with Helicobacter pylori strains expressing the CagA protein. Gastroenterology 1997;112:1482–6.
7. Wotherspoon AC, Doglioni C, Diss TC, et al. Regression of primary low-grade B-cell gastric lymphoma of mucosa-associated lymphoid tissue. Lancet 1993; 342:575–7.
8. Kolve M, Fischbach W, Greiner A, et al. Differences in endoscopic and clinicopathological features of primary and secondary gastric non-Hodgkin's lymphoma. Gastrointest Endosc 1999;49:307–15.
9. Cogliatti SB, Schmid U, Schumacher U, et al. Primary B-cell gastric lymphoma: a clinico-pathological study of 145 patients. Gastroenterology 1991;101:1159–70.
10. Radaszkiewicz T, Dragosics B, Bauer P. Gastrointestinal malignant lymphomas of the mucosa-associated lymphoid tissue. Factors relevant to prognosis. Gastroenterology 1992;102:1628–38.
11. Ruskone-Fourmestraux A, Aegerter P, Delmer A, et al. Primary digestive tract lymphoma: a prospective multicentric study of 91 patients. Gastroenterology 1993;105:1662–72.
12. Schechter NR, Portlock CS, Yahalom J. Treatment of mucosa-associated lymphoid tissue lymphoma of the stomach with radiation alone. J Clin Oncol 1998;16:1916–21.
13. Fischbach W, Dragosics B, Koelve-Goebeler ME, et al. Primary gastric B-cell lymphoma: results of a prospective multicenter study. Gastroenterology 2000; 119:1191–202.
14. Koch P, delValle F, Berdel WE, et al. Primary gastrointestinal non-Hodgkin's lymphoma: I. anatomic and histologic distribution, clinical features, and survival data of 371 patients registered in the German Multicenter Study GIT NHL 01/92. J Clin Oncol 2001;19:3861–73.

15. Koch P, Probst A, Berdel WE, et al. Treatment results in localized primary gastric lymphoma: data of patients registered within the German multicenter study (GIT NHL 02/96). J Clin Oncol 2005;23:7050–9.
16. Tsang RW, Gospodarowicz MK, Pintilie M. Localized mucosa-associated lymphoid tissue lymphoma treated with radiation therapy has excellent clinical outcome. J Clin Oncol 2003;21:4157–64.
17. Liu H, Ye H, Ruskone-Fourmestraux A, et al. T(11;18) is a marker for all stage gastric MALT lymphomas that will not respond to *H pylori* eradication. Gastroenterology 2002;122:1286–94.
18. Yeh KH, Kuo SH, Chen LT, et al. Nuclear expression of BCL10 or nuclear factor kappa B helps predict Helicobacter pylori-independent status of low-grade gastric mucosa-associated lymphoid tissue lymphomas with or without t(11;18)(q21;q21). Blood 2005;106:1037–41.
19. Fischbach W, Malfertheiner P, Hoffmann JC, et al. S3-guideline "*Helicobacter pylori* and gastroduodenal ulcer disease" of the German Society for Digestive and Metabolic Diseases (DGVS) in cooperation with the German Society for Hygiene and Microbiology, Society for Pediatric Gastroenterology and Nutrition e.V., German Society for Rheumatology, AWMF-registration-no. 021/001. Z Gastroenterol 2009; 47(12):1230–63.
20. Ruskoné-Fourmestraux A, Fischbach W, Aleman BM, et al. EGILS consensus report. Gastric extranodal marginal zone B cell lymphoma of MALT. Gut 2011; 60:747–58.
21. Wotherspoon A, Ortiz-Hidalgo C, Falzon MR, et al. Helicobacter pylori associated gastritis and primary B-cell lymphoma. Lancet 1991;338:1175–6.
22. Musshoff K. Clinical staging classification of non-Hodgkin's lymphomas. Strahlentherapie 1977;153:218–21.
23. Ruskone-Fourmestraux A, Dragosics B, Morgner A, et al. Paris staging system for primary gastrointestinal lymphomas. Gut 2003;52:912–3.
24. Nakamura S, Sugiyama T, Matsumoto T, et al. Long-term clinical outcome of gastric MALT lymphoma after eradication of *Helicobacter pylori*: a multicentre cohort follow-up study of 420 patients in Japan. Gut 2012;61:507–13.
25. Zullo A, Hassan C, Cristofari F, et al. Effects of *Helicobacter pylori* eradication on early stage gastric mucosa-associated lymphoid tissue lymphoma. Clin Gastroenterol Hepatol 2010;8:105–10.
26. Zullo A, Hassan C, Andriani A, et al. Eradication therapy for *Helicobacter pylori* in patients with gastric MALT lymphoma: a pooled data analysis. Am J Gastroenterol 2009;104:1932–7.
27. Raderer M, Streubel B, Wöhrer S, et al. Successful antibiotic treatment of *Helicobacter pylori*-negative gastric mucosa-associated lymphoid tissue lymphomas. Gut 2006;55:616–8.
28. Chung SJ, Kim JS, Kim H, et al. Long-term clinical outcome of *Helicobacter pylori*-negative gastric mucosa-associated lymphoid tissue lymphoma is comparable to that of *H. pylori*-positive lymphoma. J Clin Gastroenterol 2009;43:312–7.
29. Fischbach W, Goebeler-Kolve ME, Dragosics B, et al. Long term outcome of patients with gastric marginal zone B cell lymphoma of mucosa associated lymphoid tissue (MALT) following exclusive *Helicobacter pylori* eradication: experience from a large prospective series. Gut 2004;53:34–7.
30. Wündisch T, Thiede C, Morgner A, et al. Long-term follow-up of gastric MALT lymphoma after helicobacter pylori eradication. J Clin Oncol 2005;23(31):1–7.
31. Wündisch T, Dieckhoff P, Greene B, et al. Second cancers and residual disease in patients treated for gastric mucosa-associated lymphoid tissue lymphoma by

Helicobacter pylori eradication and followed for 10 years. Gastroenterology 2012; 143(4):936–42.

32. Fischbach W, Goebeler-Kolve M, Starostik P, et al. Minimal residual low-grade gastric MALT-type lymphoma after eradication of Helicobacter pylori. Lancet 2002;360:547–8.

33. Fischbach W, Goebeler ME, Ruskone-Fourmestraux A, et al. Most patients with minimal histological residuals of gastric MALT lymphoma after successful eradication of *Helicobacter pylori* can be safely managed by a watch-and-wait strategy. Experience from a large international series. Gut 2007;56:1685–7.

34. Copie-Bergman C, Gaulard P, Lavergne-Slove A, et al. Proposal for a new histological grading system for post-treatment evaluation of gastric MALT lymphoma. Gut 2003;52:1656.

35. Cirocchi R, Farinella E, Trastulli S, et al. Surgical treatment of primary gastrointestinal lymphoma. World J Surg Oncol 2011;9:145–51.

36. Fischbach W, Schramm S, Goebeler E. Outcome and quality of life favour a conservative treatment of patients with primary gastric lymphoma. Z Gastroenterol 2011;49:430–5.

37. Capelle LG, de Vries AC, Looman CW, et al. Gastric MALT lymphoma: epidemiology and high adenocarcinoma risk in a nation-wide study. Eur J Cancer 2008; 44:2470–6.

Gastric Carcinoids (Neuroendocrine Neoplasms)

Mark Kidd, PhD[a],*, Bjorn Gustafsson, MD, PhD[b],
Irvin M. Modlin, MD, PhD, DSc[a]

KEYWORDS

- Carcinoid • Chronic atrophic gastritis • Gastrin • Menin
- Multiple endocrine neoplasia 1 • Neuroendocrine tumor • Proton pump inhibitor
- Zollinger-Ellison syndrome

KEY POINTS

- Gastric neuroendocrine neoplasms of the stomach can be divided into the usually well-differentiated, hypergastrinemia-dependent type I and II lesions and the more aggressively behaving gastrin-independent type III lesions.
- The observed incidence has increased more than 10-fold over the past 30 years.
- Small (<15–20 mm) localized type I and II lesions, which are slowly proliferating (<2%), can usually be managed conservatively through reduction of hypergastrinemia; the use of the specific gastrin receptor antagonist YF476 or gastrin antibodies may become useful for both type I and II lesions in future protocols.
- Infiltrating and metastasized tumors and type III lesions require a more aggressive approach with surgical resection and consideration of modalities such as cytotoxics and peptide receptor–targeted treatment.
- The mutational spectrum in gastric lesions is greater than MEN-1 (eg, NF-1 and MAPK alterations occur); studying menin and its complex interrelationship with gastrin may provide insight into tumor biology at the clinical level and in terms of basic cell biology (eg, the role of the epigenome in neuroendocrine cell proliferation), and lead to potential consideration of other targets that are known candidates for molecular-based therapies in other adenocarcinomas.

INTRODUCTION

Gastric carcinoids or, as they are currently called, "neuroendocrine neoplasms" (NENs),[1] have recently become the subject of substantial clinical and investigative interest. This fact reflects global concerns regarding the consequences of prolonged

[a] Department of Surgery, Yale University School of Medicine, PO Box 208602, New Haven, CT, USA; [b] Department of Cancer Research and Molecular Medicine, Norwegian University of Science and Technology, Prinsesse Kristinas gt 1, NO-7491, Trondheim, Norway
* Corresponding author.
E-mail address: mark.kidd@yale.edu

Gastroenterol Clin N Am 42 (2013) 381–397
http://dx.doi.org/10.1016/j.gtc.2013.01.009
0889-8553/13/$ – see front matter © 2013 Elsevier Inc. All rights reserved.

hypochlorhydria, long-standing hypergastrinemia (increased use of acid-suppressive pharmacotherapeutic agents), and the proposed putative relationship between gastric adenocarcinoma and gastric NENs.[2-6] These tumors were previously considered rare lesions,[7] overall representing fewer than 2% of all gastrointestinal NENs and fewer than 1% of all gastric neoplasms. The misconception of rarity is redundant because current cancer databases indicate that gastric NENs are increasing in incidence/prevalence and that the current figures are closer to 5%.[8,9] Whether this represents increased clinical awareness, more accurate pathologic identification, or more thorough endoscopic surveillance is debatable, but nevertheless provides a far larger group of patients whose disease requires management. Delineation of the regulation of enterochromaffin-like (ECL) cell proliferation, characterization of its degree of transformation, and determination of its malignant potential are necessary adjuncts for the development of a rational strategy for clinical management. As a result of these factors, an intense clinical and scientific scrutiny of gastric neuroendocrine ECL cell tumors has developed.[8]

Gastric NENs are usually derived from the histamine-secreting ECL cell but may occasionally have a phenotype indicating an origin from other cell type, such as serotonin-secreting enterochromaffin cells, somatostatin, or ghrelin cells.[10-12] ECL cell tumors are classified as either gastrin-dependent (type I/II) or gastrin-independent (type III), although the gastrin/CCK2 receptor is expressed on both types.[13] This article reviews each type of lesion, examines the pathobiologic insights generated from animal models, and determines the translational significance of these data.

Type I Gastric NENs

Type I gastric NENs occur in patients with chronic atrophic gastritis (CAG), with hypergastrinemia caused by an absence of gastric acid. Lesions are usually located in atrophic oxyntic mucosa in the fundus in individuals with CAG with or without pernicious anemia.

Most instances (70%–80%) are seen in patients with CAG and associated hypergastrinemia, whereas pernicious anemia is common (58%).[14,15] Among 367 individuals with atrophic gastritis, the prevalence was 2.4%, with an annual incidence of 0.4% during endoscopic follow-up.[16] In general, type I NENs occur more frequently in women, and 70% to 80% are diagnosed between the fifth and seventh decades.[17,18] Because of diminished acid secretion, serum gastrin levels are significantly elevated in patients with atrophic gastritis. On the same basis, a correlation between long-term proton pump inhibitor (PPI)–induced hypergastrinemia and the development of gastric NENs is possible and supported by recent epidemiologic data and case reports.[19,20] Serum gastrin and chromogranin A (CgA) levels can be elevated in approximately 100% and 95% of patients, respectively.[21]

Lesions, when identified, are usually small (<1 cm), polypoid, and multicentric ($\approx$67% of cases). These tumors are mostly limited to the mucosa or submucosa, do not exhibit angioinvasion, and seem to be benign in behavior.[11] Larger tumors (1–2 cm) may exhibit low-grade malignant behavior, with or without angioinvasion. Tumors in this group may be either single or multiple, exhibit a low rate of lymph node invasion (3%–8%), and are rarely ($\approx$2% of cases) associated with distant metastases.[22,23] In general, irrespective of their size, lesions are classified as stage I (87%).[21]

At a histologic level, ECL cell lesions have been classified as pseudohyperplasia (cell clustering unassociated with cell proliferation), hyperplasia (diffuse, linear, micronodular, adenomatoid), dysplasia (enlarged, adenomatous or fused micronodules, microinfiltration, nodular growth), and neoplasia (intramucosal or invasive carcinoids). The entire spectrum of ECL cell proliferation, from hyperplasia to dysplasia and neoplasia, has been observed in type I tumors. Hyperplastic and pseudohyperplastic ECL alterations may also occur with some frequency in *Helicobacter pylori*–related chronic gastritis associated with ulcer disease or dyspepsia.[24] In general, ECL cell type I lesions tend to be well differentiated and are considered by World Health Organization (WHO) classification to be of benign or low-grade malignant potential. They are usually classified (>80%)[21] as G1 (**Table 1**), with a Ki-67 (if detected) of less than 1%.

At a molecular level, although germ-line mutations in the MEN-1 locus (located on 11q13) could not be identified,[25] a frequent loss of heterozygosity (LOH) within the 11q13–14 region was noted.[26] This finding suggests a potential involvement for the *MEN-1* gene and/or a more telomeric tumor suppressor gene in the pathogenesis of type I NENs. More recently, loss of methylation of long interspersed nucleotide element type 1 (*LINE1*) that has been identified in well-differentiated pancreatic NENs[27] has been examined in gastric NENs. This investigation is based on the premise that LINE1 hypomethylation may serve as a marker of tumor grade and lymph node metastasis.[28] In 11 gastric type I tumors, methylation levels were not different from normal mucosa and no difference was established for higher-grade lesions, suggesting this may not be a potential marker in these lesions. The enzyme α-methylacyl-coenzyme A racemase, which plays a role in the β-oxidation of branched-chain fatty acid and its derivatives and is used to detect prostatic adenocarcinoma,[29] has recently been examined in gastric NENs. None of the grade 1 lesions were immunoreactive, whereas 67% of grade 2 were positive, suggesting that this may be a useful marker for distinguishing between grade 1 (negative) and 2 gastric NENs.[30] The relatively high proportion of grade 1 ($\approx$90%) lesions in type I NENs limits using this enzyme as a marker, but intriguingly, given the role this enzyme plays in metabolism, differential expression could suggest metabolic differences between grade 1 and 2 lesions, suggesting a potential utility as a biomarker.

Treatment options include endoscopic and surgical resection and pharmaceutical intervention. Endoscopic resection may be appropriate for intraepithelial tumors less than 2 cm and occasionally tumors less than 1 cm invading into the lamina propria or submucosa.[31] In one study that included 16 type I NENs, complete resection was

Table 1
Clinical classification of gastric NEN

Gastric NEN Subtype	Defining Etiologic Feature	Histology
Type I	Hypergastrinemia: Diminished parietal cell function Chronic atrophic gastritis/autoimmune disorder	Well differentiated
Type II	Hypergastrinemia: Autonomous secretion by gastrinoma/MEN-1	Well differentiated
Type III (and NEC)	Normogastrinemic Sporadic	Well differentiated to poorly differentiated

Type I, II, and III disease are well-differentiated tumors associated with progressively poor prognosis. Type I gastric carcinoid is not associated with mortality, type II gastric carcinoid has an approximately 10% mortality at 5 years, and type III gastric carcinoid has a 20% to 25% mortality at 5 years. Neuroendocrine carcinomas (NECs), a subset of type III, is a poorly differentiated gastric neuroendocrine carcinoma and is an aggressive malignancy, with a 70% to 80% mortality rate at 5 years. Type I, II, and III NENs comprise approximately 75%, 5%, and approximately 20% of gastric NENs, respectively.
Data from Refs.[13,18,110]

achieved in all lesions. No procedure-related perforations and only 1 local recurrence occurred during a mean follow-up of 24.4 months.[32] In a separate study, approximately 60% of type I lesions had recurred after endoscopic resection; endoscopic management nevertheless is usually considered safe and effective.[33] Endoscopic resection or local wedge excision may also be repeated unless the lesions are excessive in number or evidence of invasion is present.[17,34] Large lesions greater than 20 mm that ulcerate or bleed may require more extensive surgical resection, particularly if the patient is young and evidence shows diffuse gastric microcarcinoidosis. In general, surgery may be effective in approximately 80% of tumors.[18,35] In selected patients at risk for metastatic disease, antrectomy to reduce gastrin levels may be considered.

Given their slow proliferation, type I NENs are not amenable to standard chemotherapeutic approaches. Instead, investigators have focused on disrupting ECL cell growth through either targeting somatostatin receptors or inhibiting the gastrin stimulus. Although somatostatin scintigraphy may be negative for small, localized tumors, receptors are readily evident on both ECL cells and ECL cell tumors, and somatostatin analogs inhibit ECL cell secretion and proliferation.[36,37] Somatostatin analogs also reduce gastrin levels, and thus gastrin's proliferative stimuli on ECL cells.[37] Therapeutic use of somatostatin analog therapy is associated with regression of lesions and reductions in circulating gastrin[37,38] and CgA,[21] the number of visible tumors, and CgA-positive immunoreactive tumor cells.[21] These effects, however, are generally short term ($\approx$ 1 year), and disease progression and even tumor dedifferentiation have been noted at 5 years after termination of therapy.[39] Treatment of benignly behaving localized type I tumors with somatostatin analogs remains controversial and, if this treatment is initiated, it should not be discontinued because of a potential risk of progression to malignant disease.[39]

The specific gastrin receptor (CCK2) antagonist YF476 is an alternative agent that has been shown to inhibit acid secretion and ECL cell proliferation, and reduce type I NEN lesions size and number.[40–42] The clinical utility of this approach was recently examined in a prospective study. Eight patients with multiple type I tumors received oral netazepide (YF476) once daily for 12 weeks, with follow-up at 12 weeks in an open-label pilot trial. All patients had a reduction in the number and size of their largest tumor, and plasma CgA was reduced to normal levels at 3 weeks, whereas gastrin levels remained unchanged.[43] This agent seemed to be well tolerated; its utility requires further assessment because CgA levels rebounded after drug withdrawal. A vaccine against gastrin (G17 molecule) was recently tested in 3 patients with CAG/type I, who were followed up endoscopically and clinically for a mean of 36 months.[44] Tumor regression was noted in 2 of the 3 patients who exhibited a significant reduction in plasma CgA levels. These pilot studies that are based on an understanding of the underlying biology of the lesion, suggest that targeting gastrin either at a receptor level or the hormone itself may be a potential therapy for type I lesions.

However, given the low mortality rate associated with these lesions, whether these pharmacologic approaches will be of utility remains unclear. Studies by Rappel and colleagues[45] in 1995 reported an observed 78% and an age-corrected 100% survival rate (Kaplan-Meier) in 88 patients with type I lesions. More recently, 5- and 10-year crude survival rates were estimated at 96.1% and 73.9%, respectively (not different from the general population), for type I tumors.[35] These data reflect an overall benign course for this disease. In general, type I tumors have survival rates that are therefore not different from the general population. The benefit of treatment must therefore be considered in conjunction with the potential morbidity associated with pharmaceutical treatment, repeated endoscopic resection, or surgery. Nevertheless, an active treatment approach is required for the more malignant tumors.[23]

Type II Gastric NENs

These ZES-MEN-1–associated hypergastrinemia-driven lesions are usually multiple, small (<1 cm), and predominantly of the ECL cell type, although some lesions contain heterogeneous cell populations.[11] Serum gastrin levels in type II NENs are usually significantly elevated.[15] A secretin test or measurement of acid secretion levels may suggest the gastrinoma origin of the type II–associated lesion. However, clinical presentations may exhibit wide variations, and include diverse symptomatology indistinguishable from peptic ulcer, gastric polyps, or even carcinoma. The clinicopathologic behavior of type II NENs occupies an intermediate position between that of the aggressive (gastrin-independent) type III sporadic lesions and the more benign type I lesions.

Like type I lesions, type II lesions range from pseudohyperplasia, hyperplasia, dysplasia, and neoplasia. Type II lesions, like type I NENs, consist mainly of ECL cells,[46] and exhibit argyrophil cell hyperplasia/dysplasia throughout the oxyntic mucosa, which, in contrast to CAG/A, is usually rugose. The cytologic characteristics of the lesion are also similar to the type I NENs. In contrast to the latter, and although they are generally considered well differentiated, local infiltration may occur at mucosal and submucosal levels and metastases occur in approximately 12% of lesions.[13] They are nevertheless characterized as WHO type 1 tumors and are considered of benign or low-grade malignant potential.

Studies show that one-third of individuals with MEN-1 develop gastric type II lesions, and LOH has been identified in 75% of ZES-MEN-1 tumor samples and 41% of MEN-1 gastrinomas.[47] The MEN-1 syndrome is an autosomal dominant disorder caused by mutations in the *MEN-1* gene.[48] The *MEN-1* gene protein product menin is a tumor suppressor involved in transcriptional regulation and genome stability.[48] Germline mutations and/or LOH are associated with disruption of menin function with a consequent loss of proliferative inhibition (perhaps through regulation of retinoblastoma expression,[49] inactivation of cell cycle inhibitors such as P16[INK4A],[50] or alterations in AKT/mTOR[51]) and development of lesions. The dysregulation of menin function during hypergastrinemia is unclear. Animal studies suggest that elevated gastrin is associated with decreased menin expression,[52] whereas cell-based assays show that menin inhibits gastrin expression.[53] Loss of menin may be associated with an elevation in gastrin transcription (secondary to elevated gastrin translation, synthesis, and secretion).

In addition to MEN-1–associated endocrine pathology, type II lesions commonly occur with a variety of other endocrine abnormalities, including hypothyroidism (39%), diabetes (19%), and Addison disease (6%).[14] Although the molecular biology is generally understood to reflect mutations in *MEN-1*, recent studies have identified 2 other loci that may be of interest: *NF1* and *CDNKB*. The *NF* gene product, neurofibromin, is a tumor suppressor and, when nonfunctional, results in activated P21ras signaling and abnormal cell proliferation. An LOH at the *NF1* locus has been demonstrated in a gastric NEN derived from a patient with *NF1* suggesting that the RAS-MAPK pathway may be associated with the proliferative regulation.[54] Progression through the cell cycle, particularly through G1, is negatively regulated by p27[KIP1] or CDKN1B. Recently, a patient with both hyperparathyroidism and a type II lesion was identified with a heterozygous GAGA deletion in the 5′-UTR of *CDKN1B* (NM_004064.3:c.-32_-29del).[55] This germline mutation falls inside the region that is responsible for *CDKN1B* transcription and is predicted to destroy a secondary stem and loop structure that includes the GAGAGA element responsible for ribosome recruitment. This function suggests that alterations in the transcription/translation rate of *CDKN1B* mRNA may be the mechanism for tumor susceptibility.[55] These results indicate that the mutational spectrum in gastric lesions is greater than *MEN-1*, and investigators could potentially consider other gene targets that are known candidates for molecular-based therapies in other adenocarcinomas (eg, MAPK inhibitors).

Although the metastatic rate (3%–12%) of ZES-MEN-1 (type II) lesions is reported to be higher than for type I lesions, the short-term prognosis is similar.[56] The long-term prognosis of type II disease, however, ultimately reflects the course of the MEN-1 gastrinoma, which itself has a 5-year survival rate of 60% to 75%.[57] Overall, the survival rate of type II lesions is therefore worse than that of type I given the increased propensity for metastasis of the gastric lesion and the additional morbidity conferred by the natural history of MEN-1.

As with type I NENs, treatment options include endoscopic and surgical resection and pharmaceutical intervention. Removal of the source of hypergastrinemia is the critical aim of surgery, and regression of type II lesions may occur after successful gastrinoma excision.[58] Endoscopic resection has also been used for gastric type II NENs, and endoscopic surveillance with extensive sampling of both the lesser and greater curvatures is recommended if the gastrinoma is inoperable.[59] More extensive surgery may be necessary for lesions greater than 20 mm and when an excessive number of lesions is evident or if deeper invasion into the muscular wall is present.[17,34]

High doses of a PPI is the preferred treatment for patients with symptoms of hyperacidity.[60] The long-acting depot formulations of somatostatin analogs can also be prescribed in the presence of symptoms,[61] and have been used to control hypergastrinemia and ulceration.[62] In addition, these analogs may decrease the gastric endocrine cell mass,[63,64] but evidence of antiproliferative efficacy is insufficient.[65]

Type III Gastric NENs

These tumors are usually large and evolve in a milieu of seemingly normal plasma gastrin levels within a "normal" gastric mucosa. Overall, type III NENs exhibit a greater similarity to neuroendocrine carcinomas than to NENs per se. In this respect, their biologic behavior is aggressive, and local invasive growth and distant metastases are predictable features of their evolution.

Tumors display a fairly uniform light microscopic appearance with typical carcinoid histopathologic features. Their growth pattern may be trabecular or gyriform, medullary or solid, glandular or rosette-like, or a combination of any of these types.[66] Lesions exhibit a spectrum from well differentiated to poorly differentiated, often demonstrate an aggressive local behavior (at diagnosis, local spread is present in approximately 15% of patients), and have a high incidence (24%–55%) of metastasis.[13]

WHO type 2 tumors include all lesions, including the traditionally annotated type III NENs, and are characterized by being greater than 2 cm in size, have invaded the muscularis propria with or without metastases and are either nonfunctional or secretory tumors. WHO type 3 tumors include the traditionally annotated "atypical" or "sporadic" gastric NENs. This subtype, which is particularly aggressive in its behavior,[61] is associated with rapid local gastric progression, distant metastases, and early death. These tumors may be identified by an increased mitotic count with nuclear polymorphism, hypochromasia, and prominent nucleoli.[17] Whether this tumor is any different from a neuroendocrine carcinoma is unclear.

LOH in the 11q13-14 region is infrequently (<25%) found in type III lesions,[26] suggesting that alterations in the MEN locus do not play a significant role in the etiopathogenesis of this gastrin-autonomous tumor type; the molecular pathogenesis of these lesions is currently unknown.

Type III lesions often display markedly aggressive local behavior, and metastasize. This poor prognosis is directly related to the high metastatic rate, and the overall 5-year survival rate is usually less than 50%.[7,13,67,68] The 5-year survival rate is significantly higher for localized disease (64.3%) and for lesions with regional metastases (29.9%) than for lesions with distant metastases (10%). Although the tendency to metastasize correlates with tumor size, minute tumors have been reported with spread.[69] Factors that predict aggressive behavior include cellular atypia, 2 or more mitoses per 10 high-powered fields, Ki-67 index greater than 2%, angioinvasion, and transmural invasion.[13,70]

These normogastrinemia-associated tumors occur more often in men older than 50 years.[17,18] They typically present as gastric adenocarcinomas with loss of appetite and weight, anemia, and evidence of local and advanced metastatic disease.[17,61] The atypical carcinoid syndrome may also be evident in some type III lesions and is characterized by cutaneous flushing, profound itching, bronchospasm, and lacrimation. This finding usually reflects the sequelae of unregulated ECL cell histamine production (though other agents, such as tachykinins, have been reported) and is often provoked by ingestion of certain kinds of foods, particularly cheeses (tyramine) and wine.[66]

Histamine 1 and 2 receptor blockade may be of benefit in suppressing skin rashes and acid hypersecretion. Whenever possible, surgical resection and lymph node dissection should be performed. If radical resection is not possible, preoperative downstaging with chemotherapy may be beneficial. Intravenous cytotoxic therapy may be used if metastases are evident.[18] In selected patients, hepatic artery perfusion, focal embolization (or chemoembolization), cryoablation, or radiofrequency ablation with or without synchronous chemotherapy may be beneficial,[34] whereas the combination of cisplatin and etoposide should be considered for anaplastic neuroendocrine carcinomas.[63,71,72] Peptide receptor radionuclide therapy (PRRT) may be considered as a treatment option, but a positive somatostatin scintigraph is a prerequisite for using this modality.[18] Neither cytotoxics nor PRRT are associated with substantial objective tumor responses (≈20%) but may increase progression-free survival.[34]

Surgically, these lesions should be managed as for gastric adenocarcinoma. Thus, the presence of solitary, large (>1 cm), or invasive tumors mandates an attempt at surgical cure.[67,69] In patients whose general condition is consistent with an acceptable operative risk, complete or partial gastrectomy (en bloc resection) with local lymph node resection is appropriate.[73] Lesions greater than 2 cm associated with local invasion require subtotal gastrectomy or extended local resection.[74]

These lesions often display markedly aggressive local behavior. The overall 5-year survival rate is usually less than 50%,[7,13,67,68] and a poor prognosis is related to metastases. Lesions with regional (29.9%) and distant metastases (10.0%) have significantly lower survivals.

INSIGHTS FROM NEN ANIMAL MODELS

In contrast to the paucity of studies that examine the pathobiology of gastric NENs, a plethora of studies in animal models have been undertaken, in both naturally occurring disease models (eg, *Mastomys* or cotton rats, knockout mice, viral vectors [eg, SV40]) and models in which acid perturbation mimics clinical conditions. The results of these studies largely highlight the important role of gastrin in the development of lesions; their translational interpretation, however, may be complicated by the underlying pathobiologic differences between these models and humans.

Natural Models

The *Mastomys* (*Praomys natalensis*) is a sub-Saharan African muroid rodent phylogenetically related to the mouse[75] that spontaneously develops gastric NENs in 20% to 50% of the population by 2 years of age.[76] The development of these tumors is caused by a gastrin receptor (CCK_2) mutant that shows ligand-independent constitutive activity for inositol phosphate formation.[77] Analysis of the *Mastomys* sequence identified 3 amino acids that, when included in the human receptor (mutagenesis studies [344]L, [353]I, and [407]D), confer ligand-independent signaling.[77] No studies have evaluated whether any of these mutations occur in humans with gastric NENs. Drug-induced hypergastrinemia consequent on acid suppression, such as after oral ingestion of histamine H_2-receptor blockers (loxtidine, cimetidine) or omeprazole (a PPI), significantly accelerates the development of ECL cell tumors.[52] Tumor development can be reversed by YF476.[41] Other growth factors involved in tumor pathobiology include CTGF/CCN2, transforming growth factor α (TNFα), and histamine.[52,78–80] The *Mastomys* is considered a model for type I/III NENs.

The female hispid cotton rats (*Sigmodon hispidus*) also spontaneously develop gastric carcinomas by approximately 10 to 16 months of age, and these tumors seem to have a neuroendocrine cell component.[81] As in the *Mastomys*, ECL cell–derived tumors can be accelerated by pharmacologic acid suppression, but this usually takes longer than 6 months.[82] The mutational spectrum of CCK2 in these animals has not been evaluated, and therefore whether this is a gastrin-mediated phenomenon remains unclear. A proportion of female cotton rats also develop spontaneous gastric hypoacidity and hypergastrinemia.[83] However, unlike the *Mastomys*, these animals develop adenocarcinomas rather than NENs. The tumors seem to develop from ECL cells of the oxyntic mucosa with hyperplasia of CgA immunoreactive cells, whereas a proportion of the adenocarcinoma tumor cells are both CgA- and Sevier-Munger–positive.[83,84] Carcinoma development can be prevented by YF476, confirming that gastrin has a role in tumorigenesis of these mixed cell lesions.[84] The cotton rat is considered a model for type III NENs and gastric neuroendocrine carcinomas.

Transgenic Models

MEN-1 model
A mouse model heterozygous for deletion in the *MEN-1* locus[85] developed a variety of tumors consistent with the human MEN-1 syndrome, but only 1 animal (3.7%) developed a gastric NEN. These animals exhibited hyperinsulinemia; gastrin levels were not documented (**Table 2**). The development of gastric NENs in humans with type II lesions requires a combination of a MEN-1 mutation and elevated gastrin levels.[25]

SV40 large T-antigen models
A transgenic mouse carrying the human SV40 large T-antigen in the *atp4b* gene[86] developed metastatic gastric neuroendocrine carcinomas that were not derived from the ECL cell but rather from increases in the progenitor oxyntopeptic cell lineage.[86] A second model, targeting CEA424, also developed neuroendocrine tumors (antral tumors that are CgA-positive and secrete serotonin).[87] Both models exhibit transcriptomes that overlap with genes considered relevant for human neuroendocrine tumor biology, suggesting that the SV40 large T antigen directly induces a neuroendocrine gene signature in gastric carcinomas. However, in both models, invasive

Table 2
Receptor knockout, transgenic mouse and bacterial models used to study ECL cell biology

Knockout/Gene Target	Physiological/Cellular Effect	Effect on ECL Cell Numbers	Effect on Serum Gastrin
MEN-1	Loss of MEN-1 locus (hyperinsulinemia)	NC	ND
SV40-*atp4b*	Atypical gastric tumors	NC	ND
SV40-CEA424	Atypical gastric tumors (hyperserotoninemia)	NC (antral enterochromaffin cell tumors)	ND
Histamine 2 receptor	Histamine 2 receptor lost	⇑	⇑
CCK₂ receptor	CCK₂ receptor lost	⇓	⇑

Abbreviations: NC, no change; ND, no data.

gastric carcinomas share expression of the transcriptional regulator gene *Etv1*, which is a master regulator of neuronally derived gastrointestinal stromal tumors and is commonly affected by gene translocations in prostate tumors, which often exhibit a neuroendocrine phenotype on progression.[88] These models likely do not generate neuroendocrine tumors from activation of neuroendocrine progenitor cells, but rather reflect transformation of cells with epithelial lineages. The relevance to gastric NENs remains unclear, although the biology suggests roles for RB1/p53 in tumorigenesis.[89] These may be models for type III lesions or, more particularly, neuroendocrine carcinomas.

Knockout Models

Several receptor knockout and transgenic models have been developed that provide insight into the relationship between receptor activation and ECL cell proliferation (see **Table 2**).

Histamine H₂-receptor knockouts

Histamine H₂ receptor deficient mice are characterized by an increase in ECL cell numbers, which is associated with both elevated histamine (+300%) and gastrin levels (+400%).[90]

CCK2 receptor knockouts

CCK2 receptor knockout mice, in contrast, exhibit a greater than 50% decrease in ECL cell numbers despite a 1000% increase in circulating gastrin levels.[91] In the absence of CCK2 expression, ECL cells do not proliferate and tumors do not develop.

Gastrin and histamine receptor activation, therefore, are required for ECL cell development, and although these studies do not examine neoplasia per se, they suggest that ECL cell differentiation in the gastric niche can be affected by activation of specific (gastrin and histamine) G protein–coupled receptors.

Bacterial Models

H pylori inoculation of transgenic mice overexpressing amidated gastrin (INS-GAS)[92] or Mongolian gerbils[93] results in the development of gastric adenocarcinoma. Infected INS-GAS mice have no evidence of ECL cell hyperplasia,[94] but male Mongolian gerbils infected with cytotoxin-associated antigen A–positive *H pylori* for longer than 24 months developed neuroendocrine cell dysplasia and NENs with marked atrophic gastritis of the oxyntic mucosa.[95] Serum gastrin levels were increased approximately

1000% in these animals. This finding suggests that *H pylori* infection is capable of producing not only gastric carcinomas but also ECL cell tumors in Mongolian gerbils, and that hypergastrinemia plays a substantial role.

Although the mechanism by which *H pylori* causes NEN development is considered to be through alterations in gastrin levels, bacterial cell wall lipopolysaccharides are bioactive and potentially mitogenic.[96] In the *Mastomys* model, *H pylori* lipopolysaccharide–induced tumor ECL cell proliferation in vitro through activation of the CD14 receptor, ornithine decarboxylase (ODC) activity, and polyamine biosynthesis.[97] Thus, alternative *H pylori*–related mechanisms may be involved in ECL cell proliferation.

Low Acid States/Hypergastrinemia

Protracted sustained acid suppression is well-known to stimulate ECL cell growth in the gastric mucosa of both mice and rats.[98,99] The mechanism for the development of ECL cell hyperplasia and neoplasia under these circumstances is an increase in serum gastrin levels with a concomitant direct proliferative effect on the ECL cells. However, in other models in which hypergastrinemia is engendered, such as after total parietal cell atrophy following oral administration of the protonophore and anti-inflammatory agent, the neutrophil elastase inhibitor DMP 777,[100] ECL cell hyperplasia does not occur. Ciprofibrate, a common lipid-lowering drug that is also a ligand for and modulator of the peroxisome proliferator-activated receptor transcription factor, also causes parietal cell loss. This function, however, is associated with both hypergastrinemia and secondary ECL cell hyperplasia.[101] The reasons for these differences are unclear, but gastric inflammation was not evident in the male rats treated with DMP 777,[100] suggesting that a combination of hypergastrinemia and gastric bacterial colonization may be required for ECL cell development.

LINKING ANIMAL STUDIES WITH CLINICAL OBSERVATIONS

In humans, low acid states, induced by either endogenous parietal cell destruction (autoimmune disease) or exogenous pharmacotherapeutic agents such as H_2-receptor antagonists or PPIs, result in G cell hypersecretion and culminate in hypergastrinemia. The association between low acid states and gastric neoplasia is well documented.[17,102] Similarly, the gastrin elevation noted in atrophic gastritis and the trophic effect of gastrin on ECL cells are consistent with the hypothesis that a low acid state with elevated plasma gastrin levels drives ECL proliferation.[6] Although it is likely that other trophic regulatory agents (TGFα, βFGF, CCN2) are implicated, gastrin seems to be the dominant effector.[17,61] Although PPIs indubitably increase plasma gastrin, most studies have shown no effect of PPIs on NEN development. This agent does, however, increases ECL cell proliferation in ZES-MEN (type II gastric NENs)[103] and has an effect on mucosal ECL cell numbers in pediatric patients.[104] Most recently, 2 patients who had been taking PPI for 12 to 13 years because of gastroesophageal reflux disease were identified on routine upper gastrointestinal endoscopy with solitary oxyntic mucosal tumors.[20] These tumors were both well-differentiated NENs that had developed in the absence of CAG. After cessation of PPI treatment, tumor regression and reversal of ECL cell hyperplasia was noted. These cases show that hypergastrinemia secondary to PPIs, like other causes of hypergastrinemia, may induce ECL cell tumors.

Autoimmune gastritis is associated with ECL hyperplasia.[105] The postulated mechanism underlying this association is that ECL cell hyperplasia develops in response to glandular damage and the resultant increased serum gastrin. Glandular damage is caused by deep or diffuse lymphocytoplasmatic infiltration within the lamina propria, which results in epithelial metaplasia and parietal cell loss, and consequently, hypergastrinemia. Long-standing pernicious anemia is also associated with hypergastrinemia and the development of multiple gastric NENs with a background of diffuse ECL cell hyperplasia.[106] These data indicate that, as in animal models, low acid states and/or chronic inflammation of the oxyntic mucosa and atrophy of the oxyntic glands are associated with the development of achlorhydria and hypergastrinemia, and results in ECL cell hyperplasia with progression to neoplasia.

SUMMARY

NENs constitute approximately 1% of all neoplastic lesions; of these, gastric NENs constitute fewer than 10%. The calculated incidence is approximately 0.33 per 100,000 people per year.[9] Although not as rare as previously thought, they remain largely understudied and are not a prominent focus of clinical attention despite that approximately 30% of cases are associated with 1 or more additional malignancies.[107] The incidence and prevalence of gastric NENs as a group have been increasing over the past 35 years (7.6% per annum).[108] The major reason for this is probably better diagnostics and an increased awareness among physicians. However, this finding may also reflect the introduction and widespread use of acid suppressive medication and secondary hypergastrinemia.[20,109] A high percentage of children (61%) receiving long-term PPI therapy continuously for up to 10.8 years (median, 2.84 years) develop minor degrees of ECL hyperplasia,[104] and the possible risk for developing NENs remains a concern, particularly given a recent case report of 2 patients who developed NENs after 12 years of PPI use.[20] Continued study of the pathobiology of human ECL cell neoplasia may yield valuable insights into the regulation of other gastric mucosal cells, particularly the relationship between histamine and/or gastrin and the development malignancies. Further studies of menin function and its complex interrelationship with gastrin may provide additional insights into tumor biology both at the clinical level and in terms of basic cell biology, such as the role of the epigenome in neuroendocrine cell proliferation. The latter may have relevance for the choice of therapy in the management of these lesions.

REFERENCES

1. Modlin IM, Oberg K, Chung DC, et al. Gastroenteropancreatic neuroendocrine tumours. Lancet Oncol 2008;9(1):61–72.
2. Smith AM, Watson SA, Caplin M, et al. Gastric carcinoid expresses the gastrin autocrine pathway. Br J Surg 1998;85(9):1285–9.
3. Modlin IM, Lawton GP, Miu K, et al. Pathophysiology of the fundic enterochromaffin-like (ECL) cell and gastric carcinoid tumours. Ann R Coll Surg Engl 1996;78(2):133–8.
4. Kitago M, Inada T, Igarashi S, et al. Multiple gastric carcinoid tumors with type A gastritis concomitant with gastric cancer: a case report. Oncol Rep 2001;8(2): 343–6.
5. Waldum HL, Haugen OA, Isaksen C, et al. Enterochromaffin-like tumour cells in the diffuse but not the intestinal type of gastric carcinomas. Scand J Gastroenterol Suppl 1991;180:165–9.
6. Modlin IM, Goldenring JR, Lawton GP, et al. Aspects of the theoretical basis and clinical relevance of low acid states. Am J Gastroenterol 1994;89(3):308–18.
7. Godwin JD 2nd. Carcinoid tumors. An analysis of 2,837 cases. Cancer 1975; 36(2):560–9.

8. Modlin IM, Lye KD, Kidd M. A 5-decade analysis of 13,715 carcinoid tumors. Cancer 2003;97(4):934–59.
9. Modlin IM, Lye KD, Kidd M. A 50-year analysis of 562 gastric carcinoids: small tumor or larger problem? Am J Gastroenterol 2004;99(1):23–32.
10. Latta E, Rotondo F, Leiter LA, et al. Ghrelin- and serotonin-producing gastric carcinoid. J Gastrointest Cancer 2012;43(2):319–23.
11. Modlin IM, Tang LH. The gastric enterochromaffin-like cell: an enigmatic cellular link. Gastroenterology 1996;111(3):783–810.
12. Bordi C. Gastric carcinoids. Ital J Gastroenterol Hepatol 1999;31(Suppl 2): S94–97.
13. Rindi G, Luinetti O, Cornaggia M, et al. Three subtypes of gastric argyrophil carcinoid and the gastric neuroendocrine carcinoma: a clinicopathologic study. Gastroenterology 1993;104(4):994–1006.
14. Gough DB, Thompson GB, Crotty TB, et al. Diverse clinical and pathologic features of gastric carcinoid and the relevance of hypergastrinemia. World J Surg 1994;18(4):473–9 [discussion: 79–80].
15. Jordan PH Jr, Barroso A, Sweeney J. Gastric carcinoids in patients with hyper-gastrinemia. J Am Coll Surg 2004;199(4):552–5.
16. Vannella L, Sbrozzi-Vanni A, Lahner E, et al. Development of type I gastric carci-noid in patients with chronic atrophic gastritis. Aliment Pharmacol Ther 2011; 33(12):1361–9.
17. Modlin IM, Lye KD, Kidd M. Carcinoid tumors of the stomach. Surg Oncol 2003; 12(2):153–72.
18. Ruszniewski P, Delle Fave G, Cadiot G, et al. Well-differentiated gastric tumors/ carcinomas. Neuroendocrinology 2006;84(3):158–64.
19. Kekilli M, Beyazit Y, Karaman K, et al. Endoscopic and pathological aspects of gastric polyps: a Turkish referral center study. Hepatogastroenterology 2012; 59(116):1147–9.
20. Jianu CS, Fossmark R, Viset T, et al. Gastric carcinoids after long-term use of a proton pump inhibitor. Aliment Pharmacol Ther 2012;36(7):644–9.
21. Thomas D, Tsolakis AV, Grozinsky-Glasberg S, et al. Long-term follow-up of a large series of patients with type 1 gastric carcinoid tumors. Data from a multi-center study. Eur J Endocrinol 2012;6:6.
22. Carcinoid tumors. International symposium on pathology, epidemiology, clinical aspects and therapy. January 13-16, 1994, Munich, Germany. Proceedings. Digestion 1994;55(Suppl 3):1–113.
23. Spampatti MP, Massironi S, Rossi RE, et al. Unusually aggressive type 1 gastric carcinoid: a case report with a review of the literature. Eur J Gastroenterol Hep-atol 2012;24(5):589–93.
24. Solcia E, Fiocca R, Villani L, et al. Hyperplastic, dysplastic, and neoplastic enterochromaffin-like-cell proliferations of the gastric mucosa. Classification and histogenesis. Am J Surg Pathol 1995;19(Suppl 1):S1–7.
25. Debelenko LV, Emmert-Buck MR, Zhuang Z, et al. The multiple endocrine neoplasia type I gene locus is involved in the pathogenesis of type II gastric carcinoids. Gastroenterology 1997;113(3):773–81.
26. D'Adda T, Keller G, Bordi C, et al. Loss of heterozygosity in 11q13-14 regions in gastric neuroendocrine tumors not associated with multiple endocrine neoplasia type 1 syndrome. Lab Invest 1999;79(6):671–7.
27. Choi IS, Estecio MR, Nagano Y, et al. Hypomethylation of LINE-1 and Alu in well-differentiated neuroendocrine tumors (pancreatic endocrine tumors and carci-noid tumors). Mod Pathol 2007;20(7):802–10.

28. Stricker I, Tzivras D, Nambiar S, et al. Site- and grade-specific diversity of LINE1 methylation pattern in gastroenteropancreatic neuroendocrine tumours. Anticancer Res 2012;32(9):3699–706.
29. Jiang Z, Woda BA, Rock KL, et al. P504S: a new molecular marker for the detection of prostate carcinoma. Am J Surg Pathol 2001;25(11):1397–404.
30. Annenkov A, Nishikura K, Domori K, et al. Alpha-methylacyl-coenzyme A racemase expression in neuroendocrine neoplasms of the stomach. Virchows Arch 2012;461(2):169–75.
31. Saund MS, Al Natour RH, Sharma AM, et al. Tumor size and depth predict rate of lymph node metastasis and utilization of lymph node sampling in surgically managed gastric carcinoids. Ann Surg Oncol 2011;18(10):2826–32.
32. Li QL, Zhang YQ, Chen WF, et al. Endoscopic submucosal dissection for foregut neuroendocrine tumors: an initial study. World J Gastroenterol 2012;18(40):5799–806.
33. Merola E, Sbrozzi-Vanni A, Panzuto F, et al. Type I gastric carcinoids: a prospective study on endoscopic management and recurrence rate. Neuroendocrinology 2012;95(3):207–13.
34. Modlin IM, Latich I, Kidd M, et al. Therapeutic options for gastrointestinal carcinoids. Clin Gastroenterol Hepatol 2006;4(5):526–47.
35. Borch K, Ahren B, Ahlman H, et al. Gastric carcinoids: biologic behavior and prognosis after differentiated treatment in relation to type. Ann Surg 2005;242(1):64–73.
36. Borin JF, Tang LH, Kidd M, et al. Somatostatin receptor regulation of gastric enterochromaffin-like cell transformation to gastric carcinoid. Surgery 1996;120(6):1026–32.
37. Fykse V, Sandvik AK, Qvigstad G, et al. Treatment of ECL cell carcinoids with octreotide LAR. Scand J Gastroenterol 2004;39(7):621–8.
38. Campana D, Nori F, Pezzilli R, et al. Gastric endocrine tumors type I: treatment with long-acting somatostatin analogs. Endocr Relat Cancer 2008;15(1):337–42.
39. Jianu CS, Fossmark R, Syversen U, et al. Five-year follow-up of patients treated for 1 year with octreotide long-acting release for enterochromaffin-like cell carcinoids. Scand J Gastroenterol 2011;46(4):456–63.
40. Boyce M, David O, Darwin K, et al. Single oral doses of netazepide (YF476), a gastrin receptor antagonist, cause dose-dependent, sustained increases in gastric pH compared with placebo and ranitidine in healthy subjects. Aliment Pharmacol Ther 2012;36(2):181–9.
41. Kidd M, Siddique ZL, Drozdov I, et al. The CCK(2) receptor antagonist, YF476, inhibits Mastomys ECL cell hyperplasia and gastric carcinoid tumor development. Regul Pept 2010;162(1–3):52–60.
42. Fossmark R, Sørdal Ø, Jianu CS, et al. Treatment of gastric carcinoids type 1 with the gastrin receptor antagonist YF476 results in regression of tumours and normalisation of serum chromogranin A. Gastroenterology 2012;36(11–12):1067–75.
43. Fossmark R, Sordal O, Jianu CS, et al. Treatment of gastric carcinoids type 1 with the gastrin receptor antagonist netazepide (YF476) results in regression of tumours and normalisation of serum chromogranin A. Aliment Pharmacol Ther 2012;36(11–12):1067–75.
44. Tieppo C, Betterle C, Basso D, et al. Gastric type I carcinoid: a pilot study with human G17DT immunogen vaccination. Cancer Immunol Immunother 2011;60(7):1057–60.
45. Rappel S, Altendorf-Hofmann A, Stolte M. Prognosis of gastric carcinoid tumours. Digestion 1995;56(6):455–62.

46. Lehy T, Mignon M, Cadiot G, et al. Gastric endocrine cell behavior in Zollinger-Ellison patients upon long-term potent antisecretory treatment. Gastroenterology 1989;96(4):1029–40.

47. Debelenko LV, Zhuang Z, Emmert-Buck MR, et al. Allelic deletions on chromosome 11q13 in multiple endocrine neoplasia type 1-associated and sporadic gastrinomas and pancreatic endocrine tumors. Cancer Res 1997;57(11):2238–43.

48. Calender A. Molecular genetics of neuroendocrine tumors. Digestion 2000;62(Suppl 1):3–18.

49. Ivo D, Corset L, Desbourdes L, et al. Menin controls the concentration of retinoblastoma protein. Cell Cycle 2011;10(1):166–8.

50. Gagrica S, Brookes S, Anderton E, et al. Contrasting behavior of the p18INK4c and p16INK4a tumor suppressors in both replicative and oncogene-induced senescence. Cancer Res 2012;72(1):165–75.

51. Hughes E, Huang C. Participation of Akt, menin, and p21 in pregnancy-induced beta-cell proliferation. Endocrinology 2011;152(3):847–55.

52. Kidd M, Hinoue T, Eick G, et al. Global expression analysis of ECL cells in Mastomys natalensis gastric mucosa identifies alterations in the AP-1 pathway induced by gastrin-mediated transformation. Physiol Genomics 2004;20(1):131–42.

53. Mensah-Osman EJ, Veniaminova NA, Merchant JL. Menin and JunD regulate gastrin gene expression through proximal DNA elements. Am J Physiol Gastrointest Liver Physiol 2011;301(5):G783–790.

54. Stewart W, Traynor JP, Cooke A, et al. Gastric carcinoid: germline and somatic mutation of the neurofibromatosis type 1 gene. Fam Cancer 2007;6(1):147–52.

55. Malanga D, De Gisi S, Riccardi M, et al. Functional characterization of a rare germline mutation in the gene encoding the cyclin-dependent kinase inhibitor p27Kip1 (CDKN1B) in a Spanish patient with multiple endocrine neoplasia-like phenotype. Eur J Endocrinol 2012;166(3):551–60.

56. Jensen RT. Management of the Zollinger-Ellison syndrome in patients with multiple endocrine neoplasia type 1. J Intern Med 1998;243(6):477–88.

57. Meko JB, Norton JA. Management of patients with Zollinger-Ellison syndrome. Annu Rev Med 1995;46:395–411.

58. Richards ML, Gauger P, Thompson NW, et al. Regression of type II gastric carcinoids in multiple endocrine neoplasia type 1 patients with Zollinger-Ellison syndrome after surgical excision of all gastrinomas. World J Surg 2004;28(7):652–8.

59. Bordi C, Azzoni C, Ferraro G, et al. Sampling strategies for analysis of enterochromaffin-like cell changes in Zollinger-Ellison syndrome. Am J Clin Pathol 2000;114(3):419–25.

60. Lew EA, Pisegna JR, Starr JA, et al. Intravenous pantoprazole rapidly controls gastric acid hypersecretion in patients with Zollinger-Ellison syndrome. Gastroenterology 2000;118(4):696–704.

61. Modlin IM, Kidd M, Latich I, et al. Current status of gastrointestinal carcinoids. Gastroenterology 2005;128(6):1717–51.

62. Campana D, Piscitelli L, Mazzotta E, et al. Zollinger-Ellison syndrome. Diagnosis and therapy. Minerva Med 2005;96(3):187–206.

63. Ruszniewski P, Ramdani A, Cadiot G, et al. Long-term treatment with octreotide in patients with the Zollinger-Ellison syndrome. Eur J Clin Invest 1993;23(5):296–301.

64. Annibale B, Delle Fave G, Azzoni C, et al. Three months of octreotide treatment decreases gastric acid secretion and argyrophil cell density in patients with Zollinger-Ellison syndrome and antral G-cell hyperfunction. Aliment Pharmacol Ther 1994;8(1):95–104.
65. Fykse V, Sandvik AK, Waldum HL. One-year follow-up study of patients with enterochromaffin-like cell carcinoids after treatment with octreotide long-acting release. Scand J Gastroenterol 2005;40(11):1269–74.
66. Creutzfeldt W, Stockmann F. Carcinoids and carcinoid syndrome. Am J Med 1987;82(5B):4–16.
67. Gilligan CJ, Lawton GP, Tang LH, et al. Gastric carcinoid tumors: the biology and therapy of an enigmatic and controversial lesion. Am J Gastroenterol 1995; 90(3):338–52.
68. Modlin IM, Sandor A. An analysis of 8305 cases of carcinoid tumors. Cancer 1997;79(4):813–29.
69. Kumashiro R, Naitoh H, Teshima K, et al. Minute gastric carcinoid tumor with regional lymph node metastasis. Int Surg 1989;74(3):198–200.
70. Moesta KT, Schlag P. Proposal for a new carcinoid tumour staging system based on tumour tissue infiltration and primary metastasis; a prospective multicentre carcinoid tumour evaluation study. West German Surgical Oncologists' Group. Eur J Surg Oncol 1990;16(4):280–8.
71. Jensen RT, Norton JA. Carcinoid tumors and the carcinoid syndrome. In: DeVita VT Jr, Hellman S, Rosenberg S, editors. Cancer: Principles Practice of Oncology. 5th edition. Philadelphia: Lippincott-Raven; 1997. p. 1704–23.
72. Moertel CG, Kvols LK, O'Connell MJ, et al. Treatment of neuroendocrine carcinomas with combined etoposide and cisplatin. Evidence of major therapeutic activity in the anaplastic variants of these neoplasms. Cancer 1991;68(2): 227–32.
73. De Vries EG, Kema IP, Slooff MJ, et al. Recent developments in diagnosis and treatment of metastatic carcinoid tumours. Scand J Gastroenterol Suppl 1993; 200:87–93.
74. Davies MG, O'Dowd G, McEntee GP, et al. Primary gastric carcinoids: a view on management. Br J Surg 1990;77(9):1013–4.
75. Jansa SA, Weksler M. Phylogeny of muroid rodents: relationships within and among major lineages as determined by IRBP gene sequences. Mol Phylogenet Evol 2004;31(1):256–76.
76. Modlin IM, Lawton GP, Tang LH, et al. The mastomys gastric carcinoid: aspects of enterochromaffin-like cell function. Digestion 1994;55(Suppl 3):31–7.
77. Schaffer K, McBride EW, Beinborn M, et al. Interspecies polymorphisms confer constitutive activity to the Mastomys cholecystokinin-B/gastrin receptor. J Biol Chem 1998;273(44):28779–84.
78. Kidd M, Modlin IM, Eick GN, et al. Role of CCN2/CTGF in the proliferation of Mastomys enterochromaffin-like cells and gastric carcinoid development. Am J Physiol Gastrointest Liver Physiol 2007;292(1):G191–200.
79. Kidd M, Schimmack S, Lawrence B, et al. EGFR/TGFalpha and TGFbeta/CTGF Signaling in Neuroendocrine Neoplasia: Theoretical Therapeutic Targets. Neuroendocrinology 2012;15:15.
80. Tang LH, Modlin IM, Lawton GP, et al. The role of transforming growth factor alpha in the enterochromaffin-like cell tumor autonomy in an African rodent mastomys. Gastroenterology 1996;111(5):1212–23.
81. Kawase S, Ishikura H. Female-predominant occurrence of spontaneous gastric adenocarcinoma in cotton rats. Lab Anim Sci 1995;45(3):244–8.

82. Fossmark R, Martinsen TC, Bakkelund KE, et al. ECL-cell derived gastric cancer in male cotton rats dosed with the H2-blocker loxtidine. Cancer Res 2004; 64(10):3687–93.

83. Waldum HL, Rorvik H, Falkmer S, et al. Neuroendocrine (ECL cell) differentiation of spontaneous gastric carcinomas of cotton rats (Sigmodon hispidus). Lab Anim Sci 1999;49(3):241–7.

84. Martinsen TC, Kawase S, Hakanson R, et al. Spontaneous ECL cell carcinomas in cotton rats: natural course and prevention by a gastrin receptor antagonist. Carcinogenesis 2003;24(12):1887–96.

85. Crabtree JS, Scacheri PC, Ward JM, et al. A mouse model of multiple endocrine neoplasia, type 1, develops multiple endocrine tumors. Proc Natl Acad Sci U S A 2001;98(3):1118–23.

86. Syder AJ, Karam SM, Mills JC, et al. A transgenic mouse model of metastatic carcinoma involving transdifferentiation of a gastric epithelial lineage progenitor to a neuroendocrine phenotype. Proc Natl Acad Sci U S A 2004;101(13):4471–6.

87. Ihler F, Vetter EV, Pan J, et al. Expression of a neuroendocrine gene signature in gastric tumor cells from CEA 424-SV40 large T antigen-transgenic mice depends on SV40 large T antigen. PLoS One 2012;7(1):e29846.

88. Chi P, Chen Y, Zhang L, et al. ETV1 is a lineage survival factor that cooperates with KIT in gastrointestinal stromal tumours. Nature 2010;467(7317):849–53.

89. Ahuja D, Saenz-Robles MT, Pipas JM. SV40 large T antigen targets multiple cellular pathways to elicit cellular transformation. Oncogene 2005;24(52): 7729–45.

90. Fukushima Y, Matsui T, Saitoh T, et al. Unique roles of G protein-coupled histamine H2 and gastrin receptors in growth and differentiation of gastric mucosa. Eur J Pharmacol 2004;502(3):243–52.

91. Chen D, Zhao CM, Al-Haider W, et al. Differentiation of gastric ECL cells is altered in CCK(2) receptor-deficient mice. Gastroenterology 2002;123(2): 577–85.

92. Fox JG, Rogers AB, Ihrig M, et al. Helicobacter pylori-associated gastric cancer in INS-GAS mice is gender specific. Cancer Res 2003;63(5):942–50.

93. Cao X, Tsukamoto T, Nozaki K, et al. Severity of gastritis determines glandular stomach carcinogenesis in Helicobacter pylori-infected Mongolian gerbils. Cancer Sci 2007;98(4):478–83.

94. Wang TC, Dangler CA, Chen D, et al. Synergistic interaction between hypergastrinemia and Helicobacter infection in a mouse model of gastric cancer. Gastroenterology 2000;118(1):36–47.

95. Kagawa J, Honda S, Kodama M, et al. Enterocromaffin-like cell tumor induced by Helicobacter pylori infection in Mongolian gerbils. Helicobacter 2002;7(6): 390–7.

96. Rudnicka W, Jarosinska A, Bak-Romaniszyn L, et al. Helicobacter pylori lipopolysaccharide in the IL-2 milieu activates lymphocytes from dyspeptic children. FEMS Immunol Med Microbiol 2003;36(3):141–5.

97. Kidd M, Tang LH, Schmid S, et al. Helicobacter pylori lipopolysaccharide alters ECL cell DNA synthesis via a CD14 receptor and polyamine pathway in mastomys. Digestion 2000;62(4):217–24.

98. Betton GR, Dormer CS, Wells T, et al. Gastric ECL-cell hyperplasia and carcinoids in rodents following chronic administration of H2-antagonists SK&F 93479 and oxmetidine and omeprazole. Toxicol Pathol 1988;16(2):288–98.

99. Poynter D, Selway SA. Neuroendocrine cell hyperplasia and neuroendocrine carcinoma of the rodent fundic stomach. Mutat Res 1991;248(2):303–19.

100. Goldenring JR, Ray GS, Coffey RJ, et al. Reversible drug-induced oxyntic atrophy in rats. Gastroenterology 2000;118(6):1080–93.

101. Bakke I, Hammer TA, Sandvik AK, et al. PPAR alpha stimulates the rat gastrin-producing cell. Mol Cell Endocrinol 2002;195(1–2):89–97.

102. McCloy RF, Arnold R, Bardhan KD, et al. Pathophysiological effects of long-term acid suppression in man. Dig Dis Sci 1995;40(Suppl 2):96S–120S.

103. Peghini PL, Annibale B, Azzoni C, et al. Effect of chronic hypergastrinemia on human enterochromaffin-like cells: insights from patients with sporadic gastrinomas. Gastroenterology 2002;123(1):68–85.

104. Hassall E, Owen D, Kerr W, et al. Gastric histology in children treated with proton pump inhibitors long term, with emphasis on enterochromaffin cell-like hyperplasia. Aliment Pharmacol Ther 2011;33(7):829–36.

105. Torbenson M, Abraham SC, Boitnott J, et al. Autoimmune gastritis: distinct histological and immunohistochemical findings before complete loss of oxyntic glands. Mod Pathol 2002;15(2):102–9.

106. Hodges JR, Isaacson P, Wright R. Diffuse enterochromaffin-like (ECL) cell hyperplasia and multiple gastric carcinoids: a complication of pernicious anaemia. Gut 1981;22(3):237–41.

107. Landry CS, Brock G, Scoggins CR, et al. A proposed staging system for gastric carcinoid tumors based on an analysis of 1,543 patients. Ann Surg Oncol 2009; 16(1):51–60.

108. Lawrence B, Gustafsson BI, Chan A, et al. The epidemiology of gastroenteropancreatic neuroendocrine tumors. Endocrinol Metab Clin North Am 2011; 40(1):1–18, vii.

109. Hodgson N, Koniaris LG, Livingstone AS, et al. Gastric carcinoids: a temporal increase with proton pump introduction. Surg Endosc 2005;19(12):1610–2.

110. DeLellis RA, Lloyd RV, Heitz PU. World Health Organization classification of tumors, pathology and genetics of tumors of endocrine organs. Lyon (France): IARC Press; 2004.

Gastrointestinal Stromal Tumors

Markku Miettinen, MD*, Jerzy Lasota, MD

KEYWORDS

- GIST • Leiomyoma • Leiomyosarcoma • Leiomyoblastoma
- Stromal tumors mesenchymal neoplasm

KEY POINTS

- What is now known as gastrointestinal stromal tumor (GIST) used to be called as gastrointestinal (GI) smooth muscle tumor: leiomyoma if benign, leiomyosarcoma if malignant, and leiomyoblastoma if with epithelioid histology.
- GISTs typically occur in older adults, and the median patient age in the major series has varied between 60 and 65 years although are rarely seen in children and young adults.
- Most GISTs, approximately 85% to –90%, contain oncogenic KIT or platelet-derived growth factor receptor alpha mutations. However, loss of function of succinate dehydrogenase complex has been identified as alternative pathogenesis, especially in GISTs in young patients.
- Most common clinical symptoms of GIST are GI bleeding and gastric discomfort or ulcer-like symptoms.
- Wedge resection is the most common surgery for a small-sized to medium-sized gastric GIST, and sufficient margins can usually be obtained.

Gastrointestinal stromal tumors (GISTs) are the most common mesenchymal tumor of the gastrointestinal (GI) tract. Soon after GIST was recognized as a tumor driven by a KIT or platelet-derived growth factor receptor alpha (PDGFRA) mutation, it became the first solid tumor target for tyrosine kinase inhibitor therapies. More recently, alternative molecular mechanisms for GIST pathogenesis have been discovered. These are related to deficiencies in the succinate dehydrogenase (SDH) complex, neurofibromatosis type 1 (NF1) gene alterations in connection with NF1 tumor syndrome, and mutational activation of the BRAF oncogene in very rare cases.

Clinically GISTs are diverse. They can involve almost any segment of the GI tract, from distal esophagus to anus, although the stomach is the most common site. From an oncologic perspective, GIST varies from a small, harmless tumor nodule to a metastasizing and life-threatening sarcoma. This article presents the clinical, pathologic, prognostic, and to some degree, oncological aspects of GISTs with attention to their clinicopathologic variants related to tumor site and pathogenesis.

This work has been supported as a part of NCI's intramural research program.
Laboratory of Pathology, NCI/NIH, 9000 Rockville Pike, Building 10, Room 2B50, Bethesda, MD 20892, USA
* Corresponding author.
E-mail address: miettinenmm@mail.nih.gov

Gastroenterol Clin N Am 42 (2013) 399–415
http://dx.doi.org/10.1016/j.gtc.2013.01.001
0889-8553/13/$ – see front matter Published by Elsevier Inc.

gastro.theclinics.com

HISTORY OF GIST AND TERMINOLOGY

What is now known as GIST, used to be called GI smooth muscle tumor: leiomyoma if benign, leiomyosarcoma if malignant, and leiomyoblastoma if with epithelioid histology. Tumors previously classified as GI autonomic nerve tumors have also turned out to be GISTs, as have many tumors historically classified as GI schwannomas or other nerve sheath tumors.

Electron microscopic studies from the late 1960s and on demonstrated that most of the "GI smooth muscle tumors" differed from typical smooth muscle tumors by their lack of smooth muscle–specific ultrastructure.[1] Immunohistochemically they lacked smooth muscle antigens, especially desmin.[2] As they also lacked Schwann cell features, GIST was then proposed as a histogenetically noncommittal term for these tumors.[3] The discovery of KIT expression and gain-of-function KIT mutations in GIST in 1998 was the basis of the modern concept of GIST – a generally KIT positive and KIT mutation-driven mesenchymal neoplasm specific to the GI tract.[4,5]

EPIDEMIOLOGY OF GIST

GIST, once considered an obscure tumor, is now known to occur with an incidence of at least 14 to 20 per million, by population-based studies from northern Europe.[6,7] These estimates represent the minimum incidence, as subclinical GISTs are much more common. In an US study, 10% of well-studied resection specimens of gastro-esophageal cancer harbored a small incidental GIST in the proximal stomach.[8] An autopsy study from Germany also found a 25% incidence of small gastric GISTs.[9]

GISTs typically occur in older adults, and the median patient age in the major series has varied between 60 and 65 years. GISTs are relatively rare under the age of 40 years, and only less than 1% occurs below age 21. Some series have shown a mild male predominance. Over half of the GISTs occur in the stomach. Approximately 30% of GISTs are detected in the jejunum or ileum, 5% in the duodenum, 5% in the rectum, and less than 1% in the esophagus. Based on our review of Armed Forces Institute of Pathology (AFIP) cases, as many as 10% of all GISTs are detected as advanced, disseminated abdominal tumors whose exact origin is difficult to determine.

Despite occasional reports to the contrary, the authors do not believe that GISTs primarily occur in parenchymal organs outside the GI tract at sites such as the pancreas, liver, and gallbladder. At the 2 first mentioned organs, GISTs are metastatic or direct extensions from gastric or duodenal or other intestinal primary tumors. The authors are skeptical about primary GISTs in the gallbladder and note that the reported evidence for this diagnosis is tenuous and that molecular genetic documentation is absent.[10,11] Furthermore, review of all gallbladder sarcomas in the AFIP failed to find any GISTs.[12] Similarly, GISTs diagnosed in prostate biopsies are of rectal or other GI and not prostatic origin.[13]

GIST IS PHENOTYPICALLY RELATED TO GI CAJAL CELLS

Almost all GISTs express the KIT receptor tyrosine kinase, similar to the GI Cajal cells that regulate the GI autonomic nerve system and peristalsis.[14] These cells have a stem cell–like character, as demonstrated by their ability to transdifferentiate into smooth muscle.[15] KIT-deficient mice lack GI Cajal cells and those with introduced KIT-activating mutations develop Cajal cell hyperplasia and GISTs, supporting the role of Cajal cells in GIST oncogenesis.[16]

KIT AND PDGFRA MUTATION AS A DRIVING FORCE OF GISTS

Most GISTs, approximately 85% to 90%, contain oncogenic KIT or PDGFRA mutations. KIT and PDGFRA are 2 highly homologous cell surface tyrosine kinase receptors for stem cell factor and platelet derived growth factors. Normally these kinases are activated (phosphorylated) up on dimerization induced by ligand binding. However, mutated receptors may self-phosphorylate in a ligand-independent manner, rendering the kinase constitutively activated, which has a critical role in cell proliferation and is considered the driving force of GIST pathogenesis. However, additional genetic changes are necessary for malignant progression as mutations are already detectable in the very small GISTs, most of which probably never grow to clinically detectable tumors.[17–20]

How KIT mutations cause increased cell proliferation has been demonstrated in several ways. KIT mutations introduced in a lymphoblastoid cell line increased cellular proliferation. Families with germline KIT or PDGFRA mutation and transgenic mouse with similar "knock-in" KIT mutations have predisposition to GIST, often developing multiple GISTs.[4] Also, it has been shown that KIT mutations are associated with constitutively phosphorylated KIT[21] and that KIT tyrosine kinase inhibitors such as imatinib mesylate can in vitro and in vivo abolish the phosphorylated status and normalize the increased cell proliferation.[21]

The clinical significance of mutation type analysis includes assessment of sensitivity to tyrosine kinase inhibitors (especially imatinib), and in some cases, mutation type, can also offer a prognostic clue.[22] The rare presence of homozygous mutation is associated with an aggressive course of disease. The main KIT mutation types and their clinical significance are summarized in **Table 1**.

Table 1
Summary of the main KIT and PDGFRA mutation types and their clinical significance

Gene	Domain	Exon	Type of Mutation	Frequency	Clinicopathologic Features
KIT	EC	9	Duplication	10%	Associated with intestinal tumors
	JM	11	Deletion Deletion/insertion Duplication Insertion Substitution	70%	Deletions and deletion/insertions associated with malignant course especially in gastric tumors Duplication associated with gastric tumors and favorable course
	TK1	13	Substitution	1%	Slightly more frequent in intestinal tumors Associated with spindle cell morphology
	TK2	17	Substitution	1%	More frequent in intestinal tumors Associated with spindle cell morphology
PDGFRA	JM	12	Deletion Deletion/insertion Duplication Substitution	1%	Associated with gastric tumors, epithelioid cell morphology and more indolent course
	TK1	14	Substitution	<1%	
	TK2	18	Deletion Deletion/insertion Duplication Substitution	5%	

KIT EXON 11 MUTANTS

Approximately 90% of KIT mutations involve exon 11, the juxtamembrane domain.[18,20] Their KIT activating potential is believed to be related to disruption of the alpha-helical structure of the juxtamembrane domain then allowing spontaneous dimerization and phosphorylation of KIT.[23] Exon 11 KIT mutations include a spectrum of in-frame deletions of 3 to 21 or rarely more base pairs, single nucleotide substitutions, internal tandem duplications, and combinations of all, and rarely true insertions of nonduplicative genomic sequences.[17–20]

Deletions in the KIT juxtamembrane domain most frequently involve the 5' portion of the exon 11 between codons 550 and 560. Tumors containing deletions in this area are clinically more aggressive than those with single nucleotide substitutions.[24,25] In large site-specific series, this was especially true for gastric GISTs.[26]

KIT exon 11 single nucleotide substitutions are generally limited to 4 codons: 557, 559, 560, and 576. Internal tandem duplications are essentially restricted to the 3' portion of exon 11 and are associated with gastric tumors and favorable course.[27] In general, most KIT exon 11 mutants are sensitive to the tyrosine kinase inhibitor imatinib mesylate, although some rare variants may show different level of resistance.[18]

OTHER KIT MUTANTS

KIT extracellular domain exon 9 mutations are rare and essentially restricted to intestinal GISTs based on Western studies.[28,29] However, in a Japanese series these mutations have also been detected in some gastric GISTs, raising the possibility of population differences.[30] Most mutations are identical 2 codon duplications introducing a tandem alanine-tyrosine pair (AY502-503). These KIT exon 9 mutant GISTs are notable for their poorer response to imatinib, so that dose escalation of imatinib from 400 mg/d to 800 mg/d or use of alternative tyrosine kinase inhibitor has been advocated.[31,32] However, in a large preimatinib series, KIT exon 9 mutant GISTs did not seem to have an inherently worse prognosis than exon 11 mutant tumors.[33]

Rarely, KIT tyrosine kinase 1 domain (exon 13) or tyrosine kinase 2 domain (exon 17) is mutated. Exon 13 mutations usually involve codon 642, whereas exon 17 mutations most often occur in codon 822.[34,35] These mutants are variably sensitive to imatinib.

PDGRFA MUTATIONS IN GISTS

PDGFRA mutations were discovered in 30% of KIT wild-type (WT) tumors. KIT and PDGFRA mutations were shown to be mutually exclusive in GISTs.[36] PDGFRA mutants are essentially restricted to gastric GISTs, comprising approximately 10% of such cases overall. Most PDGFRA-mutant gastric GISTs represent clinically indolent tumors. Also, there is some predilection to epithelioid morphology, and some of these tumors show weaker KIT expression.[37] Although they express PDGFRA, standard immunohistochemistry is not helpful for the detection of PDGFRA-mutant GISTs because PDGFRA is widely expressed in GISTs of any type and also in other tumors. PDGFRA mutations, similar to KIT mutations, include in-frame deletions, single nucleotide substitutions, and internal tandem duplications. Most of these mutations are D842V substitutions involving the PDGFRA tyrosine kinase 2 domain (exon 18), although rare mutations have been identified in juxtamembrane domain (exon 12) and tyrosine kinase 1 domain (exon 14).[37] D842V mutants are notorious for their primary resistance to imatinib. Therefore for initial therapy, if oncologically indicated, an alternative, more potent, tyrosine kinase inhibitors should be selected.[38]

CLINICAL MANIFESTATIONS OF GIST

Most common clinical symptoms of GIST are GI bleeding and gastric discomfort or ulcerlike symptoms. The bleeding varies from chronic insidious bleeding often leading to anemia to acute life-threatening episodes of melena or hematemesis. Few GISTs manifest as other abdominal emergencies, such as intestinal obstruction or tumor rupture with hemoperitoneum. Nearly one-third of GISTs are incidentally detected during surgical or imaging procedures or endoscopic screening for gastric carcinoma. Some rectal GISTs are detected during prostate or gynecologic examination.

Most of the currently detected GISTs are localized tumors less than 5 cm, but retrospective studies had larger mean tumor sizes. In general, small intestinal GISTs are larger in average, and the percentage of metastasizing tumors is higher than among gastric GISTs. Peritoneal cavity and liver are the typical sites of metastases. Rarely, GISTs metastasize into bones. In our experience, bone metastases have a predilection to axial skeleton, especially the spine. Cutaneous and peripheral soft tissue metastases are rare. In contrast to other sarcomas, malignant GISTs very rarely, if ever, metastasize to lungs, even if they have extensive other metastases. Although some GISTs metastasize in 1 to 2 years or sooner, metastatic spread is possible after a very long delay.[26,33] The longest interval from primary tumor to liver metastasis observed by us was 42 years; this indicates the need for long-term patient follow-up.

IDENTIFICATION OF GISTS

Radiologists, endoscopists, and surgeons and pathologists can suspect a GIST whenever there is a rounded to oval, circumscribed mural or extramural nonmucosa-based mass of any size that involves or is closely associated with the stomach, intestinal segments, or lower esophagus. However, in some cases such lesions prove to be other mesenchymal tumors, unusual variants of carcinomas, neuroendocrine tumors, or even lymphomas. In most cases, examination of a biopsy easily resolves the differential diagnostic problem. A GIST should also be considered for any palpable abdominal mass.

The radiologic and gross appearances of GISTs, especially the gastric ones, can be highly variable including tumors with intraluminal, intramural, external components and with pedunculated extramural and cystic appearances. Any larger GIST in the intestines typically forms an externally extending mass that is often centrally cystic and may fistulate into the lumen (**Fig. 1**). Some small intestinal GISTs form dumbbell-shaped masses with intramural and external components.[26,39]

GIST is the most common mesenchymal tumor in all segments of the GI tract with 2 exceptions: most esophageal mesenchymal tumors are true leiomyomas and not GISTs and small mucosal leiomyomas are more common in the colon and rectum than are GISTs. In the stomach, GIST is by far the most common mesenchymal tumor, as there are only 4 leiomyomas or schwannomas reported for every 100 GISTs.

Sampling of a GIST for preoperative diagnosis via endoscopic mucosal biopsy is successful in only 20% to 30% cases, including those that involve the mucosa or superficial submucosa. Endoscopic ultrasound-associated fine-needle aspiration biopsy (EUS-FNA) is more promising.[40] In a recent study, the diagnostic yield of EUS-FNA was 76%, whereas even better results were reported with Tru-cut histologic biopsies (97% yield of diagnostic material).[41] The larger GISTs especially are amenable to CT-guided needle core biopsy.

Pathologic diagnosis of GIST is based on identification of a mesenchymal neoplasm with spindle cell or epithelioid histology that is generally positive for KIT (CD117 leukocyte antigen). Common histologic features in GISTs include spindle cells with

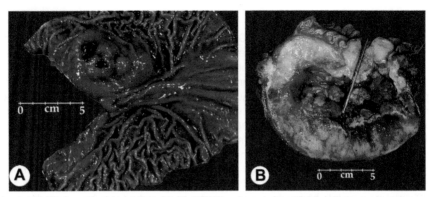

Fig. 1. (A, B) Gross features of a gastric GIST showing multinodular submucosal masses and a small intestinal GIST showing a fistula tract connecting the center of the tumor to the intestinal lumen.

sclerosing matrix, perinuclear vacuolization and nuclear palisading, epithelioid cytology, and sarcomatoid, mitotically active morphology in gastric GISTs (**Fig. 2**). Small intestinal GISTs are characterized by extracellular collagen globules and a Verocay body or neuropil-like material, reflecting complex entangled cell processes (**Fig. 3**).

Approximately 97% of GISTs are immunohistochemically positive for KIT, at least focally, but the pattern can vary from membranous and apparent cytoplasmic to

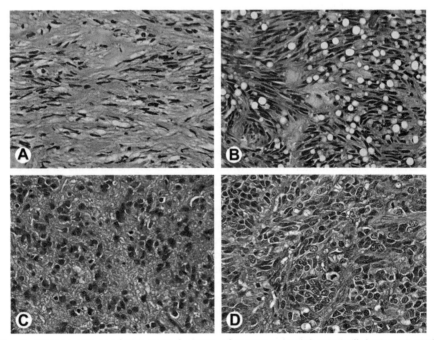

Fig. 2. Wide spectrum of histologic features of gastric GIST. (A) Paucicellular tumor with sclerosing matrix. (B) Perinuclear vacuolization and nuclear palisading. (C) Epithelioid cytology. (D) Sarcomatoid appearance with numerous mitoses.

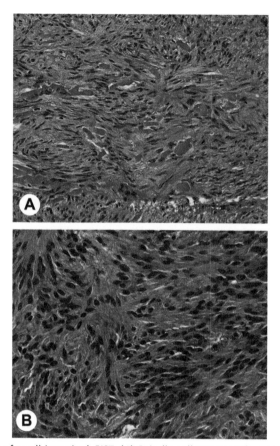

Fig. 3. Histology of small intestinal GIST. (*A*) Spindle cell tumor with extracellular collagen globules. (*B*) Nuclear zones reflecting prominent entangled cell processes.

a perinuclear dotlike pattern.[42,43] Tumors with epithelioid cytology can be only focally positive, or rarely entirely negative, which can be the cases especially with some PDGFRA-mutant GISTs.[44,45] The KIT-negative GISTs are usually positive for anoctamin-1 (Ano-1), a calcium-activated chloride channel protein also expressed in Cajal cells.[46] Ano-1 is also known under the aliases DOG1 (discovered on GIST-1) and ORAOV2 (overexpressed in oral carcinoma).[47] Approximately 97% of GISTs are Ano-1 positive including KIT-negative tumors, but some GISTs, especially small intestinal ones, are negative. Together KIT and Ano-1 capture nearly 100% of GISTs as their "shadow areas" tend to be different.[48] Other potential but less-specific and sensitive markers in the overall detection of GISTs are protein kinase C theta[49,50] and CD34. The latter is positive in 70% of GISTs and is nearly consistently detected in gastric spindle cell GISTs.[26]

For comprehensive detection of GISTs, one should consider that most GI mesenchymal tumors are GISTs, and that most intraperitoneal mesenchymal tumors are also GISTs. Even in the retroperitoneal space, a GIST is more common than a leiomyosarcoma, in our experience. GIST should also be considered in the differential diagnosis of mesenchymal or epithelioid neoplasms involving the liver, pancreas, and pelvic cavity.

GIST PROGNOSIS AT DIFFERENT SITES

The best universally applicable prognostic parameters are tumor size (maximum tumor diameter in cm) and mitotic rate per 50 high-power fields (HPFs) (corresponding to 5 mm^2). A prognostic chart (**Table 2**) has been devised by analysis of large series of gastric and small intestinal GISTs, based on AFIP cases with long-term follow-up.[26,33,51] This chart shows that gastric and small intestinal GISTs less than or equal to 5 cm with mitotic count less than or equal to 5/50 HPFs have a very good prognosis with only 3% to 5% of metastatic risk. Also, the chart shows a marked prognostic difference between gastric and small intestinal GISTs. The latter shows significant to high metastatic rates in many categories that in the gastric location have much lower rate of metastases. Other intestinal GISTs have a prognosis approximately similar to small intestinal GISTs, although less data exist, because of their rarity. Prognostic nomograms creating these parameters as continuous variables have also been devised. Based on a relatively small sample size, such a nomogram was found to offer a more accurate prognostication.[52] Addition of genetic parameters may further improve prognostication. The number and type of genomic losses and gains detected by comparative genomic hybridization[53] and genome complexity index are examples of this development. In the latter, expression of aurora kinase was found an adverse prognostic factor.[54]

Comments on GIST Surgery

Wedge resection is the most common surgery for a small-sized to medium-sized gastric GIST, and sufficient margins can usually be obtained. Results vary about the significance of microscopically negative margins after gross resection. Although in one study a microscopically positive margin was not found to be a significant adverse factor,[55] another study found it an adverse factor for survival.[56] Localized intestinal GISTs are handled with segmental resections. Laparoscopic surgery is increasingly used for small-sized or medium-sized GISTs (at least up to 5 cm). Reported series have shown excellent survival results (92%–96%),[57,58] which also reflect the fact

---

Table 2
Prognostication of GIST of different sites by tumor size and mitotic rate based on follow-up studies of more than 1700 GISTs prior to imatinib

	Tumor Parameters		Percentage of Patients with Progressive Disease During Long-term Follow-up and Quantitative Characterization of the Risk for Metastasis			
Group	Size	Mitotic Rate	Gastric GISTs	Small Intestinal GISTs	Duodenal GISTs	Rectal GISTs
1	≤2 cm	≤5/50 HPFs	0 none			
2	>2 ≤5 cm		1.9 (very low)	4.3 (low)	8.3 (low)	8.5 (low)
3a	>5 ≤10 cm		3.6 (low)	24 (moderate)	34 (high)[a]	57 (high)[a]
3b	>10 cm		12 (moderate)	52 (high)		
4	≤2 cm	>5/50 HPFs	0[a]	50[a]	[b]	54 (high)
5	>2 ≤5 cm		16 (moderate)	73 (high)	50 (high)	52 (high)
6a	>5 ≤0 cm		55 (high)	85 (high)	86 (high)[a]	71 (high)[a]
6b	>10 cm		86 (high)	90 (high)		

Abbreviation: HPF, high-power field. 50 high-power fields equal here approximately 5 mm^2.
[a] Small number of cases. Groups combined or prognostic prediction less certain.
[b] No tumors encountered with these parameters.
Data from Miettinen M, Lasota J. Gastrointestinal stromal tumors: review on morphology, molecular pathology, prognosis, and differential diagnosis. Arch Pathol 2006;130:1466–78.

that most gastric GISTs less than 5 cm are clinically favorable.[26] One study also found that laparoscopic versus open surgery offered similar 30-day morbidity and outcome but shorter hospital stay (4 vs 7 days) and slightly less blood loss with the laparoscopic group. Conversion into open surgery was often the result of a tumor location in the gastroesophageal junction or lesser curvature.[59] Larger GISTs necessitate open surgery and more extensive resections, such as distal gastrectomies for tumors involving the pyloric region or lesser curvature regions.[60,61] Total gastrectomy may be needed for very large or multiple and recurrent GISTs that include the SDH-deficient GISTs in young patients. This subgroup is discussed in detail later in this article. Tumor manipulation and rupture should be avoided, as this increases the possibility of peritoneal seeding.[62]

Surgery of metastases following imatinib treatment is practiced in selected instances. The indications include excision of metastases with developing imatinib resistance and emergency surgery for ruptured cystic metastases.[62] In CT scans, peripheral thickening and enhancing of cystic metastases can be a sign of an evolving resistance and newly progressing tumor even without size increase.[63]

Comments on Oncologic Treatment of GISTs

The KIT tyrosine kinase inhibitor imatinib mesylate, initially introduced for treatment of chronic myeloid leukemia due to its ability to inhibit ABL tyrosine kinase, was also found to inhibit KIT and to be effective in a patient with extensive hepatic and abdominal metastases.[64] Today imatinib is the treatment of choice for metastatic and unresectable GIST, and it offers prolonged survival for an average of 5 years, compared with historical controls. Orally administered imatinib is safe with few side effects. Unfortunately, tumors often develop resistance, mostly because of secondary KIT or rarely PDGFRA mutations that cluster in the tyrosine kinase domains.[65–67]

More recently imatinib has also been used as adjuvant therapy after apparently complete surgery to prevent recurrences, with several clinical trials supporting its use in this context. In general, imatinib is recommended after completely resective surgery of high-risk GISTs,[65–67] although some trials have used it with wider indications, such as GISTs greater than 3 cm.[68] In a recent randomized trial, treatment for 3 years showed a survival advantage over one-year treatment.[69]

In addition, imatinib has been used as a neoadjuvant treatment prior to surgery. In some cases, adjuvant treatment of imatinib can shrink the tumor to allow more structure-preserving surgery, and this may especially be important for GISTs at technically challenging sites such as the anorectum.[65–67]

Several newer tyrosine kinase inhibitors, such as sunitinib, nilotinib, and dasatinib, are being used to overcome imatinib resistance. These multikinase inhibitors inhibit other tyrosine kinases, such as vascular endothelial growth factor receptors, in addition to KIT and PDGFRA. Although variably effective against imatinib-resistant GISTs, these new inhibitors have a greater spectrum of side effects.[70] Additional new potential drugs currently under evaluation in in-vitro models or being used in early trials include mammalian target of rapamycin inhibitors such as everolimus,[71] heat shock protein inhibitors,[72] and the KIT transcription antagonist flavopiridol.[73]

Familial GIST Syndrome

Hereditary GIST syndrome is a rare autosomal dominant disorder characterized by germline gain-of-function KIT mutations and in rare cases by PDGFRA mutations. Structurally, these mutations are similar to those reported in sporadic tumors, although in one kindred KIT exon 8 was mutated. More than 20 families with hereditary GIST syndrome have been reported. Affected individuals develop Cajal cell hyperplasia and subsequently multiple GISTs in middle age. Dysphagia, skin hyperpigmentation, urticaria pigmentosa and mastocytosis are among other clinical features occasionally seen in the kindreds harboring KIT but not PDGFRA germline mutations. The tumors may remain stable for a long time, but often ultimately become aggressive.[16,18,74,75]

SUCCINATE DEHYDROGENASE–DEFICIENT GISTS

Approximately 7.5% of gastric GISTs, especially those in children and young adults, have tumor-specific loss of function of the SDH complex, which is considered a key factor in their pathogenesis. The SDH complex is an important metabolic enzyme complex participating both in the tricarboxylic acid cycle and in the electron transfer chain located in the mitochondrial inner membrane. SDH-deficient GISTs are restricted to the stomach, based on screening of large numbers of GIST of different locations. These tumors lack KIT and PDGFRA mutations and are not driven by activation of these oncogenes.[75–78]

The pathogenesis of SDH-deficient GISTs is related to germline loss-of-function mutations in the SDH subunit proteins, as found in 20% to 30% of extra-adrenal paragangliomas. In GIST patients, SDHA is the most commonly mutated subunit, but subunits B, C, and D can also be involved.[75–79] At least half of the patients have germline mutations, to which are added corresponding somatic mutations in the tumors, thereby leading to inactivation of the subunit and subsequently loss of function of the entire SDH-complex in the tumor. However, for patients who lack SDH-germline mutations, the underlying genetic defects are unknown, the biologic pathways affected are believed to be activated hypoxia-inducible factor signaling. Activation of the insulinlike growth factor 1 receptor (IGF1R) signaling seems to be an oncogenic signaling consequence of these changes.[75]

The practical diagnostic marker for SDH-deficient GISTs is immunohistochemically observed loss of the otherwise ubiquitously expressed SDHB (**Fig. 4**).[78,80,81] This loss occurs with the loss of any of the subunits, as has been seen in paragangliomas. SDHA-mutant tumors specifically show immunohistochemical loss of SDHA, which can also be detected immunohistochemically.[79,82–84] Currently, no reliable immunohistochemical tests are available for analysis of SDH complex subunit C and SDH complex subunit D.

SDH-deficient GISTs have a predilection to children and young adults and constitute a great majority of pediatric GISTs and half of all gastric GISTs under the age of 40 years. They may occur in older adults but with a lower frequency. The children involved are usually girls, and onset is mostly in the second decade. In rare patients, the GIST is diagnosed before the age of 10 years. Curiously, no significant familial tendency (multiple affected family members) has been observed for SDH-deficient GISTs, even though up to 50% of patients have germline mutations.[78]

Two clinical syndromes distinguished by eponyms are included among the SDH-deficient gastric GISTs. The occurrence of GIST with a paraganglioma in a patient with an SDH-subunit germline mutation defines Carney-Stratakis syndrome.[85] Occurrence of a GIST and a paraganglioma or a pulmonary chondroma or all three in the absence of an SDH-gene germline mutation defines the Carney triad.[86] In our experience, these syndromes together comprise only a minority of SDH-deficient GISTs (10%–20%), although this percentage could become higher with extended follow-up and radiologic screening for occult paragangliomas.

Clinically, the SDH-deficient GISTs are distinctive in that they often form multiple gastric tumors. There is some tendency to form regional perigastric lymph node metastases and multiple peritoneal micronodules, but neither of these seems to be

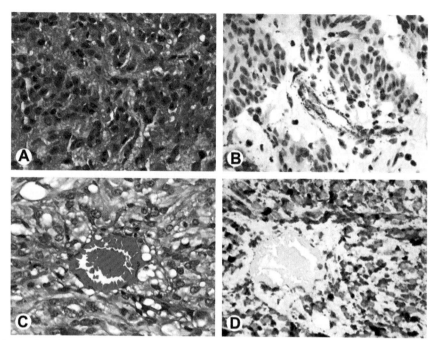

Fig. 4. (*A, B*) Succinate dehydrogenase–deficient GIST shows epithelioid cell morphology and shows loss of SDHB, which is only present in nonneoplastic vascular and stromal components. (*C, D*) A conventional GIST in comparison shows granular cytoplasmic staining for SDHB.

a prognostically adverse event. Many patients develop gastric recurrences and ultimately undergo total gastrectomy over years. Liver metastases develop in 20% to 25%, but nevertheless, the patients often survive for a long time even with these metastases – an outcome different from KIT-mutant GISTs. Tumor-related mortality was approximately 15% in a cohort with 15-year median follow-up.[78,79] In general, SDH-deficient GISTs are less predictable than KIT-mutant GISTs with the same prognostic factors. Life-long follow-up is needed as the patients continue to be at risk of development of liver metastases and other syndrome-related tumors, such as paragangliomas. The longest interval from primary tumor to liver metastasis in our study was 42 years. Similar clinicopathologic features have also been observed in Carney triad GISTs, a subgroup of SDH-deficient GISTs.[86]

Pathologically, SDH-deficient GISTs are notable for characteristic morphology: they have epithelioid cytology and multinodular gastric intramural involvement and a tendency for lymphovascular invasion and lymph node metastases. Notably, neither of the latter features are adverse prognostic factors.[78,79,86]

Optimal treatment of SDH-deficient GISTs remains to be determined. However, these tumors do not show a similar imatinib response as generally observed with KIT-mutant GISTs. Alternative tyrosine kinase inhibitors, such as sunitinib malate, have been used, but the data are relatively scant. Inhibition of IGF1R is a possible new treatment strategy for the SDH-deficient GISTs.[87,88]

GISTs in NF1 Patients

According to our estimate based on AFIP files, approximately 1% to 2% of GISTs arise in patients with NF1. GISTs belongs to the spectrum of tumors that occur in connection with this tumor syndrome, in addition to the constellation of neurofibromas, malignant peripheral nerve sheath tumors, pheochromocytomas, and other rare tumors.

An autopsy study on NF1 patients found a third of NF1 patients to harbor undiagnosed GISTs, so that the frequency of GISTs in NF1 patients is probably high.[89] Furthermore, in our review of AFIP files, the author could not identify a single malignant peripheral nerve sheath tumor in the GI tract and found that an overwhelming majority of GI mesenchymal tumors in NF1 patients are actually GISTs.

The GISTs occurring in connection with NF1 are typically located in the small intestine (or sometimes colon), and gastric GISTs in these patients are rare. These GISTs are often multiple, and most of them are incidental findings during other abdominal surgeries. However, approximately 15% to 20% of NF1-associated GISTs are clinically malignant.[89–91]

BRAF Mutant GISTs

Recently, an identical BRAF mutation (V600E) was identified in a small subset of KIT- and PDGFRA-WT GISTs. Oncogenic BRAF activation is considered to be a common driving force in malignant melanoma. Thus, V600E may represent an alternative to KIT and PDGFRA activation as a molecular mechanism of GIST pathogenesis. Although, BRAF-mutated GISTs show predilection for an intestinal location, no specific pathologic features defining this subgroup have been reported yet. BRAF inhibitors might be considered in treatment of metastatic and locally advanced BRAF-mutant GISTs.[92–95]

REFERENCES

1. Welsh RA, Meyer AT. Ultrastructure of gastric leiomyoma. Arch Pathol 1969;87: 71–81.
2. Evans DJ, Lampert IA, Jacobs M. Intermediate filaments in smooth muscle tumors. J Clin Pathol 1983;36:57–61.
3. Mazur MT, Clark HB. Gastric stromal tumors. Reappraisal of histogenesis. Am J Surg Pathol 1983;7:507–19.
4. Hirota S, Isozaki K, Moriyama Y, et al. Gain-of-function mutations of c-kit in human gastrointestinal stromal tumors. Science 1998;279:577–80.
5. Kindblom LG, Remotti HE, Aldenborg F, et al. Gastrointestinal pacemaker cell tumor (GIPACT). Gastrointestinal stromal tumors show phenotypic characteristics of the interstitial cells of Cajal. Am J Pathol 1998;153:1259–69.
6. Nilsson B, Bumming P, Medis-Kindblom JM, et al. Gastrointestinal stromal tumors: the incidence, prevalence, clinical course, and prognostication in the preimatinib mesylate era – a population-basede study in western Sweden. Cancer 2005;103:821–9.
7. Tryggvason G, Gislason HG, Magnusson MK, et al. Gastrointestinal stromal tumors in Iceland, 1990-2003: the Icelandic GIST study, a population-based incidence and pathologic risk stratification study. Int J Cancer 2005;117:289–93.
8. Abraham SC, Krasinskas AM, Hofstetter WL, et al. "Seedling" mesenchymal tumors (gastrointestinal stromal tumors and leiomyomas) are common in cidental tumors of thevesophagogastric junction. Am J Surg Pathol 2007;31: 1629–35.
9. Agaimy A, Wunsch PH, Hofstaedter F, et al. Minute sclerosing stromal tumors (GIST tumorlets) are common in adults and frequently show KIT mutations. Am J Surg Pathol 2007;31:113–20.

10. Mendoza-Marin M, Hoang MP, Albores-Saavedra J. Malignant stromal tumor of the gallbladder with interstitial cells of Cajal phenotype. Arch Pathol Lab Med 2002;126:481–3.

11. Park JK, Choi SH, Lee S, et al. Malignant gastrointestinal stromal tumor of the gallbladder. J Korean Med Sci 2004;1:763–7.

12. Al-Daraji WI, Makhlouf HR, Miettinen M, et al. Primary gallbladder sarcoma: a clinicopathologic study of 15 cases, heterogeneous sarcomas with poor outcome, except pediatric botryoid rhabdomyosarcoma. Am J Surg Pathol 2009;3:826–34.

13. Herawi M, Montgomery EA, Epstein JI. Gastrointestinal stromal tumors (GISTs) on prostate needle biopsy: a clinicopathologic study of 8 cases. Am J Surg Pathol 2006;30:1389–95.

14. Huizinga JD, Thuneberg L, Kluppel M, et al. W/kit gene required for interstitial cells of Cajal and for intestinal pacemaker activity. Nature 1993;373:347–9.

15. Torihashi S, Nishi K, Tokutomi Y, et al. Blockade of kit signaling induces transdifferentiation of interstitial cells of Cajal to a smooth muscle phenotype. Gastroenterology 1999;117:140–8.

16. Kitamura Y, Hirota S. Kit as a human oncogenic tyrosine kinase [review]. Cell Mol Life Sci 2004;61:2924–31.

17. Fletcher JA, Rubin BP. KIT mutations in GIST. Curr Opin Genet Dev 2007;17:3–7.

18. Lasota J, Miettinen M. Clinical significance of oncogenic KIT and PDGFRA mutations in gastrointestinal stromal tumors. Histopathology 2008;53:245–66.

19. Corless CL, Barnett CM, Heinrich MC. Gastrointestinal stromal tumours: origin and molecular oncology. Nat Rev Cancer 2011;1:865–78.

20. Taniguchi M, Nishida T, Hirota S, et al. Effect of c-kit mutation on prognosis of gastrointestinal stromal tumors. Cancer Res 1999;59:4297–300.

21. Rubin BP, Singer S, Tsao C, et al. KIT activation is a ubiquitous feature of gastrointestinal stromal tumors. Cancer Res 2001;61:8118–21.

22. Demetri GD. Targeting c-kit mutations in solid tumors: scientific rationale and novel therapeutic options. Semin Oncol 2001;28(5 Suppl 17):19–26.

23. Longley BJ, Reguera MJ, Ma Y. Classes of c-KIT activating mutations: proposed mechanisms of action and implications in disease classification and therapy. Leuk Res 2001;25:571–6.

24. Wardelmann E, Losen I, Hans V, et al. Deletion of Trp-557 and Lys-558 in the juxtamembrane domain of the c-kit protooncogene is associated with metastatic behavior of gastrointestinal stromal tumors. Int J Cancer 2003;106:887–95.

25. Martín J, Poveda A, Llombart-Bosch A, et al. Deletions affecting codons 557-558 of the c-KIT gene indicate a poor prognosis in patients with completely resected gastrointestinal stromal tumors: a study by the Spanish Group for Sarcoma Research (GEIS). J Clin Oncol 2005;23(25):6190–8.

26. Miettinen M, Sobin LH, Lasota J. Gastrointestinal stromal tumors of the stomach: a clinicopathologic, immunohistochemical, and molecular genetic studies of 1765 cases with long-term follow-up. Am J Surg Pathol 2005;29:52–68.

27. Lasota J, Dansonka-Mieszkowska A, Stachura T, et al. Gastrointestinal stromal tumors with internal tandem duplications in 3' end of KIT juxtamembrane domain occur predominantly in stomach and generally seem to have a favorable course. Mod Pathol 2003;16:1257–64.

28. Antonescu CR, Sommer G, Sarran L, et al. Association of KIT exon 9 mutations with nongastric primary site and aggressive behavior: KIT mutation analysis and clinical correlates of 120 gastrointestinal stromal tumors. Clin Cancer Res 2003;9:3329–37.

29. Lasota J, Kopczynski J, Sarlomo-Rikala M, et al. KIT 1530ins6 mutation defines a subset of predominantly malignant gastrointestinal stromal tumors of intestinal origin. Hum Pathol 2003;34:1306–12.

30. Sakurai S, Oguni S, Hironaka M, et al. Mutations in c-kit gene exons 9 and 13 in gastrointestinal stromal tumors among Japanese. Jpn J Cancer Res 2001;92: 494–8.

31. Debiec-Rychter M, Sciot R, Le Cesne A, et al. KIT mutations and dose selection for imatinib in patients with advanced gastrointestinal stromal tumours. Eur J Cancer 2006;42:1093–103.

32. Marrari A, Trent JC, George S. Personalized cancer therapy for gastrointestinal stromal tumor: synergizing tumor genotyping with imatinib plasma levels. Curr Opin Oncol 2010;22:336–41.

33. Miettinen M, Makhlouf HR, Sobin LH, et al. Gastrointestinal stromal tumors (GISTs) of the jejunum and ileum – a clinicopathologic, immunohistochemical and molecular genetic study of 906 cases prior to imatinib with long-term follow-up. Am J Surg Pathol 2006;31:477–89.

34. Lux ML, Rubin BP, Biase TL, et al. KIT extracellular and kinase domain mutations in gastrointestinal stromal tumors. Am J Pathol 2000;156:791–5.

35. Lasota J, Corless CL, Heinrich MC, et al. Clinicopathologic profile of gastrointestinal stromal tumors (GISTs) with primary KIT exon 13 or exon 17 mutations: a multicenter study of 54 cases. Mod Pathol 2008;21:476–84.

36. Heinrich MC, Corless CL, Duensing A, et al. PDGFRA activating mutations in gastrointestinal stromal tumors. Science 2003;299:708–10.

37. Lasota J, Miettinen M, Lasota J, et al. A great majority of GISTs with PDGFRA mutations represent gastric tumors with low or no malignant potential. Lab Invest 2004;84:874–83.

38. Corless CL, Schroeder A, Griffith D, et al. PDGFRA mutations in gastrointestinal stromal tumors: frequency, spectrum and in vitro sensitivity to imatinib. J Clin Oncol 2005;23:5357–64.

39. Levy AD, Remotti HE, Thompson WM, et al. Gastrointestinal stromal tumors: radiologic features with pathologic correlation. Radiographics 2003;23:283–304.

40. Vander Noot MR 3rd, Eloubeidi MA, Chen VK, et al. Diagnosis of gastrointestinal tract lesions by endoscopic ultrasound-guided fine-needle aspiration biopsy. Cancer 2004;102:157–63.

41. DeWitt J, Emerson RE, Sharman S, et al. Endoscopic ultrasound-guided trucut biopsy of gastrointestinal mesenchymal tumor. Surg Endosc 2011;25:192–202.

42. Sarlomo-Rikala M, Kovatich A, Barusevicius A, et al. CD117: a sensitive marker for gastrointestinal stromal tumors that is more specific than CD34. Mod Pathol 1998;11:728–34.

43. Hornick JL, Fletcher CD. Immunohistochemical staining fo KIT (CD117) in soft tissue sarcomas is very limited in distribution. Am J Clin Pathol 2002;117: 188–93.

44. Medeiros F, Corless CL, Duensing A, et al. KIT-negative gastrointestinal stromal tumors: proof of concept and therapeutic implications. Am J Surg Pathol 2004; 28:889–94.

45. Lasota J, Stachura J, Miettinen M. GISTs with PDGFRA exon 14 mutations represent subset of clinically favorable gastric tumors with epithelioid morphology. Lab Invest 2006;86:94–100.

46. Hwang SJ, Blair PJ, Britton FC, et al. Expression of anoctamin 1/TMEM16A by interstitial cells of Cajal is fundamental for slow wave activity in gastrointestinal muscles. J Physiol 2009;587:4887–904.

47. West RB, Corless CL, Chen X, et al. The novel marker, DOG1, is expressed ubiquitously in gastrointestinal stromal tumors irrespective of KIT or PDGFRA mutation status. Am J Pathol 2004;165:107–13.

48. Miettinen M, Wang ZF, Lasota J. DOG1 antibody in the differential diagnosis of gastrointestinal stromal tumors: a study of 1840 cases. Am J Surg Pathol 2009; 33:1401–8.

49. Duensing A, Joseph NE, Medeiros F, et al. Protein kinase C theta (PKCtheta) expression and constitutive activation in gastrointestinal stromal tumors (GISTs). Cancer Res 2004;64:5127–31.

50. Motegi A, Sakurai S, Nakayama H, et al. PKC theta, a novel immunohistochemical marker for gastrointestinal stromal tumors (GIST), especially useful for identifying KIT-negative tumors. Pathol Int 2005;55:106–12.

51. Miettinen M, Lasota J. Gastrointestinal stromal tumors: pathology and prognosis at different sites. Semin Diagn Pathol 2006;23:70–83.

52. Gold JS, Gönen M, Gutiérrez A, et al. Development and validation of a prognostic nomogram for recurrence-free survival after complete surgical resection of localised primary gastrointestinal stromal tumour: a retrospective analysis. Lancet Oncol 2009;10:1045–52.

53. El-Rifai W, Sarlomo-Rikala M, Andersson L. DNA sequence cop number changes in gastrointestinal stromal tumors tumor progression and prognostic significance. Cancer Res 2000;60:3899–903.

54. Lagarde P, Perot G, Kauffmann A, et al. Mitotic checkpoints and chromosome instability are strong predictors of clinical outcome in gastrointestinal stromal tumors. Clin Cancer Res 2012;18:826–38.

55. McCarter MD, Antonescu CR, Ballman KV, et al. Microscopically positive margins for primary gastrointestinal stromal tumors: analysis of risk factors and tumor recurrence. J Am Coll Surg 2012;215:53–9.

56. Catena F, DiBattista M, Ansaloni L, et al. Microscopic margins of resection influence primary gastrointestinal stromal tumor survival. Onkologie 2012;35:645–8.

57. Novitsky YV, Kercher KW, Sing RF, et al. Long-term outcomes of laparoscopic resection of gastric gastrointestinal stromal tumors. Ann Surg 2006;243:738–45.

58. Otani Y, Furukawa T, Yoshida M, et al. Operative indications for relatively small (2-5 cm) gastrointestinal stromal tumor of the stomach based on analysis of 60 operated cases. Surgery 2006;139:484–92.

59. Karakousis GC, Singer S, Zheng J, et al. Laparoscopic varsus open gastric resections for primary gastrointestinal stromal tumors (GISTs): a size-matched comparison. Ann Surg Oncol 2011;18:1599–605.

60. Pucci MJ, Berger AC, Lim PW, et al. Laparoscopic approaches to gastric gastrointestinal stromal tumors: an institutional review of 57 cases. Surg Endosc 2012; 26:3509–14.

61. Sasaki A, Koeda K, Obuchi T, et al. Tailored laparoscopic resection for suspected gastri gastrointestinal stromal tumors. Surgery 2010;147:516–20.

62. Rutkowski P, Ruka W. Emergency surgery in the era of molecular treatment of solid tumours. Lancet Oncol 2009;10:157–63.

63. Mabille M, Vanel D, Albiter M, et al. Follow-up of hepatic and peritoneal metastases of gastrointestinal stromal tumors (GIST) under imatinib therapy requires different criteria of radiologic evaluation (size is not everything!!!). Eur J Radiol 2009;69:204–8.

64. Joensuu H, Roberts PJ, Sarlomo-Rikala M, et al. Effect of tyrosine kinase inhibitor STI571 in a patient with metastatic gastrointestinal stromal tumor. N Engl J Med 2001;344:1052–6.

65. Reichardt P, Blay JY, Boukovinas I, et al. Adjuvant therapy in primary GIST: state of the art. Ann Oncol 2012;23:2776–81.
66. Casali PG, Fumagalli E, Gronchi A. Adjuvant therapy of gastrointestinal stromal tumors (GIST). Curr Treat Options Oncol 2012;13:277–84.
67. Demetri GD, von Mehren M, Antonescu CR, et al. NCCN task force report: update on the management of patients with gastrointestinal stromal tumors. J Natl Compr Canc Netw 2010;8(Suppl 2):S1–41.
68. Dematteo RP, Ballman KV, Antonescu CR, et al. Adjuvant mesylate after resection of localised, primary gastrointestinal stromal tumor: a randomized, double-bling, placebo-controlled trial. Lancet 2009;373:1097–104.
69. Joensuu H, Eriksson M, Sundby Hall K, et al. One vs. three years of adjuvant imatinib for operable gastrointestinal stromal tumor: a randomized trial. JAMA 2012;307:1265–72.
70. Demetri GD. Differential properties of current tyrosine kinase inhibitors in gastrointestinal stromal tumors. Semin Oncol 2011;38(Suppl 1):S10–9.
71. Shoffski P, Reichardt P, Blay JY, et al. A phase II study of evelolimus (RAD001) in combination with imatinib in in patients with imatinib-resistant gastrointestinal stromal tumors. Ann Oncol 2010;21:1990–8.
72. Smyth T, van Looy T, Curry JE, et al. The HSP inhibitor, AT13387, is effective against imatinib-sensitive and resistant gastrointestinal stromal tumor models. Mol Cancer Ther 2012;11:1799–808.
73. Sambol EB, Ambrosini G, Geha RC, et al. Flavopiridol targets c-KIT transcription and induces apoptosis in gastrointestinal stromal tumor cells. Cancer Res 2006; 66:5858–66.
74. Veiga I, Silva M, Vieira J, et al. Hereditary gastrointestinal stromal tumors sharing the KIT Exon 17 germline mutation p.Asp820Tyr develop through different cytogenetic progression pathways. Genes Chromosomes Cancer 2010;49:91–8.
75. Janeway KA, Kim SY, Lodish M, et al. Defects in succinate dehydrogenase in gastrointestinal stromal tumors lacking KIT and PDGFRA mutations. Proc Natl Acad Sci U S A 2011;108:314–8.
76. Stratakis CA, Carney JA. The triad of paragangliomas, gastric stromal tumours, and pulmonary chondromas (Carney triad), and the dyad of paragangliomas and gastric stromal sarcomas (Carney-Stratakis syndrome): molecular genetics and clinical implications. J Intern Med 2009;266:43–52.
77. Pasini B, McWhinney SR, Bei T, et al. Clinical and molecular genetics of patients with the Carney-Stratakis syndrome and germline mutations of the genes coding for the succinate dehydrogenase subunits SDHB, SDHC, and SDHD. Eur J Hum Genet 2008;16:79–88.
78. Miettinen M, Wang ZF, Sarlomo-Rikala M, et al. Succinate dehydrogenase-deficient GISTs: a clinicopathologic, immunohistochemical, and molecular genetic study of 66 gastric GISTs with predilection to young age. Am J Surg Pathol 2011;35:1712–21.
79. Miettinen M, Killian JK, Wang ZF, et al. immunohistochemical loss of succinate dehydrogenase subunit a (sdha) in gastrointestinal stromal tumors (GISTs) signals SDHA germline mutation. Am J Surg Pathol 2013;37:234–40.
80. Gill AJ, Chou A, Vilain R, et al. Immunohistochemistry for SDHB divides gastrointestinal stromal tumors (GISTs) into 2 distinct types. Am J Surg Pathol 2010;34: 805–14.
81. Gaal J, Stratakis CA, Carney JA, et al. SDHB immunohistochemistry: a useful tool in the diagnosis of Carney-Stratakis and Carney triad gastrointestinal stromal tumors. Mod Pathol 2011;24:147–51.

82. Pantaleo MA, Astolfi A, Indio V, et al. SDHA loss-of-function mutations in KIT-PDGFRA wild-type gastrointestinal stromal tumors identified by massively parallel sequencing. J Natl Cancer Inst 2011;103:1–5.

83. Dwight T, Benn DE, Clarkson A, et al. Loss of SDHA expression identifies SDHA mutations in succinase dehydrogenase-deficient gastrointestinal stromal tumors. Am J Surg Pathol 2013;37(2):226–33.

84. Wagner AJ, Remillard SP, Zhang YX, et al. Loss of SDHAS predicts SDHA mutations in gastrointestinal stromal tumors. Mod Pathol 2013;26:289–94.

85. Carney JA, Stratakis CA. Familial paraganglioma and gastric stromal sarcoma: a new syndrome distinct from the Carney triad. Am J Med Genet 2002;108:132–9.

86. Zhang L, Smyrk TC, Young WF, et al. Gastric stromal tumors in Carney triad are different clinically, pathologically, and behaviorally from sporadic gastric gastrointestinal stromal tumors: findings in 104 cases. Am J Surg Pathol 2010;34:53–64.

87. Agaram NP, Laquaglia MP, Ustun P, et al. Molecular characterization of pediatric gastric gastrointestinal stromal tumors. Clin Cancer Res 2008;14:3204–15.

88. Pappo AS, Janeway K, Laquaglia M, et al. Special considerations in pediatric gastrointestinal stromal tumors. J Surg Oncol 2011;104:928–32.

89. Andersson J, Sihto H, Meis-Kindblom JM, et al. NF1-associated gastrointestinal stromal tumors have unique clinical, phenotypic, and genotypic characteristics. Am J Surg Pathol 2005;29:1170–6.

90. Kinoshita K, Hirota S, Isozaki K, et al. Absence of c-kit gene mutations in gastrointestinal stromal tumours from neurofibromatosis type 1 patients. J Pathol 2004; 202:80–5.

91. Miettinen M, Fetsch JF, Sobin LH, et al. Gastrointestinal stromal tumors in patients with neurofibromatosis 1. A clinicopathologic study of 45 patients with long-term follow-up. Am J Surg Pathol 2006;30:90–6.

92. Agaram NP, Wong GC, Guo T, et al. Novel V600E BRAF mutations in imatinib-naive and imatinib-resistant gastrointestinal stromal tumors. Genes Chromosomes Cancer 2008;47:853–9.

93. Agaimy A, Terracciano LM, Dirnhofer S, et al. V600E BRAF mutations are alternative early molecular events in a subset of KIT/PDGFRA wild-type gastrointestinal stromal tumours. J Clin Pathol 2009;62:613–6.

94. Hostein I, Faur N, Primois C, et al. BRAF mutation status in gastrointestinal stromal tumors. Am J Clin Pathol 2010;133:141–8.

95. Daniels M, Lurkin I, Pauli R, et al. Spectrum of KIT/PDGFRA/BRAF mutations and Phosphatidylinositol-3-Kinase pathway gene alterations in gastrointestinal stromal tumors (GIST). Cancer Lett 2011;312:43–54.

Index

Note: Page numbers of article titles are in **boldface** type.

A

ACCORD trial, 362
ACTS-GC trial (Adjuvant Chemotherapy Trial of TS-1 for Gastric Cancer), 361
ADAMTS9 gene mutations, 249
Adherens junctions, *Helicobacter pylori* action on, 291
Adhesins, *Helicobacter pylori,* 289
Adhesion proteins, *Helicobacter pylori,* 213
Adjunctive therapies, **359–369**. *See also* Chemotherapy; Radiation therapy.
Adjuvant Chemoradiation Therapy in Stomach Cancer (ARTIST) trial, 360–361
Adjuvant Chemotherapy Trial of TS-1 for Gastric Cancer (ACTS-GC trial), 361
Alcohol consumption, as cancer risk, 232–233
ALDOC protein, 251
Angiogenesis inhibitors, 363
Ann Arbor classification, for MALT lymphoma, 374
Ano-1, in GISTS, 405
Antibiotics, for *Helicobacter pylori* infections, 231
Apatinib, 364
APC gene mutations, 244, 248, 272
Apical-junctional complex, in *Helicobacter pylori* infections, 290–291
Apoptosis, 247–248, 287
ARIDA gene mutations, 248
ARTIST (Adjuvant Chemoradiation Therapy in Stomach Cancer) trial, 360–361
Aspirin, for cancer prevention, 307–312
ATM gene mutations, 244
Atrophic gastritis, 266, 382
Autoimmune gastritis, 266
Autonomic nerve tumors, 400

B

BabA protein, *Helicobacter pylori,* 213
Barium radiography, for screening, 322
Barrett metaplasia, 278
BAX gene mutations, 246–248
B-cell lymphomas, 371
Bevacizumab, 363, 365
Biomarkers, 251–252
Biopsy
    for early cancer, 329–330
    for GISTs, 403–405
    for MALT lymphoma, 373–374
Bleeding, in GISTs, 403
Blood group antigen-binding adhesin, *Helicobacter pylori,* 289

Gastroenterol Clin N Am 42 (2013) 417–427
http://dx.doi.org/10.1016/S0889-8553(13)00039-3
0889-8553/13/$ – see front matter © 2013 Elsevier Inc. All rights reserved.

gastro.theclinics.com

Printed and bound by CPI Group (UK) Ltd, Croydon, CR0 4YY

03/10/2024

01040439-0004